Palgrave Macmillan Studie:

Titles include:

Graham Allan, Graham Cro...
STEPFAMILIES

Harriet Becher
FAMILY PRACTICES IN SOUTH ASIAN MUSLIM FAMILIES
Parenting in a Multi-Faith Britain

Elisa Rose Birch, Anh T. Le and Paul W. Miller
HOUSEHOLD DIVISIONS OF LABOUR
Teamwork, Gender and Time

Ann Buchanan and Anna Rotkirch
FERTILITY RATES AND POPULATION DECLINE
No Time for Children?

Deborah Chambers
SOCIAL MEDIA AND PERSONAL RELATIONSHIPS
Online Intimacies and Networked Friendship

Robbie Duschinsky and Leon Antonio Rocha (*editors*)
FOUCAULT, THE FAMILY AND POLITICS

Jacqui Gabb
RESEARCHING INTIMACY IN FAMILIES

Stephen Hicks
LESBIAN, GAY AND QUEER PARENTING
Families, Intimacies, Genealogies

Clare Holdsworth
FAMILY AND INTIMATE MOBILITIES

Rachel Hurdley
HOME, MATERIALITY, MEMORY AND BELONGING
Keeping Culture

Peter Jackson (*editor*)
CHANGING FAMILIES, CHANGING FOOD

Riitta Jallinoja and Eric Widmer (*editors*)
FAMILIES AND KINSHIP IN CONTEMPORARY EUROPE
Rules and Practices of Relatedness

Lynn Jamieson, Ruth Lewis and Roona Simpson (*editors*)
RESEARCHING FAMILIES AND RELATIONSHIPS
Reflections on Process

David Morgan
RETHINKING FAMILY PRACTICES

Eriikka Oinonen
FAMILIES IN CONVERGING EUROPE
A Comparison of Forms, Structures and Ideals

Róisín Ryan-Flood
LESBIAN MOTHERHOOD
Gender, Families and Sexual Citizenship

Sally Sales
ADOPTION, FAMILY AND THE PARADOX OF ORIGINS
A Foucauldian History

Tam Sanger
TRANS PEOPLE'S PARTNERSHIPS
Towards an Ethics of Intimacy

Elizabeth B. Silva
TECHNOLOGY, CULTURE, FAMILY
Influences on Home Life

Lisa Smyth
THE DEMANDS OF MOTHERHOOD
Agents, Roles and Recognitions

Yvette Taylor
EDUCATIONAL DIVERSITY
The Subject of Difference and Different Subjects

Palgrave Macmillan Studies in Family and Intimate Life
Series Standing Order ISBN 978–0–230–51748–6 hardback
978–0–230–24924–0 paperback
(*outside North America only*)

You can receive future titles in this series as they are published by placing a standing order. Please contact your bookseller or, in case of difficulty, write to us at the address below with your name and address, the title of the series and the ISBN quoted above.

Customer Services Department, Macmillan Distribution Ltd, Houndmills, Basingstoke, Hampshire RG21 6XS, England

---

Fertility Rates and Population Decline

NO TIME FOR CHILDREN?

Edited by

Ann Buchanan
University of Oxford, UK

and

Anna Rotkirch
Population Research Institute, Finland

palgrave
macmillan

Softcover reprint of the hardcover 1st edition 2013 978-1-137-03038-2

First published 2013 by
PALGRAVE MACMILLAN

Palgrave Macmillan in the UK is an imprint of Macmillan Publishers Limited, registered in England, company number 785998, of Houndmills, Basingstoke, Hampshire RG21 6XS.

Palgrave Macmillan in the US is a division of St Martin's Press LLC, 175 Fifth Avenue, New York, NY 10010.

Palgrave Macmillan is the global academic imprint of the above companies and has companies and representatives throughout the world.

Palgrave® and Macmillan® are registered trademarks in the United States, the United Kingdom, Europe and other countries.

ISBN 978-1-349-44041-2 ISBN 978-1-137-03039-9 (eBook)

DOI 10.1057/9781137030399

This book is printed on paper suitable for recycling and made from fully managed and sustained forest sources. Logging, pulping and manufacturing processes are expected to conform to the environmental regulations of the country of origin.

A catalogue record for this book is available from the British Library.

A catalog record for this book is available from the Library of Congress.

Transferred to Digital Printing in 2013

Contents

Figures and Tables

Figures

Tables

Contributors

Editors

Ann Buchanan is currently senior research associate and director of the Centre for Research into Parenting and Children in the Department of Social Policy and Intervention at the University of Oxford. She is a social worker/psychologist by training. For the last 17 years, through her studies on parenting, fathering, divorce and grand-parenting, children in state care, and children at risk of social exclusion, she has been central to research on child and family well-being. She has been a frequent contributor to all party discussions on family policy. In 2009, she was invited to talk about 'Preparing children for the 21st century' to the Cabinet Office Strategy Unit. In recent years she has been a regular visitor to China at the invitation of the Chinese Academy of Social Science in Beijing and also to Shanghai. She is a visiting professor to the State University of St Petersburg and has travelled widely on all five continents. She was appointed to the Council of the ESRC in 2007 and reappointed to the Council for a further three years in 2010. She became an academician of the Academy of Social Sciences in 2009 and council member in 2011. She was awarded an M.B.E. for services to social science in 2012.

Anna Rotkirch is director of the Population Research Institute, Väestöliitto – Finnish Family Federation and Docent in Social Policy and Women's Studies at the University of Helsinki. She has conducted comparative research in Europe related to families, sexuality and childbearing behaviour. She has co-authored or edited ten books, including *Living Through Soviet Russia* and *Women's Voices in Russia Today*. Her work has appeared in nine languages. Her current research focuses on pathways to above-average fertility and the popular phenomenon of 'baby lust'. During the academic year of 2010–11, she was visiting scholar at the Oxford Population Centre, Department of Social Policy and Intervention, University of Oxford.

Contributors

Jennifer S. Barber is a professor in the Department of Sociology and a research professor within the Institute for Social Research at the University of Michigan. Her research is at the intersection of family sociology, demography and social psychology. The 'Relationship Dynamics and Social Life' project, described in this edited volume, explores the types of attitudes, relationships and contraceptive practices that produce unintended pregnancies. The project is collecting and analyzing multiple types of longitudinal data – including surveys, semi-structured interviews, observation and administrative data – from a cohort of 18- and 19-year-old women. The project is funded by the National Institute of Child Health and Human Development (NICHD). Recently, Dr Barber received a Distinguished Fellows award from the William T. Grant Foundation, which will allow her to work at a family planning clinic and a teen pregnancy prevention centre, in order to increase the extent to which her research is relevant to prevention and intervention efforts.

Stuart Basten is a research fellow in demography and social policy in the Department of Social Policy and Intervention at the University of Oxford, and a research fellow at the Social Policy Research Centre, National Taiwan University. His primary research interest lies in the future of global fertility patterns and the uncertainty surrounding population projections. His work has a strong regional focus on Eastern Asia in general, and Taiwan, Hong Kong SAR and the People's Republic of China in particular. His theoretical work concerns the general question of 'Why do people have children in the 21st century?' He has sought to approach this question in a truly interdisciplinary and multidisciplinary sense and has written on the contribution of research from both the natural and social sciences to our understanding of contemporary fertility.

David Coleman has been professor of demography at the University of Oxford since 2002. Between 1985 and 1987, he worked for the British government as special adviser to the home secretary, and then to the ministers of housing and of the environment. His research interests include the comparative demographic trends in the industrial world, the future of fertility, the demographic consequences of migration and the demography of ethnic minorities. International collaborative work continues on these topics at the Vienna Institute of Demography. He was the joint editor of the *European Journal of Population* (Paris) from 1992 to 2000, and in 2001 was elected to the Council of the International Union for the Scientific Study of Population.

Gøsta Esping-Andersen is professor of sociology at the Universitat Pompeu Fabra, where he directs the DEMOSOC research unit. In 2009, he was nominated ICREA-academia professor. Born in Denmark, he studied economics and sociology at Copenhagen University and at the University of Wisconsin–Madison, where he received his PhD. His scientific work centres on life course dynamics, social stratification and comparative social policy. Before coming to Pompeu Fabra, he taught at Harvard University, the University of Trento and the European University in Italy. Among his major academic publications are numerous books, including *The Three Worlds of Welfare Capitalism*, for which he was awarded the APSA's Aaron Wildavsky Enduring Contribution Award in 2005; *The Social Foundations of Postindustrial Economies, The Incomplete Revolution* (2009) and, most recently, *Trois Lecons sur L'Etat Providence*. He is a member of the American Academy of Arts and Sciences, Doctor *Honoris Causa* at Roskilde University and honorary professor at the University of Aalborg. He is member of the scientific board of numerous scientific institutions including the Danish National Institute for Social Research and the CEACS of the Juan March Institute and IMDEA. He has been actively engaged in applied policy relevant work for international organizations, including the United Nations, the OECD, ISSA and the European Union. He participated in the preparation for the EU's Lisbon Summit in 2000 and co-authored a report on welfare state reform for the Belgian presidency of the EU in 2002. He has been actively involved in the design of early childhood policies in several countries, and is member of EU President Baroso's social policy advisory group.

Heather H. Gatny is a research director within the Institute for Social Research at the University of Michigan. She specializes in both survey methodology and family demography, with an advanced degree in survey data collection methodology and multiple publications on these topics. She has worked for more than ten years on the execution of large-scale, interdisciplinary data collection projects with family demographers. Ms Gatny is the project director of the 'Relationship Dynamics and Social Life' project, described in this edited volume.

Anne H. Gauthier is senior researcher at the Netherlands Interdisciplinary Demographic Institute (NIDI) and professor of sociology at the University of Calgary. She completed her doctorate at the University of Oxford in 1992 and has since held academic positions in Britain, Canada and the United States. Between 2001 and 2010, she was the Canada Research Chair in Comparative Family Policy at the University of Calgary. She has published widely in the area of family policies including a recent literature review on the impact of family policies on fertility in industrialized countries (published in *Population Research and Policy Review* 26.3: 323–46). Her Comparative Family Policy Database is available online: http://www.demogr.mpg.de/cgi-bin/databases/FamPolDB/index.plx

Sarah Harper is professor of gerontology at Oxford University and director of the Oxford Institute of Population Ageing. Her current research concerns globalization and global population ageing. In particular, she considers the impact at the global, societal and individual level of the age-structural shift from predominantly young to predominantly older societies, addressing such questions as the implications of the widespread falls in fertility and growth in extreme longevity. Sarah has strong research interests in the Asia-Pacific Region. She has worked and lectured in Japan, China, Korea, Singapore, Hong Kong, Australia and New Zealand and was the first holder of the International Chair in Old Age Financial Security established at the University of Malaya. She was an author of the Royal Society report on population change, *People and the Planet*, and serves as on the Advisory Board of Population Europe, the World Demographic Association, the English Longitudinal Study of Ageing and the Scientific Board of Natural England. Sarah presented the 2012 Oxford London Lecture, an annual lecture series hosted by the Vice-Chancellor of the University of Oxford, speaking on 'The 21st Century – the last century of youth?' She is co-editor of the *Journal of Population Ageing* and author of *Ageing Societies* (2006) and *Population Challenges for the 21st Century* (forthcoming).

John Haskey has been a visiting senior research fellow at the University of Oxford for the past 12 years, and was, until recently, head of the Family Demography Unit within the Population and Demography Division of the Office for National Statistics. He has published a variety of statistical studies, analyses and commentaries on the subjects of marriage, divorce, cohabitation, living apart together, ethnicity, adoption, families – including one-parent families and step-families – as well as households and relationships, including kin relationships. One particular interest is the influence of legal regulations and legislative changes upon subsequent demographic behaviour. He has recently contributed to family law on: trends in divorce; the potential for court information to be better used for research purposes; and on profiles of surviving kin of different kinds of family member who die – the latter being a report of research carried out for the Law Commission for their work and recommendations on changing the law on intestacy. John recently contributed a chapter on measuring household and family variables in social surveys to a book called *Measurement Through Social Surveys: An Applied Approach*. He is a past president of the British Society for Population Studies, and an assistant editor for the demographic journal *Population Studies*.

Olga Isupova is a sociologist and a senior researcher at the Institute of Demography, National Research University Higher School of Economics in Russia, and has published extensively on fertility and the cultural importance of motherhood. Currently, the main focus of her interest is the social and cultural implications of assisted reproductive technologies, the changing meanings and cultural practices in the area of motherhood in her home country, and the impact of modern Russian social policies on fertility.

Gavin W. Jones is currently a professor at the Asia Research Institute at the National University of Singapore. His academic career has been closely linked with consultancy assignments in the areas of population and development, educational planning and urban planning. After completing his PhD at the Australian National University in 1966, he joined the Population Council, where he worked first in New York, then in Thailand and Indonesia, before returning to Australia. He was with the Demography and Sociology Program at Australian National University for 28 years, serving as head of program for six years.

Yasamin Kusunoki is an assistant research scientist in the Population Studies Center and Survey Research Center within the Institute for Social Research at the University of Michigan. Dr Kusunoki's research focuses on understanding the sources of gender, racial/ethnic and socio-economic disparities in health and demographic behaviours during adolescence and the transition to adulthood. She is particularly interested in the social contexts in which young people are embedded such as their families, neighbourhoods, and romantic and sexual relationships. Current investigations include the influence of multiple, dynamic social contexts on young women's risk of unintended pregnancy; the ways in which neighbourhoods shape young people's relationship experiences; and the role of gender and relationship characteristics on condom use. She is one of the co-investigators on the 'Relationship Dynamics and Social Life' project, described in this edited volume.

Marie-Louise Newell, a maternal and paediatric epidemiologist, is director of the Africa Centre for Health and Population Studies, a UKZN facility located in northern KwaZulu-Natal. Seconded from the Institute for Child Health at University College London, where she is professor of Paediatric Epidemiology, she is a strong advocate of international collaboration and is a co-founder of the International Ghent Group on HIV-infected women and children. At the Africa Centre she directs a large programme of work evaluating the impact of HIV and its treatment on the population. Lorna Benton is currently her doctoral student from the Institute of Child Health and is working on her thesis on fertility and family planning for HIV-positive women accessing ART in KwaZulu-Natal.

Brienna Perelli-Harris has been a lecturer in social statistics and demography at the University of Southampton since 2011. She received her PhD in sociology in 2006 at the University of Michigan and held a post-doc at the University of Wisconsin. She then worked as a research scientist at the Max Planck Institute for Demographic Research. She has studied Eastern European fertility with quantitative and qualitative methods and has been especially interested in the impact of socio-economic and subjective factors. Her current research compares changes in the family across countries and over time, with a particular focus on childbearing within cohabitation.

David S. Reher is professor of population studies at the Facultad de Ciencias Politicas y Sociologia, Universidad Complutense de Madrid and director of the Grupo de Estudios Población y Sociedad (GEPS). He has written widely on the history of the family and demography. In 2011, together with Ronald D. Lee, he edited the supplement to Volume 37 of *Population and Development Review* on *Demographic Transition and Its Consequences*, including a co-authored article on 'The landscape of demographic transition and the aftermath' (2011). He has also written 'Population and the Economy during the Demographic Transition', which appeared recently in *Economic Affairs* (32(1), 2012).

Justine Roberts is one of the founders of Mumsnet, which was set up in 2000. The idea was to create a website where parents 'could swap advice about holidays, pushchairs and last night's TV'. In 2011, it received 4 million visits per month (Mumsnet website 2011) and has been credited as one of the most influential forces in the UK. Kate Williams is a member of the Mumsnet Campaign team.

Robert Rowthorn is emeritus professor of economics at the University of Cambridge in the Faculty of Economics and Politics. His research interests are economic growth, employment and inequality and the economics of the family.

Jennifer Yarger is a sociologist and public policy researcher in the Bixby Center for Global Reproductive Health and the Philip R. Lee Institute for Health Policy Studies at the University of California, San Francisco. She received her PhD in public policy and sociology from the University of Michigan in 2011, where she participated in the doctoral training programme in the Population Studies Center. Her research is focused broadly on the relationship between social context and fertility attitudes and behaviour in the United States. She is particularly interested in studying socio-economic disparities in unintended pregnancy and how government policies influence reproductive health.

Zhenzhen Zheng is professor of demography at the Institute of Population and Labor Economics at the Chinese Academy of Social Science. Before that she was associate professor at Peking University. Her current research focuses on fertility intention and childbearing behaviour, migration and rural women's development, migration and health vulnerability. She is also involved in an evaluation of the Youth Reproductive Health Project.

Acknowledgements

Ann Buchanan would like to say a special thank you to Professor Zhenzhen Zheng who invited her to Beijing to take part in a conference on Family Change in the Wake of Demographic Transition, Beijing, China, on 17–18 September 2010. The proceedings from the conference were the inspiration for this book. As indeed was Anna Rotkirch, who arrived in Oxford on sabbatical in Michaelmas Term 2010 and first spoke to the Department about 'Baby Fever'.

Chapter 5 by Coleman and Rowthorn is a shortened and adapted version of a paper that originally appeared in a supplement to Volume 37, 2011, of *Population and Development Review*. Adapted and reprinted here with the permission of the Population Council.

In Chapter 1, Figures 1.1 and 1.2 are reprinted with permission of OECD Family Database www.oecd.org/social/family/database

Part I

What Is Happening to Fertility Behaviour?

1
No Time for Children? The Key Questions

Ann Buchanan and Anna Rotkirch

While many are concerned about global overpopulation and its impact, this book takes another view. Silently, with little fanfare, a dramatic change is taking place: people are having fewer children. The UN World Fertility Patterns (2007) note that in the world the total fertility rate (TFR), or the lifetime number of children women are calculated to have, has declined from 4.5 in 1970–75 to 2.6 in 2000–05. In 2010 it was 2.5 (see Table 1.1). The decline affects all regions of the world, but it started in Europe where, in all but three countries, the TFR has fallen below two. In recent years, a particularly dramatic decline has been seen in some Asian countries.

The main focus of this book is the reasons for declining fertility rates across the globe and the possibility of population decline. The secondary focus is that in a world with fewer children it will be important to maximize the potential of all children, including those who stayed at the margins of society in the past. Children will become a nation's most valuable asset in maintaining and sustaining economic well-being. Childbearing is a complex phenomenon, which has been approached from varying angles by different scientific disciplines. Typically, demographers describe what is going on, psychologists study individual motivations and well-being and the social scientist analyses the structures, norms and policies that link micro and macro levels. This book engages insights from all these disciplines to provide a comprehensive and accessible overview of the *what, why* and *how* in contemporary childbearing behaviour.

Table 1.1 Total fertility rate (children per woman)

Country or area	Subgroup	Year	Unit	Value
Africa	**Total**	**2010**	**Births per woman**	**4.5**
Asia	**Total**	**2010**	**Births per woman**	**2.2**
Central African Republic	Total	2010	Births per woman	4.6
China	Total	2010	Births per woman	1.6
Eastern and Southern Africa	Total	2010	Births per woman	4.6
Latin America and Caribbean	Total	2010	Births per woman	2.2
Middle East and North Africa	Total	2010	Births per woman	2.8
Russian Federation	Total	2010	Births per woman	1.5
South Africa	Total	2010	Births per woman	2.5
South Asia	Total	2010	Births per woman	2.7
Sub-Saharan Africa	Total	2010	Births per woman	4.9
United States of America	Total	2010	Births per woman	2.1
Western and Central Africa	Total	2010	Births per woman	5.4
World	**Total**	**2010**	**Births per woman**	**2.5**

The State of the World's Children (2010); United Nations Population Division.
Source: Derived from UN data. Population Statistics, 2011.

The key questions

First, what is happening to fertility rates across the world? How low is the current fertility decline likely to go, and why is fertility modestly growing again in some countries? How is the increase in childlessness and the one-child family shaping fertility trends?

Next, why are parents having fewer children? Is it because, with the availability of contraception and careers, women have more choices, or are economic and policy constraints impinging? Case studies around the world give differing perspectives.

Thirdly, what will be the consequences of lower fertility rates? If indeed lower fertility means smaller populations, what will be the impact on adults and children? What is happening to less fortunate children who in some cases lack any effective parenting? Since the relations and obligations between generations affect childbearing, we also consider the effect of the growing number of elderly. To what extent can and should the older generation fill the parenting gap in time-poor societies? Will adults be willing to take care of their parents, and will this conflict with their own childbearing? In many parts of the world, particularly in Confucian societies, it is a moral imperative for the younger generation to provide for their parents, sometimes so that one of them renounces the opportunity to have a family of his or her own. Finally, we ask social policy scholars how we should respond to a world with fewer children. Can policy initiatives influence parental ambivalence about having babies by giving them more help? How can we make more time for children and improve their well-being?

What is happening to fertility rates?

In Part I, the demographers discuss the implications of the raw facts given here. If we look at data across the developed world we see dramatic changes. The following chart (Figure 1.1) highlights the decline in fertility across the industrialized countries of the Organisation for Economic Co-operation and Development (OECD). The dotted line plots the level that is theoretically necessary for a population to replace itself. That is, on average, two people need to produce just over two children (allowing for mortality). Figure 1.1 shows that in 2009 TFRs were well below the replacement rate in most countries, but exceeded two children per woman in Iceland, Ireland, Israel, Mexico, New Zealand, Turkey and the United States. Particularly, dramatic drops can be seen in Mexico, Turkey and Korea between 1970 and 2009.

However, while no country had higher fertility in 2009 than in 1970, a few have higher levels now than they did in 1995. In the last census, the UK Fertility Rates were the highest since 1972. In 2010, the

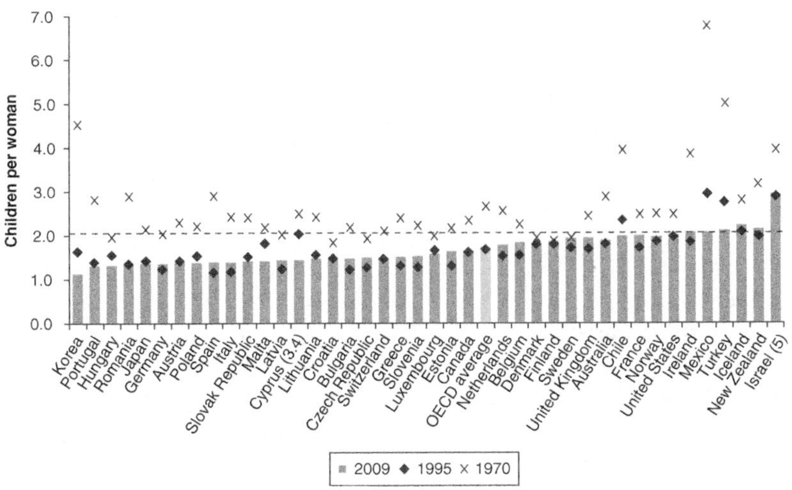

Figure 1.1 Total fertility rates (TFRs) in 1970, 1995 and 2009
Source: OECD Family Database (2010a).

census reported a TFR of 1.98. This was felt to be due mainly to increases in the numbers of foreign born women as well as some mothers who had previously delayed having children completing their families (ONS 2011). Indeed, many European societies appear to have reached the end of the almost uninterrupted fertility decline they have experienced for over a century. The most developed countries, like the United Kingdom, are exhibiting a modest rise in fertility today and may be approaching replacement levels (Myrskylä et al. 2009). Many believe that this surprising turn in fertility decline is related to gender equality and family policies facilitating both women's wage work and parenthood. Although the evidence is mixed, long-term, family-friendly policies do appear to boost fertility at least above very low levels (Bradshaw and Attar-Schwartz 2010, pp. 185–212; Gauthier – chapter 16; Rønsen and Skrede 2010). However, shifts in TFRs are also influenced by changes in the timing and spacing of children. Since women are having children increasingly later in life, postponement of births may create a gap between estimated fertility rates and actual childbearing (Billari et al. 2006). The actual number of children born to any generation, or completed cohort fertility, can be known only after women have reached the end of their childbearing years. Thus we cannot yet tell for sure to what extent fertility rates have really stopped declining in some countries.

Looking more widely across the world, TFRs are dropping below the replacement level in many countries. Higher fertility rates are seen mainly in Africa. Table 1.1 looks at a broad range of fertility rates across the globe. The highest rate shown is in sub-Saharan Africa.

Average fertility rates conceal the polarization of childbearing between different families. The proportion of childless people is growing in most societies. In some nations, such as Germany or China, the one-child family is an increasingly popular choice. In other countries, such as the United Kingdom, TFRs are rising because more parents are choosing to have three or four children.

Within countries, there are significant differences in fertility rates between ethnic groups. For example in the United States, since 1980, fertility rates have been relatively stable, remaining between 64 and 71 births per 1000 women but in the last few decades, fertility rates have declined substantially among non-Hispanic blacks and among American Indian and Native Alaskan women. Fertility rates have declined slightly overall among non-Hispanic whites, but have increased among Hispanics (Child Trends DataBank 2007).

Immigrant workers who have just arrived in a country have, as we have recently seen in the United Kingdom, an important impact on

TFRs. In Scotland, for example, the proportion of births to non-Scots born mothers has increased from 13 per cent in 1977 to 24 per cent in 2009. In recent years (from 2004 to 2007) Scots-born mothers accounted for 40 per cent of the increase in births, other UK-born mothers a further 5 per cent of the increase, while mothers born elsewhere accounted for 55 per cent of the increase. However, research suggests that the fertility behaviour of migrants tends to converge with that of the resident population over time (Scottish Government 2010).

Population statistics are fraught with controversies. The demographers in Part I of this book will argue these various viewpoints.

What difference does contraception make?

One of the key drivers to declining fertility is, of course, the availability of contraception. While in the past women spent most of their lives rearing the next generation and caring for the family's vulnerable members, the arrival of reliable methods to control fertility meant, for the first time, that women were freer to consider a life outside the home.

Although attempts to control fertility date back to the earliest times in China, ancient Greece and Rome, it was not until the twentieth century that the first birth control clinics were set up for married women. In 1910, only 13 per cent of English married couples used birth control; however, by 1982 in the United States nearly 70 per cent of married couples practised birth control (Quarini 2005).

Contraception use is strongly affected by religious and moral beliefs. The aim of the early pioneers, such as Marie Stopes and Margaret Sanger in the United States, was to alleviate poverty and improve women's health. But access to contraception will not automatically translate into contraceptive use, even among poor women. Behavioural ecologists have shown how strongly contraceptive uptake can differ even between neighbouring villages and how it is mediated by broader changes in well-being and women's life course (Mace and Colleran 2009). The fascinating social and psychological variation of contraceptive use is further analysed by Barber in Chapter 7, *Young Women's Relationships, Contraception and Unintended Pregnancy in the United States*, of this book.

Table 1.2, derived from UN statistics, gives an overview of the availability of contraception globally in 2007. The extremely low rates of availability are particularly notable in parts of Africa and Melanesia.

It is interesting that although declining fertility rates reflect the availability and use of contraception, the proportion of unwanted

Table 1.2 United Nations: Department of Economic and Social Affairs, *World Contraceptive Use 2007*

Country or area	Thousands	Year(s)	Any method (%)	Total (%)
World	1,134,650	2003	63.1	56.1
More developed regions	154,469	1999	67.4	56.1
Less developed regions	980,181	2004	62.4	56.1
Africa	148,108	2003	28.0	21.4
Sub-Saharan Africa	122,951	2003	21.5	14.8
Northern Africa (excl. Sudan)	25,157	2004	60.0	53.8
Eastern Africa	45,156	2004	25.4	20.3
Northern Africa	30,327	2005	51.0	45.6
Middle Africa	18,729	2002	24.2	5.9
Southern Africa	6,074	2003	57.5	57.3
Western Africa	47,823	2003	13.6	8.6
Asia	750,671	2004	67.9	61.7
Eastern Asia	290,335	2004	87.6	86.4
South-Central Asia	321,376	2005	54.2	45.8
South-Eastern Asia	103,337	2003	59.9	51.0
Western Asia	35,623	2002	54.5	34.4
Europe	96,762	1997	67.5	52.5
Eastern Europe	44,336	1996	63.7	41.7
Northern Europe	9,878	2001	77.3	74.1
Southern Europe	19,571	1999	62.6	45.5
Western Europe	22,977	1995	74.8	70.2
Latin America and the Caribbean	94,780	2001	71.4	64.5
Caribbean	6,344	2002	60.4	55.9
Central America	24,341	2005	68.2	63.0
South America	64,095	1999	73.7	65.8
North America	40,194	2001	73.0	68.6
Oceania	4,134	1995	52.9	48.9
Australia/New Zealand	2,588	1995	68.3	65.5
Melanesia/Micronesia/Polynesia	1,545	1996	27.1	21.0

Source: Derived from United Nations (2008)

pregnancies remains high. An estimated 41 per cent of all contemporary pregnancies worldwide and 44 per cent in Western Europe are thus reported to be either mistimed or unwanted (Singh et al. 2010).

In some areas abortion is used as a means of controlling fertility, and this is not recorded in Table 1.2. Obtaining accurate data on the number of induced abortions is difficult. However, it is estimated that approximately 26 million legal and 20 million illegal abortions were performed worldwide in 1995, resulting in a worldwide abortion rate of 35 per 1000 women aged 15–44. Eastern Europe had the highest abortion rate (90 per 1000) and Western Europe the lowest (11 per 1000). Abortion rates are lower overall in areas where abortion is generally restricted by law (and where many abortions are performed under unsafe conditions) than in areas where abortion is legally permitted (Henshaw et al. 1999). Where abortion is restricted by law, there is another concern. Children born from unwanted pregnancies, after abortion has been refused, have much less favourable life outcomes. In the Prague Study of Subjects born of Unwanted Pregnancies, Kubička et al. (1995) showed at age 30, the unwanted children had significantly poorer outcomes compared to children from wanted pregnancies.

Has women's employment influenced fertility behaviour?

A key feature in declining fertility is the increased range of choices parents have, and the choices they perceive that their children should have. Central to these is income and employment.

In most societies, a man's higher income and social status is related to also having more children (Nettle and Pollet 2008). This is especially because men with low education and income are more likely to remain childless. By contrast, highly educated women often remain without children. It would be a mistake, however, to divide women everywhere into career-oriented women with few or no children and family-centred women with many children. Rather, most women opt for both interesting employment and children – given the choice. As a result, although there is an uncertain relationship between employment and low fertility in the developing world, the association is more certain in OECD countries.

As can be seen in Figure 1.2, there is a fairly strong relationship between female employment rates and TFRs, and this has switched from negative to positive in just three decades. Today, societies with a high level of female employment, and usually also a longer history of full-time working women, have had to adapt to dual earner families and have higher fertility rates (McDonald 2006). In the Scandinavian countries with high gender equality, mothers have fairly equal numbers of children across all educational groups (Kravdal and Rindfuss 2008). By contrast, societies where women have entered the labour market, without a corresponding change in family values and family policies,

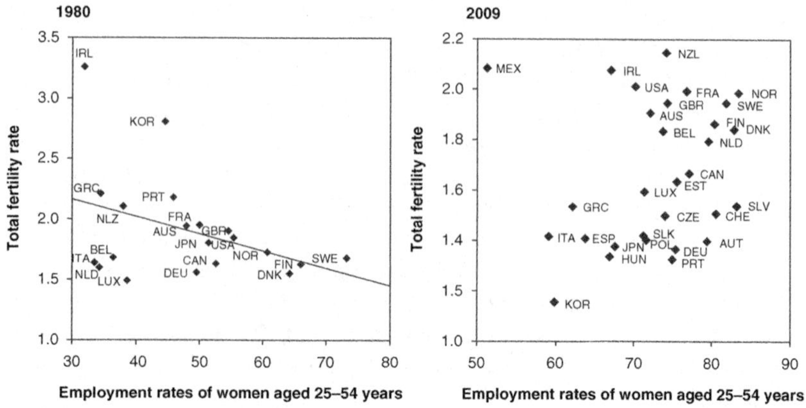

Figure 1.2 Cross-country relation between female employment rates and total fertility rates, 1980 and 2009

Source: Permission to reproduce from 'Employment rates – OECD Employment Outlook', *UN World Statistics Pocketbook, 2010*, and 'Fertility rates – National statistical authorities, UN Statistical Division and Eurostat Demographic Statistics, 2010' (OECD 2010b).

witness the sharpest reductions in childbearing. Particularly dramatic is the situation in Korea and the changes between 1980 and 2009.

Economic opportunities are also related to the timing of the first child. The transition to parenthood is happening increasingly late in most countries, especially among those with higher education (Billari et al. 2006). Having children later in life has usually been seen as contributing to lower fertility. However, in many highly developed countries, such as Europe's Nordic societies, average age at first birth is quite high, while fertility is also relatively high. In an analysis of 166 countries, Nettle (2011) found that a woman's expected longevity and income explained 74 per cent of the variation in age at first birth between countries. It seems as if improving health and living standards stimulate women to time their children later in life. Indeed, it appears that postponement of maternity need not be a major factor of concern, as long as the average age does not reach beyond 30. However, on the individual level postponing may increase involuntary childlessness or having fewer children than one would like to due to unforeseen life events.

Maximizing the potential of children

Considerable consternation was caused in the United Kingdom when Bradshaw et al. (2007) in a UNICEF study placed the United Kingdom at the bottom of the list of child well-being in rich countries. Well-being in children is important because there is considerable evidence that there are strong links between childhood well-being and later economic prosperity. The first editor, in discussing her 16 years of research in this area, argued to the UK Cabinet Office (Buchanan 2009), that there is considerable evidence that children's well-being is associated with better attainment in school, better relationships with parents and partners and better outcomes in adulthood. Indeed, promoting their well-being is central to better outcomes for children. Lack of well-being, in particular among children with conduct disorders, is very expensive, both for the cost of treating their disorder (Scott et al. 2001) and for the possible association with later dependence on benefits and loss of earning capacity.

Interestingly, it is as if middle-class parents sense this too: behind the shift to fewer children is often their desire to concentrate time and resources on one or two offspring, so that they will do well in life (Mace 2008). Thus, promoting the well-being of our future children in a changing world may strengthen the trust parents feel towards society and encourage them to have the children they ideally would like to have.

Originally, it was assumed that, as people became richer, their sense of well-being would increase. Recent syntheses of international studies have shown that this is a myth (e.g. Layard 2011). There is a growing realization that, in measuring the well-being of society, we need to think beyond GDP and consider personal and social well-being as well as happiness (Layard 2011).

> Seventy-five years ago the original architects of systems of national accounts were clear that welfare could not be inferred from measures of national income alone..... A myopic obsession with growing the economy has meant that we have tended to ignore its negative impacts on our well-being.
>
> (Michaelson et al. 2009, p. 2)

Michaelson et al. (2009) highlight factors which they consider should be included in national well-being accounts: absence of emotional or negative feelings, satisfying life, resilience and self-esteem, positive functioning, supportive relationships and trust and belonging. More recently, further systems to measure child well-being are being developed (Thompson and Aked 2009).

Michaelson et al. (2009) from the New Economics Foundation have, among others, been working on ways to measure child well-being more accurately. Globally, the United Nations Development Project (UNDP) has long been collecting indicators of better lives but more recently it, too, has been concerned about developing measures of subjective well-being (Conceição and Bandura 2008). Although harder to grasp, well-being can be a stronger indicator than 'mere' poverty. Finland, the country of the second editor, scores very well on the UNICEF's list of children's well-being and has among the best results for child poverty, health and education in the world. However, on measures of subjective well-being, such as satisfaction with school and social life, Finns score worse, and the loneliness and frustration of youth can in a worst-case scenario express itself in events such as the school shootings by marginalized young men in 2007 and 2008.

Outline of book chapters

The issues highlighted earlier are explored in separate chapters written by some of the leading international and inter-disciplinary experts from the major world regions.

What is happening to fertility behaviour?

The book opens with Part I examining the evidence of declining fertility and the controversies surrounding the issues. In Chapter 2, *Demographic Transitions and Familial Change: Comparative International Perspectives,* David S. Reher, a US demographer based in Spain, takes a historical look at demographic transitions and family change. He explores plausible scenarios for the future, including the possibility of future population stagnation or decline. World population decline will happen, he posits, first in the developed world, but it will likely affect the entire world during the second half of the twenty-first century. Given this, we should start preparing for it now.

In Chapter 3, *The Growth of the One-child Family and Other Changes in the Low Fertility Countries of Asia,* Gavin W. Jones, a demographer, originally from Australia, but now working at the National University of Singapore, Singapore, considers the growth of the one-child norm and other family changes in the low fertility countries of Asia. Jones, living and working in the area, may be nearer to the reality of population decline. Fertility rates in East Asia, he reports, are now the lowest in the world, and this appears likely to remain the case. The one-child family is actually even more characteristic of other East Asian countries than of China. In his chapter, he remarks on the irony of the situation:

> The very pressures to prioritize economic growth and the factors that can contribute to it – long hours of work, involvement of women in the workforce on much the same terms as men, strong pressure on children to perform outstandingly in school, and the extra tuition and coaching that is considered indispensible for reaching this goal – contain the seeds of an inability of the population to replace itself. Thus the successful East Asian economies are placed at risk by a shortage of people to continue to power the economies and enjoy their fruits, generated by the very factors that have resulted in the growth of these economies in the first place.
>
> (Jones Chapter 3, p. 58)

John Haskey, in Chapter 4, *Childlessness: Choice and Circumstances*, focuses on the phenomenon of increasing childlessness. He hypothesizes that the opening up of equal opportunities is the key to understanding fertility – and childlessness. Whether a woman can achieve her employment goals may depend upon whether her available resources are sufficient for raising a family, as well as for realizing her other ambitions.

Finally in Chapter 5, *Population Decline – Facing an Inevitable Destiny?* David Coleman, a demographer, and *Bob Rowthorn*, an economist, argue that populations have 'overshot' their sustainable or comfortable limits. Although there may be major impacts on national economies, there are also advantages in having a stagnant or declining population. While it is clear that the process of decline has numerous drawbacks, these are only important if the decline is fast and protracted. Smaller population size, they feel, has social, economic and environmental advantages. And, in any case, it may be forced on us, as a requirement for our survival, if the fears about climate change come to pass.

What are the reasons for women having fewer children?

Part II starts to identify the triggers for the decline in fertility. We provide case studies from Western and Eastern Europe, the United States, Asia, South America and South Africa in order to illustrate how the reasons influencing fertility are shaped in different contexts. These factors are women's subjective experiences and ambivalence towards childbearing (the United Kingdom and the United States), rapid socio-economic change (Russia and China), policies to limit fertility (legislation in China), less direct media influences in South America and a health epidemic (South Africa).

The opening chapter of this part, Chapter 6, *Why Are Women Having Fewer Babies? The Views of Mumsnet Users*, collated by – Justine Roberts, Kate Williams and Ann Buchanan – vividly illustrates the decisions Western parents, and mothers in particular, are making regarding having or not having more children. Demographers may dispute what is happening and the possible consequences of the current decline in fertility, but mothers who are currently making decisions about their families are more direct. These mothers from Mumsnet probably represent an upwardly mobile sector of UK society. Their views are interesting because, given similar levels of education and well-being, they may reflect the aspirations of less fortunate mothers and, as such, predict future trends.

Mumsnet mothers may sound as if every child born was planned for and wanted. In thinking about declining fertility, we also need to remember those children who may have been born 'by mistake'. In Chapter 7, *Young Women's Relationships, Contraception and Unintended Pregnancy in the United States*, we start to identify those children who may be at the other end of the spectrum. George Albee, the late distinguished psychologist, commented that, if there was one intervention that would improve the well-being of children worldwide, it was that every child should be born to a financially secure couple who had planned for, and wanted the child (Albee et al. 1992). Jennifer S. Barber, Yasamin Kusunoki, Heather H. Gatny and Jennifer Yarger, who are from the United States, in Chapter 7, show us that many pregnancies are not planned, and indeed many may be unwanted. Ninety-five per cent of young women reported no general desire to get pregnant but almost 20 per cent of respondents reported during the study that they forgot to use birth control. Nineteen per cent of respondents reported a pregnancy and about 9 per cent of respondents had a baby during the study. Around three-quarters of these women were not married, engaged or cohabiting. Contraception may be readily available, but when it comes to day-to-day use, mothers often remain ambivalent about its use.

The scene then moves to the first of the country studies. As we noted at the start of this chapter, extraneous events can strongly influence women's private decisions. Social scientists *Brienna Perelli-Harris* and *Olga Iussupova* from the United Kingdom and St Petersburg, Russia, discuss in Chapter 8, *Crisis and Control: Russia's Dramatic Fertility Decline and Efforts to Increase It*, how, in Russia, massive political, social and economic changes collided with long-held cultural traditions and love of children, resulting in extremely low fertility with a preponderance of single children. Some mothers hoped things would get better, so they put off having children only to find later that they were no longer able to conceive. During the post-Soviet period, the demographic situation became so acute that the government reacted by instituting ambitious pro-natalist policies, including the maternity capital payment.

The stage then shifts to China. Indeed, it was Ann Buchanan's attendance at a conference on Family Demography, organized by the Chinese Academy of Social Sciences in Beijing in 2010, which was the inspiration for this book. The conference was organized to commemorate the 30th anniversary of the One Child Policy. Participants included some of the most distinguished family and demographic scholars in China and a few scholars from elsewhere. With a population in China estimated at over 1.3 billion, it was surprising to hear that one of the main concerns of the country was depopulation. As scholars pointed out, among other issues, there was concern, already becoming critical, about who was to care for the elderly. Zhenzhen Zheng's essay in Chapter 9, *The Choice of Having a Second Child and Its Implication for Future Family Structure in China*, is particularly illuminating. She confirms that, as a result of the birth policy, most couples, particularly in towns, have only one child. Her more recent research shows that despite relaxation of the policy, many couples who had themselves been single children are choosing to have only one child. The Lone Child Policy appears to have become imprinted in these lone-child parents' psyche so that, taking into account the economic constraints of the Chinese middle class, they have now decided that one child is 'about right' for a family. This phenomenon, however, as Gavin Jones shows in Chapter 3, is not restricted to China.

In yet another shift across the world, we come to Africa, and in particular, to South Africa, where doctors have been struggling to contain the AIDS epidemic. An estimated 5.6 million people were living with human immunodeficiency virus (HIV) and acquired immunodeficiency syndrome (AIDS) in South Africa in 2009, more than in any other country (UN AIDS 2010). In 2009, it is believed an estimated 310,000 South Africans died of AIDS. Prevalence is 17.8 per cent among those aged 15–49, with some age groups being particularly affected. Almost one in three women aged 25–29, and over a quarter of men aged 30–34, are living with HIV. In Chapter 10, *Childbearing and the Impact of HIV: The South African Experience*, Marie-Louise Newell, an internationally renowned maternal and paediatric epidemiologist from the Africa Centre, South Africa, and *Lorna Benton* from London explore the relationship between fertility and the impact of AIDS. They report that, following the evidence of the Demographic Transition elsewhere, there is conflicting evidence surrounding the much-awaited African transition. They note that a limited number of sub-Saharan countries have observed declining birth rates in the past 20 years. There has been a swift reduction in fertility rates in Zimbabwe, Botswana, Nigeria, Kenya and South Africa. This was felt to be due to increased urbanization, improved education, health services, higher prevalence of contraceptives and access to reproductive health care. This effect is most pronounced in South Africa, where fertility rates of 2.4 births per woman in 2009 were exactly half of those in 1980 and are now the lowest in sub-Saharan Africa.

Newell and Benton report that, although the impact of HIV on both child and adult mortality in sub-Saharan Africa is well known, the impact of HIV on fertility is less well understood. They hypothesize that the epidemic may influence population fertility rates through increased mortality amongst reproductive age groups, reduced fecundity of HIV-infected women and men or changes in reproductive behaviour to avoid pregnancy and prevent the spread of the disease. In South Africa, where 5.6 million people are currently living with HIV, the effects are likely to be most pronounced.

The situation in China and elsewhere has shown that changing cultural norms can powerfully influence fertility behaviour. Stuart Basten, with his multidisciplinary background in anthropology and historical and contemporary demography, brings an innovative perspective and discusses in Chapter 11, *Declining Fertility, Television and the (Mis)representation of Motherhood,* how the media can affect fertility behaviour. In the developing world (Mexico and Brazil), he shows how soap operas have been important in delivering family planning messages. In the developed world, he shows how childbearing models can be influenced by soap operas and celebrities. NGOs, media and peers spread the 'fashion' that it is desirable to have either fewer or more children. This impacts on what is felt to be the ideal family and on behaviour, which can change quite rapidly. With the growth of media technologies and Internet chatting, these influences are likely to become more important in the future.

What will be the impact of women having fewer babies?

In Part III, we start to untangle some of the possible consequences. In Chapter 12 *What Will Be the Impact on the Well-being of Children,* by Ann Buchanan, we consider the central actors in this book. What impact will changing trends have on children? In a world where there are more lone children or children with only one brother or sister how will this impinge on their development? What role do siblings play in family life and what will be missing if they do not have them? What stresses will they bear as they carry the aspirations of their parents and grandparents and how will this affect their mental health?

More worrying, in the transition to lower fertility, is the growing evidence of a divide between the 'privileged' children and the more disadvantaged: those children for whom times are harder. The story for most children in smaller families is generally positive. Most children thrive in small families, especially when this means there are more assets per child than there would be in a large family. This is aptly demonstrated by the hard facts from the *United Nations Development Report*. Where fertility is lower, there are fewer infant deaths, less child mortality and better education. But hidden behind the good news is a darker picture: gender preference leading to selective abortion and even forced sex change, poor care for girls and unequal opportunities. Extreme pressure on the child to fulfil the expectations of parents and grandparents may be associated with rising mental health rates and even suicide. Of considerable importance is the growing gap between more prosperous families and those at the other end of the spectrum, poor families both within nations and internationally.

A second central impact is the imbalance caused by declining fertility and the rise in the number of elderly. As the Chinese girl who was Buchanan's guide in Beijing explained: 'I cannot get married because my future husband and I would have to provide for all our grandparents and we need to save up a lot of money before we could have a child'. The burden on young couples, in having to support and care for up to eight grandparents, can be extremely heavy. As life expectancy increases, so do the challenges of care. In developing economies where little exists in the way of pensions or state welfare, it is harder still. In Chapter 13, *Falling Fertility, Ageing and Europe's Demographic Deficit*, Sarah Harper, at the Oxford Institute of Ageing, who over the last 20 years has brought international scholars together to study ageing, notes how falling fertility and ageing have led to a 'demographic deficit', with large numbers of the elderly needing care from a diminishing number of young people. She highlights future dependency ratios and the importance of keeping elders fit and healthy, and indeed continuing to contribute in the workforce, for as long as possible. This has led to many women finding themselves in 'the sandwich generation'. As Ann Buchanan demonstrates, in Chapter 14, *The Impact on Mothers: Managing the Competing Needs*, more women across the globe are employed in full-time wage work. While working, time-poor parents can be drawn in both ways: simultaneously caring for their elderly parents and for their children, many of whom, once into adulthood, may be reluctant to leave the family home in these hard economic times.

While healthy, many grandparents are often motivated to take care of their (increasingly few) grandchildren. However, there are also drawbacks to 'grandchildren carers', especially when the grandparent care is full-time and they take on more than their health and financial well-being allow. In the United States, some grandparents are overburdened by the pressures of caring for young children. Both grandparents and grandchildren become depressed (Tan et al. 2010). Grandparents have also taken on some children who have been 'left behind' while their parents migrate to other towns or countries for work. Questions have been raised whether this is good for children? There is growing evidence that 'left-behind' children are often lonely and sad.

A fourth consequence is that by delaying parenthood and having to opt for the 'right time' to become a parent many men and women long for children they feel they do not have, or should not yet have, or that they lack a suitable partner or face the challenges of infertility. As Anna Rotkirch discusses, in Chapter 15, *Baby Fever and Longing for Children,* in connection with the earlier chapter by John Haskey on childlessness, more people are childless for longer parts of their lives, even within unions. This contributes to new psychological and social trends such as the discourse around 'baby fever' and longing for children. Rotkirch argues that with falling fertility rates, both for social and human benefit, more advice and support is needed for people hesitating about childbearing or facing involuntary childlessness. Infertility treatments are increasingly used and have a higher success rate, yet many couples hesitate to use them or cannot afford them. By contrast, international adoption is an increasingly difficult solution to childlessness. A few decades ago, Westerners started travelling to the developing world to find the babies they so desperately wanted. Today, developing countries are growing richer and starting to worry about their own decline in fertility, and international adoption opportunities have become much more restricted.

A look into the crystal ball: possible responses

The final part of the book looks into the crystal ball and considers possible responses. As David Coleman posits in Chapter 5, do we need to worry about population decline? Certainly a world with fewer people may be beneficial for the environment and sustainability. David Reher's comment in Chapter 2 is perhaps more to the point. Whatever the controversies, population decline is likely to happen by the middle of the twenty-first century and since life expectancy is rising everywhere, even if some countries revert to about the replacement level of fertility, societies need to start preparing now for a world with a lower proportion of children.

The first chapter in this part of the book, Chapter 16, *Family Policy and Fertility: Do Policies Make a Difference?* by Anne H. Gauthier, a demographer and comparative social policy authority, in her analysis of European welfare regimes, questions whether pro-natalist policies make a difference. She outlines, across the European Union, the availability and length of maternity leave and various benefits for women and children. The conclusion is that although they do not make a huge difference, family-friendly work and social policies can and do impact on women's decisions to have babies. But, as noted in other chapters, when parents choose to have children, other factors also impinge on this choice: the availability of contraception, economic considerations, current lifestyle and work–life balance, availability of support and care for the children, health, family relationships and cultural factors, to name but a few. In Europe women and families have benefited enormously from legislation to protect their jobs when they become pregnant, longer maternity leave, paternity leave, family allowances and the like.

The next chapter, Chapter 17, *Investing in Early Childhood*, written by the distinguished social policy scholar Gøsta Esping-Andersen, argues that we need to invest more in our existing children in the early years. He highlights the large number of children living in poverty. As the population structure shifts and the economy has an increased need for highly skilled workers, we need to maximize the productive potential of contemporary youth. He evidences the research that has been important in fostering better early years' care and demonstrates that the investment in more excluded children has an important economic return.

The final chapter, Chapter 18, *Making Time for Children*, by the editors Ann Buchanan and Anna Rotkirch, 'Making Time for Children', sums up some of the key findings and seeks a possible direction in a fast-changing scenario.

References

Albee, G., Bond, L. and Cook, T. (1992) *Improving Children's Lives: Global Perspectives on Prevention* (Newbury Park, CA: Sage Publications).

Bradshaw, J., Hoelscher, P. and Richardson, D. (2007) An overview of child well-being in rich countries, *Innocenti Report Card* 7, 2007, UNICEF Innocenti Research Centre, Florence. The United Nations Children's Fund.

Bradshaw, J. and Attar-Schwartz, S. (2010) Fertility and social policy, in N. Takayama and M. Werding (eds) *Fertility and Public Policy: How to Reverse the Trend in Declining Birth Rates* (Cambridge, MA and London, UK: MIT-Press), pp. 183–202.

Billari, F. C., Liefbroer, A. C. and Philipov, D. (2006) The postponement of childbearing in Europe: driving forces and implications, *Vienna Yearbook of Population Research,* 1–18, doi:10.1553/populationyearbook2006s1.

Buchanan, A. (2009) *Preparing Children for the 21st Century* (London: Cabinet Office Strategy Unit Seminar, 28 September 2009).

Conceição, P. and Bandura, R. (2008) *Measuring Subjective Wellbeing: A Summary Review of the Literature.* United Nations Development Project. http://www.undp.org/developmentstudies/docs/subjective_wellbeing_conceicao_bandura.pdf, date accessed 12 March 2012.

Child Trends DataBank (2007) http://www.childtrendsdatabank.org/pdf/79_PDF.pdf, date accessed 12 March 2012.

Henshaw, S., Singh, S. and Haas, T. (1999) The incidence of abortion worldwide, *International Family Planning Perspectives, 1999,* 25(Supplement): S30–3.

Kravdal, Ø. and Rindfuss, R. R. (2008) Changing relationships between education and fertility: a study of women and men born 1940–64, *American Sociological Review,* 73: 854–73.

Kubička, L., Matějček, Z., David, H., Dytrych, Z., Miller, W. and Roth, Z. (1995) Children from unwanted pregnancies in Prague, Czech Republic revisited at age thirty, *Psychiatrica Scandinavica,* 91(6): 361–9.

Layard, R. (2011) *Happiness: Lessons from a New Science* (London: Penguin).

Mace, R. (2008) Reproducing in cities, *Science,* 319: 764–6.

Mace, R. and Colleran, H. (2009) Kin influence on the decision to start using modern contraception: a longitudinal study from rural Gambia, *American Journal of Human Biology* 21(4): 472–7, doi: 10.1002/ajhb.20940.

McDonald, P. (2006) An assessment of policies that support having children from the perspectives of equity, efficiency and efficacy, *Vienna Yearbook of Population Research,* 213–34, http://hw.oeaw.ac.at/0xc1aa500d_0x00144e27.

Michaelson, J., Abdallah, S., Steuer, N., Thompson, T. and Marks, N. (2009) *Working Model for National Accounts of Well-Being* (London: New Economics Foundation (nef)).

Myrskylä, M., Kohler, H-P. and Billari, F. (2009) Advances in development reverse fertility declines, *Nature,* 460: 741–3.

Nettle, D. (2011) Flexibility in reproductive timing in human females: integrating ultimate and prozimate explanations, *Philosophical Transactions of The Royal Society B,* 366: 357–65.

Nettle, D. and Pollet, T. V. (2008) Natural selection on male wealth in humans, *The American Naturalist,* 172(5): 658–66.

Office for National Statistics (2011) Frequently asked questions: births and fertility, www.ons.gov.uk/ons/rel/vsob1/...of.../2010/faq-births-and-fertility.pdf

Organisation for Economic Co-operation and Development (OECD) (2010a) Family Database OECD – Social Policy Division – Directorate of Employment, Labour and Social Affairs, www.oecd.org/els/social/family/database, date accessed 18 March 2012.

Organisation for Economic Co-operation and Development (OECD) (2010b). *Employment Rates – Employment Outlook,* UN World Statistics Pocketbook,

2010; Fertility rates – National statistical authorities, UN Statistical Division and Eurostat Demographic Statistics, http://www.oecd.org/dataoecd/37/59/40192107.pdf, date accessed 12 March 2012.

Quarini, C. (2005) History of contraception, *Women's Health Medicine*, 2(5): 28–30.

Rønsen, M. and Skrede, K. (2010) Can public policies sustain fertility in the Nordic countries? Lessons from the past and questions for the future, *Demographic Research*, 22: 3, http://www.demographic-research.org/volumes/vol22/13/, date accessed12 March 2012.

Scott, S., Knapp, M., Henderson, J. and Maughan, B. (2001) Financial cost of social exclusion: follow-up study of antisocial children into adulthood, *British Medical Journal*, 323: 191–4.

The Scottish Government (2010) Demographic change in Scotland, http://www.scotland.gov.uk/Publications/2010/11/24111237/6, date accessed 18 March 2012.

Singh, S., Sehgh, G. and Hussain, R. (2010) Unintended pregnancy: worldwide levels, trends, and outcomes, *Studies in Family Planning*, 41(4): 241–50.

Tan, J-P., Buchanan, A., Flouri, E., Attar-Schwartz, S. and Griggs, J. (2010) Filling the parenting gap? Grandparent involvement with UK adolescents, *Journal of Family Issues*, published online before print 24 February 2010, doi: 10.1177/0192513X09360499.

Thompson, S. and Aked, J. (2009) *A Guide to Measuring Children's Well-Being* (London: New Economics Foundation (nef)).

United Nations AIDS (2010) *UNAIDS Report on the Global AIDS Epidemic*, United Nations.

United Nations Data Statistics (2011) UN: Total fertility Rate. The State of the World's Children. UN_United Nations Population Division, http://data.un.org/Data.aspx?d=SOWCandf=inID%3A127, date accessed 5 October 2012.

United Nations Department of Economic and Social Affairs – Population Division (2007) *World Fertility Patterns*, http://www.un.org/esa/population/publications/worldfertility2007/worldfertility2007.htm, date accessed 18 March 2012.

United Nations Department of Economic and Social affairs (2008) *World Contraceptive Use 2007*, http://www.un.org/esa/population/publications/contraceptive2007/contraceptive2007.htm, date accessed 12 March 2012.

2

Demographic Transitions and Familial Change: Comparative International Perspectives

David S. Reher

This chapter deals with the way demographic transitions throughout the world have proved to be an important source of social, economic and familial change. The chapter has different parts. After an initial overview of the role played by the family in social organization and continuity in the past, as well as of the basic dynamics of the demographic transition, the different ways in which demographic change triggers medium- and long-run social and economic change will be assessed. Age structures, migration trends, reproductive efficiency and familial strategies as well as adult health are all ways in which the transformational effects of demographic transition are felt. The end result of these changes hinges in part on the rate of change of vital rates, which has been far faster in the developing world. This chapter discusses the way the demographic transition leads to significant change in the role of the family in those countries undergoing the historic transition as well as the likelihood that this sort of pattern of social change will spread to countries where the demographic transition started not so long ago. In the final section of this chapter, plausible scenarios for the future are mentioned, including the possibility of future population stagnation or decline, the potentially conflictive pattern of familial and social change in parts of the world characterized by strong religions and equally strong family systems, and the overall duration of the grand cycle of the demographic transition throughout the world.

Introduction

Throughout history, the family has been a cornerstone of society. It has been the source of demographic and social reproduction, the context for most intergenerational transmission of goods and services, the main guarantor of care and support for its vulnerable members, and the main vehicle for the education of the young and thus a key source of transmission of ideas, ideals and attitudes from one generation to the next. The family by its very nature is a conservative institution because its entire existence is predicated on guaranteeing stability between one generation and shielding family members from the potentially pernicious effects of the outside world. Family forms and family systems have varied widely throughout the world and over time, but everywhere the family has fulfilled these functions. If we are to judge from historical records, it is safe to say that the family has been successful even though the paths used to assure social reproduction may have differed in important aspects. At present, the ability of the family to continue carrying out these functions satisfactorily may be in doubt, at least in some parts of the world. The reasons for this nascent pessimism about the family are rooted in many ways in the demographic transition and its long-term effects on society. The purpose of this chapter is to comparatively explore some of the issues involved from a historical perspective.

The relationship between the family and historical change has long attracted the interest of researchers. The extent to which family systems can condition historical outcomes, intriguing as it is, has not received the attention it might warrant from scholars. The way history and historical change affects the family, on the other hand, is a central aspect of much of the literature on the subject. The appearance of the 'modern' family is an underlying source of enquiry. The advent of wage-labour, the urbanization of once-rural populations, the increasing participation of the State in the education of the young, the advent of a working-class movement and of democracy and many other aspects of the enormous historical changes that have taken place during the last two centuries have been considered components of this 'modernization' process. Despite this, however, it has also been shown that in contemporary society the distinguishing traits of family systems are still quite readily recognizable, despite the evidently profound changes that have taken place. The prediction whereby the modernizing process in society was going to lead to a uniform, rather monotonic, family is just not the case (see, e.g. Roussel 1992). The changes have been deep and pervasive, but the identifying characteristics persist (Reher 1998).

The purpose of this chapter is to evaluate some of the effects of the demographic transition on family systems and social organization. This transition is a part of the general process of modernization but, unlike other characteristics of this, it directly alters the fundamentals of one of the key functions of the family: assuring human reproduction. Other changes affecting society, such as the growth in formal education, wage-labour, urbanization, also have implications for family life, but in a more indirect way. As we will see, this process of demographic change has ended up eviscerating a large part of what the family meant traditionally, though it has been more benign with some of the cultural aspects of this institution.

A time line for the demographic transition

The demographic transition refers to a process through which mortality typically begins to decline first, followed some decades later by fertility decline, leading to a series of changes in population growth rates, size and age distribution that continues for many decades. This pivotal process started in many European and some American nations well over a century ago and is currently under way in most of the world. No country in the world has completed this process, since fertility and mortality continue to change, and population ageing will mainly be in the future even for countries like Japan, which are farthest along this path. The transition transforms the demography of societies from many children and few elderly to few children and many elderly; from short life to long; from life-long demands on women in raising young children to the concentration of these demands in a small part of adulthood; from horizontally rich kin networks to vertically rich ones. The transition made possible the radical change in women's economic and social roles, the invention of retirement as the third stage of life, and a demographic efficiency that fostered heavy investment in the human capital of fewer but longer-lived births. Some of these implications were visible nearly immediately after the transition began, while others have only become apparent many years later. Some of these effects have been beneficial for the societies involved, while others are much less so. In many ways, a number of the major challenges facing societies today can be considered as a direct or indirect consequence of the demographic transition. The term 'demographic transition' often refers to the period in which fertility and mortality moved from high and sharply fluctuating levels to low and stable ones. It also refers to the period of history in which traditionally low population growth rates first began to increase at rates unknown previously and subsequently returned to the low levels characteristic of all historic societies. Since these changes in population growth rates result from the actual pattern of change in vital rates, with mortality typically declining several decades before fertility, they both refer to the same overall process, though from slightly different angles. The entire world has ended up participating in this transition, though this would have been difficult to forecast in the middle decades of the twentieth century when fertility was fairly low in some countries and still quite high in others (Reher 2004). With a certain lag, the changes in reproductive dynamics taking place over the last half century have confirmed one of the underlying premises of demographic transition theory that it would eventually affect the entire world.[1] This process ranks as one of the most important changes affecting human society in the last half millennium, which is in many ways on par with the spread of democratic government, the Industrial Revolution, the increase in urbanization, the Protestant Reformation or the progressive increases in the educational levels of human populations.

In very general global terms, this open-ended and as yet largely incomplete process has had a number of different phases. The first phase stretches from the middle of the eighteenth century until the second half of the nineteenth century and the trend was seen mainly in Europe.[2] This initial period of demographic transition was characterized by a gradual decline in mortality caused mainly by the progressive reduction in the importance of mortality crises (Flinn 1974; Livi Bacci 2000, pp. 50–2; Wrigley and Schofield 1981)[3] and, at least in some societies, a very gradual reduction in fertility by means of restrictions to nuptiality. With the exception of France, there is little indication of fertility control within marriage.[4] The ultimate consequence of these changes was an acceleration in population growth rates, the beginnings of large-scale interregional migrations and, during the central decades of the nineteenth century, the onset of the mass international migration flows that were to characterize both European and non-European societies for nearly a century.[5] This period of gradual demographic change drew to a close during the second half of the nineteenth century when declines in both fertility and mortality slowed and, in some areas, even reversed. This last trend change, never adequately explained by historical demographers, gives this preliminary phase of demographic transition a distinct ski-jump appearance.

The next phase of transition in Europe started towards the end of the nineteenth century and lasted until the middle of the twentieth century. It corresponds to a period of sharp reductions in infant and child mortality accompanied by a nearly simultaneous drop in fertility. This period shows very distinct patterns from the preceding phase, as mortality change was mostly unrelated to crisis mortality and was achieved through the reduction of infectious diseases among the young, thanks largely to more efficient maternal care and infant-feeding practices, accompanied by improved levels of nutrition (Riley 2005a, 2005b). Public health was also important during the period, though its educational inputs regarding infant hygiene and care may have been more important than public works and vaccination programs, at least in the initial stages (Schofield and Reher 1991). Fertility reduction was no longer achieved by restricting marriage; rather reduction was based on parity-specific fertility control within marriage. Initially, though this control appeared to have been the mechanism that offset increasing numbers of surviving children, it became apparent fairly quickly that people were aiming for, and achieving, smaller family sizes (Reher and Sanz 2007). The reductions in vital rates were achieved with relatively low levels of technical sophistication, in sharp contrast to the changes that were to characterize the subsequent phase of the transition. Since, at least initially, mortality tended to decline more rapidly than fertility, population growth rates increased as did net family size. By the late Inter-War Period, however, fertility was already quite low – often near replacement – and population growth had begun to decline in many of the historic transitional societies (van Bavel 2010). This period came to an end in the two decades after the Second World War as fertility once again rose or at least ceased its decades-long decline. For these historic transitions, this second phase of transitions once again has ski-jump appearance.

In much of the rest of the world, the process of change was quite different. From the early years of the twentieth century, there appears to have been significant improvements in mortality in some countries and by the 1940s this process seems to have affected most of the world.[6] Indeed, the 1940s and 1950s generally marks the period of fastest improvement in health during childhood throughout the world, and in many countries of the developing world, gains in life expectancy at birth during this period were in excess of 10–12 years per decade. Unlike the earlier transitions, these changes in health were achieved to a large extent through public health programmes (including maternal education) and initiatives as well as through the increasingly effective dissemination of vaccinations and antibiotics. Surprisingly, in many countries total fertility rates actually increased during this period of massive improvements in life-expectancy. The result was a jump in population growth that peaked in most societies in the late 1950s or 1960s and sometimes exceeded 2.5 or 3.0 per cent per year.

The delayed reaction of fertility to the initial improvement of mortality, with disastrous consequences for much of the world, has never been satisfactorily explained, though the following factors may have been important: (1) In historic transitions, both mortality and fertility change was non-technical in nature and emanated from changes inherent in those societies, whereas in the developing world they stemmed from technologically sophisticated interventions that originated elsewhere, in the developed world, and were imported into these societies. (2) The 1950s and 1960s was a period in which out-migration was a readily available mechanism that enabled families to fend off some of the potentially negative effects of the growing numbers of surviving children. (3) The traditional economic constraints on family size, praised by Malthus and which had always existed in Europe, may have been much weaker in other parts of the world where family systems were different and population densities lower. (4) The effect of the baby boom may have made itself felt in the developing world as well. On this last point it is worth noting that the period of continued high or even growing fertility in the developing world coincides to a large extent with the baby boom in the more developed world, though any connections between the two have never been explained adequately (Dyson and Murphy 1985, 1986). (5) It could also reflect, at least in part, the improving health of women of reproductive age.

The third phase of the demographic transition began in the 1960s and has lasted until very recently. During this period, unquestionably the most important fact has been the decline of fertility almost everywhere in the world. The first countries to show important rates of decline in the late 1950s were societies that were regional leaders or had more or less important populations of European origin (Reher 2004, p. 24). By the 1960s, this was no longer the case as sharp reductions in fertility spread to much of the world, with fertility decline commencing between 1955 and 1990 in nearly 150 countries. Even in sub-Saharan Africa, decline in fertility in most countries dates from this period. Everywhere the pace of decline in fertility was far faster than it ever was historically. This can be explained by the pent-up demand for fertility control in the face of rapidly improving mortality together with the widespread availability of effective birth control. The end result of this process was the declining population growth rates in much of the world, an incipient process of ageing in many societies and the ability of a growing number of countries to take advantage of the demographic dividend often associated with the demographic transition (Bloom et al. 2003; Lee and Mason 2010; Reher 2011). In many of these countries, fertility is currently near or even below replacement.

Among countries pioneering the historic transition, after the baby boom, fertility began to decline rapidly once again and low fertility became the norm, often at levels far below replacement. It was also a period in which a wide array of social changes related directly or indirectly to the demographic transition also appeared in society: delayed marriage, widespread cohabitation, births out of wedlock, divorce, changes in family structure with decreases in parental authority and a profound transformation in the role of women in society. From a strictly demographic standpoint, in many countries the ultimate result of these changes was a significant decline in the aggregate number of births, which started in the 1960s and 1970s and continues today. However, in some societies these numbers have stabilized or even increased marginally but remain at levels below those held just a few decades ago. As a result, the pace of ageing has accelerated, currently dominating the political and social agenda in most countries, and may well be an important handicap for pension systems, economic growth and living standards in the decades to come.

The fourth phase of the demographic transition is only just now beginning. It promises to be one of low fertility and intense ageing nearly everywhere in the world. Population age structures, which at present show an excess of population of working age in the developing world and an incipient shortage of these same age groups in the developed world, will become top-heavy the world over, as ageing becomes an issue for the entire world and not just for those countries participating in the historic demographic transition. While significant rebounds in fertility are possible and may be currently affecting many low fertility nations (Goldstein et al. 2009; Myrskylä et al. 2009) at this stage, it is quite unlikely that fertility will once again rise in most countries to above-replacement levels. Should that occur, however, it will only slow the process of ageing but is unlikely to reverse it. Population growth rates will continue to decline and eventually will turn negative in many countries. For the world as a whole, population growth will be attenuated but should continue until the central decades of the twentieth century. After that, population decline appears to be in store for much of the world, according to the recent long-run population projections of the United Nations (2008).[7]

Long-range implications of demographic transition and the pace of change

From a strictly demographic standpoint, the entire process of transition has generated a number of changes that have deep and lasting effects for society, which can be summed up in the following points.

(1) Any reduction in fertility will lead to lasting changes in population age structures. Initially these changes affect the relative weight of the very young in society and lead to an increase in the relative importance of working age population, generating the first demographic dividend. Further on, however, low fertility reduces the growth rate of labour and brings about a top-heavy age structure and rising old age and total dependency. The pace of ageing is particularly rapid whenever there are prolonged declines in the aggregate number of births. The process of ageing may be one of the most important effects of the demographic transition as it has multiple and extremely important social and economic implications for society.

(2) The period of relatively high population growth characterizing all demographic transitions tends to coincide with intense migratory pressure that has done much to shape the world we know today both ethnically and economically. Mass migration was the fellow traveller of the demographic transition both among the forerunners and during the more recent period of fertility decline in the developing world. While the international atmosphere for migration was different in each period, many of the effects are similar (Hatton and Williamson 1998, 2005).

(3) Reductions in fertility coupled with increasing life expectancy have an important and very direct effect on kin groups: they shrink the overall size of the network, reduce its breadth and lengthen its generational depth, much as happened with age structures: before the demographic transition, kin-networks were bottom-heavy, and more distant kin (cousins, uncles, aunts, etc.) played an important role for family life. Once fertility and mortality declines, family size shrinks, the number of lateral kin declines substantially, and parents and especially grandparents and even great grandparents become increasingly important for family life (Murphy 2011).

(4) By definition, increasing reproductive efficiency leads to a massive liberation in the time spent by mothers in bearing and rearing their children (Lee 2003). This fundamental alteration in women's lives leads to a whole host of changes affecting women and their role in society, their children and men everywhere.

(5) Longer life expectancy achieved during the demographic transition couples with greater investments in human capital to produce a better-educated, healthier and more productive working life. Dramatically longer life raises the return to investments in human

capital and greatly expands the years spent at older ages where labour supply is diminished or there is outright retirement.

(6) A longer life coupled with a sharply reduced duration of the reproductive period also tends to change the locus of life-long decision-making, substituting certain types of behaviour that once were considered essential for a successful life with others whose ultimate goal may only be realized much later on in life. There are many important examples of this last aspect including the stability of marriage as a life-long institution, the reassessing of certain aspects of intergenerational relations or the time horizon for given life strategies (Keyfitz 1987).[8]

All of these effects have important social and economic implications. Taken together they appear to be essential for the emergence of modern, individual-oriented societies (Dyson 2010; Reher 2011). It is safe to say that modern society would never have emerged as we know it today without the demographic transition. It is also true, however, that the demographic transition has not been uniform throughout the world, and this promises to condition the way it affects society. The demographic transition opens a *window of opportunity* for economic, social and familial changes. It is a period in which demographic change can work in favour of change, rather than against it as was often the case in earlier periods. It becomes, so to speak, a fellow traveller of change and progress. Just how beneficial its effects will be and how long they will last is related to the 'size' of this window. These benefits are constrained by three factors: (1) the speed of demographic change; (2) the population growth rates that are reached during the key period following initial mortality declines; and (3) the mechanisms available for population regulation at key moments of the transition.

On all these points, the earlier demographic transitions appear to have been much better situated than the more recent ones to take full advantage of the implications of demographic change (Reher 2011, pp. 21–9). Among them, the speed of decline of vital rates was far slower than it has been in the transitions of the developing world. The reason for this is that the reduction of mortality and the limitation of fertility in more recent transitions have benefited from technological inputs (antibiotics, vaccinations, artificial contraception, etc.) that were unavailable in historic transitions together with what was probably a far greater pent-up demand than that in historic transitions. Secondly, the population growth rates reached after the initial decline of mortality have been far greater in more recent transitions, often 2.0–2.5 per cent per year or even higher, than those reached historically (seldom much above 1 per cent per year). Finally, the mechanisms aimed at containing the effects of rapid population growth historically (principally mass migration to countries with very low population densities) are simply no longer available. A by-product of this last reality is that migration policies in receiving nations are no longer as benign and migration-friendly as they were in many parts of the world between 1850 and 1960 or even more recently.

For newcomers, the pace of change is far faster than it ever was historically, and it has often been accompanied by adverse economic and political realities, many of which are related to extraordinary population growth rates lasting for at least two to three decades. As the decline of fertility has accelerated in the past two decades, these population growth rates have also diminished to a point where population is now the fellow traveller of social and economic change in much of the developing world, with the exception of sub-Saharan Africa. These nations have entered, so to speak, the window of opportunity for a period of benign change. Unfortunately, this period may not last very long because the intensity of decline of fertility is such that the process of ageing in many of the countries, only in its initial stages at the moment, promises to be far more intense than it ever was in the countries undergoing the historic transition. Whether or not the time available will be sufficient to reap the full benefits of the demographic transition remains to be seen and is certainly a question of enormous importance for these nations.

The demographic transition also has its negative side, one that has no uncertain implications for economies, societies and the family. The historic transitions are entering this phase right now, and it is difficult to find optimistic voices regarding the prospects for future society in these countries. At least, however, they are rich and have consolidated institutions and fully developed political systems that should enable them to address the changes with wisdom and social stability. That does not brighten the prospects, but at least it suggests that societies have instruments available to them should they be needed. For the newcomers, it is not at all clear that this will be the case. The success stories are brilliant, in some cases even luminous, but so are those indications that many societies continue to be far from sufficiently developed to confront the new situation with confidence.

Social and political implications of the forces of change

Beyond the contribution of the demographic transition to economic growth or overall social change, other often vexing issues warrant our attention. Over the long run, the demographic transition unleashes a series of forces that end up changing the very nature of the family and the way it functions in society. Some of them emerge more or less directly from the interplay of demographic variables during the period of transition and in the decades following, and these affect the structural context of family life and the way it carries out its traditional tasks in society. Others affect the ability or the willingness of the family to carry out these tasks. Here the links to the demographic transition are less direct, and second-stage consequences of the changes are under way. Both of these effects are essential to family life and family forms, and the ultimate implications of the demographic transition for the family comes from the interaction of both.

The consequence of this process is a sea change for society and for the role played by the family both in society and in the lives of its members. A convenient way of envisioning the potential consequences for society is to look at the characteristics, either currently held or expected to hold, in many countries that are at advanced stages of their own transitions, which can be attributed directly or indirectly to the demographic transition. These are portrayed schematically in Table 2.1 and are grouped into several general areas. In all of them the forces of change are evident,

Table 2.1 Some characteristics of societies currently at advanced stages of the demographic transition

General population characteristics

- Low or negative population growth rates; relatively stagnant or declining numbers of births
- Extreme population ageing. Doubts about the sustainability of pension systems and costs of health care
- Problems with the supply of labour
- High levels of international migration (wherever supply of potential immigrants in sending countries is sufficient)

Mortality

- Extremely reduced mortality, increasing longevity even at very old ages
- Increases in both healthy and dependent life expectancy

Marriage and reproduction

- Below replacement fertility
- Widespread use of contraception
- High levels of abortion and of adoption
- Delayed childbearing; partial recovery of fertility at older ages
- High levels of permanent celibacy
- Growth in importance of partnering, cohabitation
- Children out of wedlock

Family and family life

- The family as we know it (especially coresident domestic group) is no longer the locus of social and demographic reproduction
- Significant decrease in parental authority
- Reduction in economic importance of family, especially with respect to intra-familial wealth transfers
- Shrinking kin networks coupled with an increase in the generational depth of these networks; the beanpole family
- Increases in single-person households, reduction in mean household size and drastic decreases in large and multi-familial households.
- Ability to care for vulnerable members stretched to the limit
- Parental concern about quality of life available for offspring. This concern constrains reproductive choices.
- Persistence of many traditional ways of understanding family life, together with changes in the way these are shown

Social and cultural characteristics

- Generally high levels of education
- A significant role for women in the labour force and in society. Increasing female autonomy
- Difficulties for gender relations in many societies, as men attempt to adapt and are often not successful
- Decline in traditional religion and religious values; increased secularization

On the horizon

- Potential difficulties in maintaining living standards
- The role of migration called into question
- Pervasive changes in the family, weakening its position and affecting its ability to successfully complement and cushion social trends and policy defects
- Long-term population decline

---

as is the fact that these societies appear to be entering a darker side of the demographic transition.

With regard to general population characteristics, the period of abundance of population and human capital has been replaced by one of scarcity: low growth, extreme ageing, a shrinking supply of labour and the high levels of migration needed to compensate for it. With respect to mortality, the changes set in motion by the demographic transition continue, with remarkably strong advances in general life expectancy among elderly populations though not necessarily of healthy life expectancy (Crimmins and Saito 2001; Crimmins et al. 1989, 1994; Molla et al. 2004).

Many of the traditional aspects of marriage and reproduction have been turned on their heads with a strikingly weakened and delayed institution of marriage, below replacement fertility and the progressive appearance of partnering as an alternative to marriage. The family and family life have changed to the point of hardly being recognizable. The family is no longer the locus of social and demographic reproduction; parental authority has declined enormously; kin networks are smaller, narrower and generationally deeper; households have shrunk, with far fewer large households and an abundance of persons living alone; the ability of families to come to the aid of their own vulnerable members is subject to severe doubt; and the concern of parents for the future social and economic situation of their offsprings is growing and has become a reason for keeping the numbers of children down (Dalla Zuanna 2007). Despite these changes, however, it is also possible to detect the persistence of many traditional ways of understanding family life, even though everywhere the change in different family variables is in the same direction (Reher 1998).

Society as a whole has also experienced important changes linked to the demographic transition with important implications for family life. The most important of these affects the role of women in society, which has undergone a revolutionary change over the last half century, that is 30–60 years. Women's labour force participation rates are now similar to those of men, their educational attainment is equal to or even higher than those of men, and their autonomy as persons has changed dramatically. In many societies this has led to difficulties in gender relations as men have found it hard to cope. The starting point of this trend differed widely by society (from the late 1950s to the mid-1980s), but everywhere the long-term trends have coincided. These changes have been accompanied by societies with high levels of education and where traditional religious values and organized religion have been in decline for decades.

The change in the role of women in society is one of the main outcomes of the revolution in reproductive efficiency which characterized the demographic transition and led to a massive reduction of the time women spent bearing and raising children together with important increases in per capita investment in the human capital of their children. Both of these effects became especially visible once the initial increases in family size due to the intrinsic dynamics of the demographic of transition explained earlier began to transform into smaller net family size. This happened in the historic transitions two to three decades after the onset of fertility change and was to have a pervasive effect on society and family life. Even during the baby boom, increases in family size were modest compared to levels held earlier, and so the overall process of liberation of women's time coupled with greater investments in the quality of their children and, eventually, relatively high educational levels among women themselves continued for decades. All of these became prerequisites for the eventual entry of women into the labour market. Other aspects of contemporary family life, such as delayed marriage and the ascendancy of individual-oriented values, were also linked to the changing locus of decision making brought on by sharply increased longevity and, as said before, increased reproductive efficiency. Both processes went hand in hand with other social and economic changes maturing during the Post-War period, many of them also triggered by the demographic transition, to completely alter many of the fundamental focal points of family life in developed countries.

Many of the elements of the scenario proposed earlier are also components of the Second Demographic Transition (SDT) theory so brilliantly set forth by Dirk van de Kaa and Ron Lesthaeghe among others.[9] For these authors, many of the strikingly different ways of understanding the family, marriage and reproduction in contemporary societies are the product, to a large extent, of shifts in values, away from group-oriented values (family, nation) and towards individual, often post-materialist ones in which self-fulfilment is a key goal for most people who are willing and able to predicate their behaviour on these ideas. For the SDT to take place, the following social realities must exist: postponement of marriage and childbearing, the importance of individual autonomy for marriage choice, the social acceptability of premarital cohabitation and value orientations that are able to influence demographic behaviour (Lesthaeghe 2010, p. 234). The proponents of this theory eschew the possibility that all of these characteristics might be the consequences set in motion by an earlier historical process, in this case the demographic transition. This is not the proper venue to polemicize with much-respected colleagues, but it is worth noting that by negating the historical origins of these characteristics, SDT theory ends up being a savvy description of current social reality but ultimately is incapable of explaining how and why those changes came to be, other than in an immediate way. In the long run, negating history severely limits the explanatory and the predictive power of SDT theory (Lesthaeghe 2010, p. 219). When understanding these changes as the by-product of the demographic transition, however, this limitation disappears.

Is this sort of social and familial change in store for much of the developing world?[10] In his recent paper, Ron Lesthaeghe (2010) shows, cautiously but convincingly, that at least with respect to marriage behaviour and certain aspects of ideational change, the SDT has spread to Southern and Eastern Europe and, more recently and partially, to a number of countries in East Asia. While not a good example of the 'developing world', this diffusion of the SDT from its original roots in Northwestern Europe is noteworthy. Will something similar happen to other countries in South Asia, the Middle East, Northern Africa or Latin America? Throughout these regions fertility is declining precipitously, in many nations it is close to or below replacement, and in some places the aggregate number of births has also begun to decline. Everywhere the demographic transition is in full swing and, as a result, population growth rates are also declining very quickly and the process of population ageing is under way. The demographic transition was a prerequisite for the changes described by the SDT framework wherever it happened, and there is no reason to believe that something similar will not also take place throughout much of the rest of the world. If we look at individual case studies, important heterogeneity emerges, but everywhere the trends are similar. The basic underlying demographic dynamics are undeniable in many countries, and there are also changes in many social variables: age at marriage, educational attainment especially of women and the female labour force participation levels are on the rise in many contexts. Recent increases in cohabitation in many Latin American countries may be a harbinger of an unfolding SDT in that world region (Esteve et al. 2012). This is only the beginning of the type of change we can expect throughout much of the world. As Arland Thornton puts it, much of the world appears to have bought into the developmental idealism so aggressively promoted by the West (Thornton 2001, 2005).

Everything will take place at a far faster pace than it did in historic Europe because here the pace of decline of vital rates has been far faster than it was in the historic transitions. In some aspects, this may be good indeed because the economic growth and societal transformation may also be much faster than it ever was historically. It may, however, have unwanted side effects because the window of opportunity for the beneficial effects of the transition may be too short for many developing countries to fully assimilate its meaning and reap its benefits. This is because the darker side of the transition, which is currently coming front and centre in the developed world, with rampant ageing, a shrinking supply of labour and serious problems in maintaining many of the social benefits that have accrued over many decades, may well show up in the developing world fairly soon. In this sense, in countries where the transformation has been less than complete – the case in much of the developing world – more difficult times may arrive all too soon, and processes of growth and transformation may be cut off before they can fully mature.

From a strictly social standpoint, one affecting the family and the way it interacts with its members and with society, the pace of change in the developing world promises to be very rapid indeed. In the historic transitions, the time between the initial onset of fertility change (the onset of the demographic transition) and entry into the most recent phase characterized by SDT spanned as much as eight decades. In the developing world, estimates of entry into the SDT phase are still premature, though we can expect that it will happen soon. In these regions, for the most part, fertility began to decline between the mid-1960s and the mid-1980s, and at present, there is growing evidence that the new phase of social change has already commenced in many countries. In other words, somewhat speculatively, the time between these two key transformations promises to be about one half as long as it was in the historic transitions. Change has been intense in Europe in recent decades and in many countries there are severe problems of adjustment. The dizzying nature of the pace of change in much of the rest of the world will be far greater than it ever was in the developed world, at least if the pace of social change keeps up with the pace of demographic change. The ability of these countries to experience this sort of change in a complete and relatively un-traumatic way is certainly open to question.

On the horizon: plausible scenarios for the future

As presented earlier, the developed regions of the world appear to have entered the darker side of the demographic transition. Nearly a century of largely positive effects have come to an end. The bellwether for the change is unquestionably the issue of ageing, but there are many other aspects as well that suggest that the times ahead may become increasingly difficult ones for society (Reher 2007). These changes can be summed up very generally in four main points: (a) long-term population decline or at least stagnation, below (or near) replacement fertility as a structural aspect of society and extreme ageing; (b) potential difficulties in maintaining economic growth and living standards in societies with dysfunctional age structures; (c) increasing importance of migration for the maintenance of living standards, increasingly multi-ethnic societies (with their attendant problems and advantages) and a major threat on the horizon as the sending societies begin to have labour shortages of their own; (d) pervasive changes in family life, weakening its position in society and affecting its ability to successfully complement and cushion adverse social trends and care for its own vulnerable members.

The extent to which the developing world can escape this type of scenario is an open question. In a sense, many areas of this vast world are already characterized by some aspects of this pattern of change. In particular, very low fertility, slowing population growth and rapid ageing with labour shortages visible in the not-so-distant future appear to be very much on course for the developing world unless, of course, there is another trend change in fertility. A new baby boom, however, appears unlikely, though in theory it is possible. Despite considerable intra-regional disparities, fertility is declining precipitously throughout the world – far faster than ever envisioned – and in many countries it is now near or below replacement. We expect that most of the rest of the less developed countries will follow suit, though there is no way of knowing just how far fertility will fall.

Other long-term implications of the demographic transition, especially those involving massive social change, are more difficult to confidently forecast. There is little doubt that these types of changes have taken place in societies undergoing the historic demographic transition. The results are everywhere to be seen. For these sort of changes to spread to the newcomers at this banquet of demographic change, serious obstacles in different societies will have to be overcome. The most important of these are cultural and are linked to the way the family and society function. Will the Islamic, Buddhist or Hindu regions of the world be able to resist the forces of social and cultural change unleashed by the demographic transition, or will they too succumb to a tidal wave of individualism, below replacement fertility, weakening marriage ties, female autonomy and secularization as much of the West has? It is, of course, impossible to say, but it is worth remembering that the forces of change in the historic demographic transitions over the past 50–60 years have been monumental, far beyond anything imaginable at the early stages of this process. With all due humility, we suspect that the forces of change will also affect the rest of the world as other demographic transitions mature and educational levels increase. Just how this will happen is unclear, but we also suspect that it will be a fairly traumatic process, much as it has been in the West.

If we look at the big historical picture, the *longue durée* in the words of Fernand Braudel, it can be said that the demographic transition gave rise to the enormous breakaway population growth that characterized much of the nineteenth and twentieth centuries. It also appears that the demographic transition will bring this period of growth to an end, as slow even negative population growth increasingly appears to be the most likely final outcome of the changes in due course. First this will happen in the developed world, but will quite likely affect the entire world during the second half of the twenty-first century. World population decline, should it happen, will not start any time soon, but it surely will if fertility continues to remain at the levels it is nearly everywhere at present. Is this a bad thing or not? Here there are many potential answers (Coleman and Rowthorn 2011; Reher 2007 and Chapter 5). Whatever they are, we had best get ready for it because increasingly it appears to be the end goal of the process under way. Ultimately the long-term implications of the demographic transition will only end when this downward phase of the world population cycle comes to an end. Like all demographic cycles in the past, inherent in the period of growth are the corrective mechanisms that are destined to bring that period to an end and to restore some sort of balance. In the final analysis, the complete cycle of the demographic transition will have spanned three centuries or more.

Will this balance be reached at world population levels of 1800 or 1900, below them or above them? We of course do not know. Our hunch is that the equilibrium state, itself transitory, will be reached at population levels considerably higher than those holding in 1900, mostly because the technological advances of the past two centuries have gone far to guaranteeing that world resources will be able to sustain considerably higher levels of population than those held 100 years ago. This idea is premised, of course, on the basically Malthusian belief that the carrying capacity of the world economy is the prime determinant of population size. Should this not be the case – and it may not be –, there is no telling where, when and how the downward trend in population will come to an end.

Notes

1. In his seminal article on the demographic transition, when referring to those countries with 'high growth potential' Frank Notestein (1945, p. 52) stated

   > If, on the other hand, a period of peace, order, and rapidly rising production were to be accompanied by a thorough and balanced modernization, we could expect the same or even faster immediate growth but a different termination. If such developments brought urbanization, industrialization, rising levels of living, popular education, and popular participation in political life, the same forces that eventually induced a declining fertility in the West would probably come into play. The population

would then undergo transitional growth, perhaps tripling in the process. If events marched swiftly and studied efforts were made to induce declining fertility, perhaps only a doubling of present populations would be involved.

2. For this period, basically there are only data for European and for a limited number of non-European societies, and thus our knowledge of the period is mostly restricted to this region.
3. For a lively debate on the role of famine mortality for population growth some years ago in *Population and Development Review*, see Watkins and Menken (1985, 1988), Palloni (1988) and Komlos (1988).
4. For France there is evidence of very significant reductions in both childhood mortality and marital fertility beginning just before or around the time of the French Revolution. The demographic change in France was much more like that which was going to occur a century later in much of Europe, leaving it 'alone in Europe' as Etienne van de Walle so eloquently termed (1978).
5. The fact that countries like Japan and China also participated in a similar pattern of relatively intense trans-oceanic migration suggests, at least indirectly, that some of the same demographic mechanisms existing in Europe were also at work in areas of East Asia, especially with respect to population growth.
6. In Costa Rica, for example, Pérez Brignoli (2010) has found that the initial improvement in mortality dates from the 1920s. In other countries initial declines may have taken place even earlier.
7. The plausible scenario is quite different for sub-Saharan Africa where fertility continues to be high and decline more recent, coupled with an AIDS epidemic, low levels of education, a different cultural mix and scant development, though here too population decline may be in store in the more distant future for most nations. Just when this period of population decline will end is anyone's guess.
8. For a more detailed account of many of these effects, see Lee and Reher (2011, pp. 1–2) and Reher (2011, pp. 13–21, 30).
9. On the SDT, see van de Kaa (1987), Lesthaeghe (2010), Ariès (1980) and Surkyn and Lesthaeghe (2004).
10. For the purposes of simplicity, it is best to leave the sub-Saharan region out of this discussion because in this region the demographic transition is only in its initial phase.

References

Ariès, P. (1980) 'Two successive motivations for the declining birth rates in the West', *Population and Development Review,* 6(4): 645–50.

Bloom, D. E., Canning, D. and Sevilla, J. (2003) *The Demographic Dividend: A New Perspective on the Economic Consequences of Population Change,* Population Matters Monograph MR-1274 (Santa Monica: RAND).

Coleman, D. and Rowthorn, R. (2011) 'Who's afraid of population decline? A critical examination of its consequences', in R. Lee and D. S. Reher (eds) *Demographic Transition and Its Consequences, Population and Development Review* (Supplement to Volume 37 of *Population and Development Review*), pp. 217–48.

Crimmins, E. M., Hayward, M. D. and Saito, Y. (1994) 'Changing mortality and morbidity rates and the health status and life expectancy of the older population', *Demography*, 31: 159–75.

Crimmins, E. M. and Saito, Y. (2001) 'Tends in healthy life expectancy in the United States, 1970–1990: gender, racial, and educational differences', *Social Science & Medicine*, 52: 1629–841.

Crimmins, E. M., Saito, Y. and Ingegneri, D. (1989) 'Changes in life expectancy and disability-free life expectancy in the United States', *Population and Development Review*, 15: 235–67.

Dalla Zuanna, G. (2007) 'Social mobility and fertility', *Demographic Research*, 17(article 15): 441–64.

Dyson, T. (2010) *Population and Development. The Demographic Transition* (London/New York: Zed Books).

Dyson, T. and Murphy, M. (1985) 'The onset of fertility transition', *Population and Development Review*, 11(3): 399–440.

Dyson, T. and Murphy, M. (1986) 'Rising fertility in developing countries', in R. Woods and P. Rees (eds) *Population Structures and Models: Developments in Spatial Demography* (London: Allen & Unwin), pp. 68–94.

Esteve, A., Lesthaeghe, R. and López-Gay, A. (2012) 'The Latin American cohabitation boom, 1970–2007', *Population and Development Review*, 38(1): 55–81.

Flinn, M. W. (1974) 'The stabilization of mortality in pre-industrial Western Europe', *Journal of European Economic History*, 3(2): 285–318.

Goldstein, J. R., Sobotka, T. and Jasilioniene, A. (2009) 'The end of "lowest-low" fertility?', *Population and Development Review*, 35(4): 663–99.

Hatton, T. J. and Williamson, J. G. (1998) *The Age of Mass Migration: Causes and Economic Impact* (New York/Oxford: Oxford University Press).

Hatton, T. J. and Williamson, J. G. (2005) *Global Migration and the World Economy: Two Centuries of Policy and Performance* (Cambridge, MA: MIT Press, 2006).

Keyfitz, N. (1987) 'Form and substance in family demography', in J. Bongaarts, T. K. Burch and K. W. Wachter (eds) *Family Demography. Methods and Their Application* (Oxford: Clarendon Press), pp. 4–16.

Komlos, J. (1988) 'On the role of crises in historical perspective: comment', *Population and Development Review*, 14(1): 159–64.

Lee, R. (2003) 'The demographic transition: three centuries of fundamental change', *Journal of Economic Perspectives*, 17(4): 167–90.

Lee, R. and Mason, A. (2010) 'Fertility, human capital, and economic growth over the demographic transition', *European Journal of Population*, 26(2): 159–82.

Lee, R. and Reher, D. S. (2011) 'Introduction. The landscape of the demographic transition and its aftermath', in R. Lee and D. S. Reher (eds) *Demographic Transition and Its Consequences*, Supplement to Vol. 37 of *Population and Development Review*, 1–7.

Lesthaeghe, R. (2010) 'The unfolding story of the second demographic transition', *Population and Development Review*, 36(2): 211–51.

Livi Bacci, M. (2000) 'Mortality crises in historical perspective: the European experience', in G. A. Cornia and R. Paniccià (eds) *The Mortality Crisis in Transitional Economies* (Oxford: Oxford University Press), pp. 38–58.

Molla, M., Madans, J. H. and Wagener, D. K. (2004) 'Differentials in adult mortality and activity limitation by years of education in the United States at the end of the 1990s', *Population and Development Review*, 30(4): 65–647.

Murphy, M. (2011) 'Long-term effects of the demographic transition on family and kinship networks in Britain', in R. Lee and D. S. Reher (eds) *Demographic Transition and Its Consequences, Population and Development Review* (Supplement to Volume 37 of *Population and Development Review*), pp. 55–80.

Myrskylä, M., Kohler, H.-P. and Billari, F. C. (2009) 'Advances in development reverse fertility declines', *Nature*, 460(7256): 741–3, doi: 10.1038/nature08230.

Notestein, F. (1945) 'Population, the long view', in T. W. Schultz (ed.) *Food for the World* (Chicago: University of Chicago Press), pp. 36–57.

Palloni, A. (1988) 'On the role of crises in historical perspective: an exchange – comment', *Population and Development Review*, 14(1): 145–58.

Pérez Brignoli, H. (2010) *La población de Costa Rica, 1750–2000. Una historia experimental* (San José: Editorial de la Universidad de Costa Rica).

Reher, D. S. (1998) 'Family ties in Western Europe: persistent contrasts', *Population and Development Review*, 24(2): 203–34.

Reher, D. S. (2004) 'The demographic transition revisited as a global process', *Population, Space and Place*, 10: 19–41.

Reher, D. S. (2007) 'Towards long-term population decline: a discussion of relevant issues', *European Journal of Population*, 23: 189–207.

Reher, D. S. (2011) 'Economic and social implications of the demographic transition', in R. Lee and D. S. Reher (eds) *Demographic Transition and Its Consequences, Population and Development Review* (Supplement to Volume 37 of *Population and Development Review*), pp. 11–33.

Reher, D. S. and Sanz-Gimeno, A. (2007) 'Rethinking historical reproductive change: longitudinal data for a Spanish town', *Population and Development Review*, 33(4): 703–28.

Riley, J. C. (2005a) 'Estimates of regional and global life expectancy, 1800–2001', *Population and Development Review*, 31(3): 537–43.

Riley, J. C. (2005b) 'The timing and pace of health transitions around the world', *Population and Development Review*, 31(4): 741–64.

Roussel, L. (1992) 'La famille en Europe occidentale: divergences et convergences', *Population*, 47(1): 133–52.

Schofield, R. and Reher, D. S. (1991) 'The decline of mortality in Europe', in R. S. Schofield, D. Reher and A. Bideau (eds) *The Decline of Mortality in Europe* (Oxford: Oxford University Press), pp. 1–17.

Surkyn, J. and Lesthaeghe, R. (2004) 'Value orientations and the Second Demographic Transition (SDT) in Northern, Western and Southern Europe: an update', *Demographic Research*, special collection 3(article 3): 45–86.

Thornton, A. (2001) 'The developmental paradigm, reading history sideways, and family change', *Demography*, 38(4): 449–65.

Thornton, A. (2005) *Reading History Sideways: The Fallacy and Enduring Impact of the Developmental Paradigm on Family Life* (Chicago: University of Chicago Press).

United Nations (2008) *World Population Prospects Database. The 2008 Revision*, http://esa.un.org/unpp/

van Bavel, J. (2010) 'Subreplacement fertility in the West before the baby boom: past and current perspectives', *Population Studies*, 64(1): 1–18.

van de Kaa, D. J. (1987) 'Europe's second demographic transition', *Population Bulletin*, 42: 1 (Washington, DC: Population Reference Bureau Inc).

van de Walle, E. (1978) 'Alone in Europe: the French fertility decline until 1850', in C. Tilly (ed.) *Historical Studies of Changing Fertility* (Princeton, NJ: Princeton University Press).

Watkins, S. and Menken, J. (1985) 'Famines in historical perspective', *Population and Development Review*, 11(4): 647–75.

Watkins, S. and Menken, J. (1988) 'On the role of crises in historical perspective: reply', *Population and Development Review*, 15(1): 165–70.

Wrigley, E. A. and Schofield, R. (1981) *The Population History of England, 1541–1871: A Reconstruction* (Cambridge: Cambridge University Press).

3
The Growth of the One-child Family and Other Changes in the Low Fertility Countries of Asia

Gavin W. Jones

Introduction

In this chapter, I will concentrate on the low fertility countries of Asia – those with Total Fertility Rate (TFR) of 1.5 or below. Which countries are we talking about? Essentially all of East Asia (except for North Korea and Mongolia), as well as Singapore and Thailand[1] in Southeast Asia. Trends in TFR for the countries for which annual estimates are available are given in Table 3.1. Although the exact level of fertility in China is still a highly contested issue, for our purposes, China can be considered one of these low fertility countries. If its TFR is not as low as 1.5, it is certainly not very much higher.

Fertility in East Asia is now the lowest in the world, and this appears likely to remain the case for some time (Frejka et al. 2010). TFRs of around 1.1–1.3 in Japan, South Korea and Singapore mean that the one-child family, which in international public perception is characteristic of China because of the publicity given to the 'one-child policy', is actually even more characteristic of other East Asian countries than of China. Indeed, Taiwan's fertility (a TFR of 0.895 in 2010) was the lowest ever recorded in a country with a population exceeding 10 million. Thus all these countries have to deal with the consequences of very low fertility – children lacking the traditional 'baggage' of family – siblings and cousins, and over time, also aunts and uncles.

Revised version of paper prepared for the Conference on Family Change in the Wake of Demographic Transition, Beijing, 17–18 September 2010.

Table 3.1 Trends in total fertility rates, East Asia

Year	Japan	South Korea	Taiwan	Singapore	Hong Kong SAR
1995	1.42	1.64	1.78	1.67	n.a.
1996	1.43	1.70	1.76	1.66	1.19
1997	1.39	1.54	1.77	1.61	1.12
1998	1.38	1.47	1.47	1.47	1.02
1999	1.34	1.42	1.56	1.47	0.98
2000	1.36	1.47	1.68	1.60	1.04
2001	1.33	1.30	1.40	1.41	0.93
2002	1.32	1.17	1.34	1.37	0.94
2003	1.29	1.17	1.24	1.25	0.90
2004	1.29	1.16	1.18	1.24	0.93
2005	1.25	1.08	1.12	1.25	0.97
2006	1.32	1.13	1.12	1.26	0.98
2007	1.34	1.26	1.12	1.29	1.02
2008	1.37	1.19	1.05	1.28	1.06
2009	1.37	1.21	1.03	1.22	1.04
2010	1.39	1.22	0.89	1.16	1.04

Source: Jones (2007), Table 3.1, updated from official sources for each country.

Fertility and changing family and household composition

The size and composition of households is a dynamic process, changing over the life cycle as children are born, grow up and leave the family. Migration affects household composition, as does the decreasing prevalence of extended family forms where these were once more prominent. Household composition, however, is not the same as family composition. Absent members are not necessarily uninvolved in family matters, especially in this age of the ubiquitous cell phone. Indeed, maintenance of the role of absent members – including those who live overseas for lengthy periods – both in household functioning and decision making is increasingly observed and accepted as part of the reality of a globalizing world with mobile populations (see, e.g. Douglass 2011; Fan 2011).

Whether we focus on the residential household or the family, however, the sharp decline in fertility in East Asian countries clearly makes for smaller family size. Even in the case of Indonesia, where fertility is still slightly above the replacement level, the declining size of households over time is quite clear (Jones 2002, pp. 219–20). In Thailand, the average household size declined from 5.8 in 1970 to 4.6 in 1990 and is expected to continue to fall steadily to 3.3 in 2015 (Mason et al.

1993, p. 70). Extended family contacts will, of course, widen the network of interaction, but not to anything like the extent in the past, when an average individual had 5 siblings, 6 children, 30 nieces and nephews, 10 uncles and aunts, 60 first cousins, 120 first cousins of his parents and 720 second cousins.

Non-marriage

Low fertility throughout East Asia has partly been achieved through an increasing proportion of women who will never marry (Jones 2007). This raises many issues about the way such women will fit into the family structure and the need for traditional conceptions of the family to change. In 2005, the most recent year for which data for all countries are available, the percentage of women aged 35–39 remaining never married was 18 in Japan, 8 in South Korea, 16 in Taiwan, 15 in Singapore, 20 in Hong Kong SAR and 8 in South Korea.[2] Not only were these percentages very high by international standards, but also they had continued to rise since 2000, except in Singapore (Jones and Gubhaju 2009). Census data for 2010 show continuing increases for Taiwan (to 21 per cent) and Singapore (to 17 per cent).

It is important to note that at this stage, China does not fit into the East Asian pattern of rising proportions of women who will never marry, as marriage for women remains nearly universal by age 30. In 2000, at age 30, less than 2 per cent of Chinese women remained single, compared with 20 per cent in Thailand, more than 25 per cent among Chinese women in Singapore and about 25 per cent among Chinese women in Malaysia. And in 2005, only 0.7 per cent of Chinese women aged 35–39 remained never married, compared with the much higher figures (11–28 times higher!) for the other countries listed in the previous paragraph. While the proportion of women remaining single into their 30s does seem to be rising in cities such as Beijing and Shanghai, the non-conformity of China to the pattern of delayed and non-marriage sweeping other parts of East and Southeast Asia remains a paradox. However, marriage seems certain to be increasingly delayed in China, notwithstanding the increasing imbalance in the sex ratio that will develop over the coming decade in the marrying age groups, which will both place increasing pressure on women to marry and widen their choice of partners. The reason for expecting that marriages will be delayed despite this countervailing force is that some of the social and economic trends making for delayed marriage among women in China are following much the same path as in other East Asian countries – difficulties of combining work and raising a family (even of one child); rising educational levels; and 'marriage squeeze' issues for educated women, given the strength of hypergamy.

Family sizes of children

Fertility in East Asian countries is very low, with an average TFR of just over one child per woman. In countries where fertility has fallen to really low levels – TFR below 1.5 – half of all women have at most one child (Le Bras 1979). Does this mean that most children are growing up as only children? Not necessarily. Singularly, children are born to a cohort of women whose average number of children is currently higher than suggested by the cross-sectional snapshot provided by period fertility rates. But this aside, many women are not marrying at all – the figures are likely to reach 20 per cent for recent cohorts in Japan (Ogawa 2003), and probably also in Taiwan and Hong Kong – and some of those who marry are not having children.[3] Though an increasing proportion of adults are remaining childless, it is important to bear in mind that *no children grow up in no-children families.* Among women who have children, many have just one, while others have two or more. Taking into account childless women, this can still average out at just above one per woman. As Preston (1976, p. 105) and Le Bras (1979) noted, women with large families contribute disproportionately to the average family size of children.[4] Other East Asian countries probably differ substantially from China in the distribution of family size of children, because of universal marriage and the one-child policy in China, which could be expected to make for a higher proportion of Chinese children growing up in one-child families.

Length of generation

Another point to bear in mind is the increased length of generation, because of the increase in the average age of childbearing. Increased length of generation is normally related to issues of population growth; it slows the rates of population growth, even if women end up bearing as many children as in the past when women bore their children at an earlier age. But a longer time to 'turn over' generations has other implications at the family level. In East Asian countries, women are now typically bearing their first child at an age that is four or five years older than their mothers' generation did, and some of them are having their first (and perhaps only) child in their late 30s. This may have a number of implications. It no doubt means that women are psychologically more mature when they are bearing their children. It may also mean, however, that they and their husbands are more settled in 'child-free' ways, and therefore the adjustment necessary when the first child comes along is greater than would be the case for couples who had had less time to settle into child-free life styles. There is also the greater risk of birth abnormalities occurring when the mother and/or father are older. With ultrasound checks, such abnormalities are more likely to be detected in advance these days, but this still means wrenching decisions for potential parents about whether to terminate the pregnancy, perhaps with the knowledge that there may be no further chance to produce another child.

Benefits and costs of small family size

There are significant differences between the families of five or six children, typical of earlier generations, and those of one or two children, in the way children are raised and the social dynamics within the family. Typically, in large families, the older children play a role from a young age in assisting with the raising of their younger siblings, and perhaps later in financing their education. With low fertility, parents' attention is focused on just one or two children. This has positive implications for human capital, as the investment of money and time by the parents will no doubt assist their one or two children achieve better results in school and in career-related activities. Indeed, all the evidence points to the trade-off between the quantity and quality of children, which has been resoundingly resolved in favour of quality in the East Asian countries (Montgomery et al. 2000), and to the fact that this is a major reason for the very low fertility they are now experiencing. The smaller cohorts of children should also enable government investment in education to achieve more per child.

Are there downsides to small family size? In China, both parents and the government fear the so-called 4-2-1 syndrome: the ratio of four grandparents and two parents per one child. This can be interpreted in two alternative ways: a great deal of attention focused on the one child by two parents and four grandparents, or as a weighty responsibility placed on the one child for the care of two parents and four grandparents as they age. As noted by Xin Yuan (2004), family intergenerational analysis suggests that the situation may not be as dire as is often argued.

> Before '1' (one-child) becomes an adult, he or she will be raised with his/her parents' help, which means '2' (parents) and '4' (grandparents) support one child, that is to say, '2+4' support '1'. When the child reaches maturity, he/she can assist the parents in supporting

> the grandparents, that is, '2+1' support '4'. Moreover, not all elders need external support and not all survive to old age.

However, he also notes that when two only children marry, they will be responsible for four parents and eight grandparents. They can only live with one set of parents, which means that the other half of their parent and grandparent families will be empty nesters. What proportion of families is in this situation? It has certainly risen substantially, though further careful studies are needed on the exact amount of increase. Moreover, the issue is certainly not unique to China. There are many single-child families throughout East Asia, despite the absence of a one-child policy. However, as noted earlier, in the other East Asian countries ultra-low fertility is due to a much larger extent than in China to non-marriage, and therefore in most cases the number of childless women is increasing even more rapidly than the number of women with one child (Frejka et al. 2010, pp. 583–7).

The issue of 'self-centredness' of only children is also frequently raised – the 'little emperor' syndrome. It seems to be frequently speculated in China that divorce rates will rise with the clash of wills and personalities when two 'little emperors' marry each other. Inherently plausible as these speculations may be, they require evidence and research to back them up.

There are, however, other twists to this story in the East Asian setting. The general East Asian family-raising context in the early twenty-first century needs to be kept in mind. Tremendous pressure is placed on the parents (especially the mother) to ensure that children perform well in the high-pressure educational competition that characterizes these societies (Ochiai and Molony 2008; Retherford and Ogawa 2006; Yi et al. 2009). It is speculated that the extent of this pressure is one of the factors contributing to the low rates of marriage and childbearing, as some potential parents, despite their general interest in having children, find the pressure of expectations on them as parents more than they are willing to undergo (Jones 2007, p. 470; Hirao 2007).

Extended adolescence and the family role of singles

In East Asia, there is a continued tradition of living at home until marriage. Indeed, there is some explaining to be done to parents by any unmarried person despite being in his or her late 20s and 30s who chooses to leave the family home while remaining in the same city. Because of delayed marriage, there is therefore a tendency for young people to stay at home longer, and this tendency is strongly reinforced by the high cost of owning or renting a house and the convenience of living at home without paying for one's board (on Japan, see Retherford and Ogawa 2006, pp. 17–19).

Are there value changes in these societies that are closely related to the rise in singlehood and the decline in fertility? Atoh (2001) argues that in Japan, individualism has increased, but only slowly, while gender role attitudes have changed much more markedly. Lee (2009) and Eun (2006) seem to agree over the trend in South Korea. Women's attitude changes appear to be more related to dissatisfaction with the dilemmas and the conflicts that traditional gender roles pose for educated women in a rapidly changing economy than with 'individualism' per se. As expressed by Eun (2007, p. 61):

> Unlike the sea change occurring in women's social status and economic capacity, Korean family values and attitudes are still very conservative and traditional in many respects.... Though women's public participation in education and the labor force has grown by leaps and bounds, family norms regulating family life remain within a male-centred and female-subordinated structure. For example, working mothers are expected to fulfill the roles of a full-time housewife after returning from work. 'Second shift' is mandatory for Korean women regardless of their educational achievement or professional careers.

However, Lesthaeghe (2010) argues that Japan now demonstrates the major characteristics of the Second Demographic Transition. A 2004 survey revealed that a fifth of Japanese men and women aged 25–29 had ever experienced cohabitation, and the mean duration of premarital cohabitation is close to two years. Premarital conceptions and the divorce rate are also rising. 'The only missing ingredient so far is parenthood among cohabiting couples' (Lesthaeghe 2010, p. 239). World Values Survey data also 'demonstrate that the demographic dimension of postponement of parenthood can be linked to the same value orientations as those associated with the SDT in Europe' (Lesthaeghe 2010, pp. 241–2).

If young people in East Asia are increasingly displaying the elements of individualism, consumerism and distaste for traditional authority structures, this can be expected to lead to strong reactions from more conservative elements in these strongly patriarchal societies. And indeed a pejorative attitude is evident in many commentaries on the role of singles in Japan and South Korea. The terms 'parasite singles' and 'gold misses' have become widespread in Japan and South Korea, respectively, emphasizing their selfish lifestyles and their willingness to continue being subsidized by their parents. What is the actual role of the large non-married population in their households and in society? We know that in Japan, 64 per cent of unmarried men and 71 per cent of unmarried women in their 20s were living with parents in 2005 (Bumpass et al. 2009, p. 225). Are they, and singles into their 30s, contributing financially or in other ways to their households or extended families? Are many 40-something singles playing caring roles for elderly or disabled in the family?

There is need for more research into the lives of singles in these countries. Should they be condemned? Pitied? Or simply accepted as a new reality? The proportion of singles is now so high that they can no longer be regarded as a 'fringe' or deviant group, but rather very much part of the mainstream. We need to understand why they remain single – whether it is through choice or circumstance – and the context in which they plan their future.

There is likely to be an association between the changing attitudes of singles in these societies and the increased proportion of one-child families. Is the proclaimed self-centredness of only children founded on any stronger evidence than of the 'selfishness' of the non-married who remain in the family home and enjoy the benefits of doing so? In what ways will growing up as single children affect the orientation to marriage or to enjoying the supposed benefits of single life?

Ageing and support for the dependant elderly

There is little doubt that issues related to population ageing will be central, not only to national policy reactions to ultra-low fertility, but also to family level adjustments needed to cope with radically altered population structures. At an aggregate level, the issues can be well illustrated by trends in ageing support ratios – that is, the ratio of the population aged 20–64 to the population aged 65+. Admittedly, the precise age limits used for this calculation do not accurately reflect the actual dependency situation, which depends on the ages at which people actually enter and withdraw from the labour force, and on the proportion of the elderly requiring various kinds of support (in the case of physical support, the requirement is usually quite small). But as a general indicator, the ageing support ratio does give the sense of the trends which are so dramatic that modification of these ages will not alter the general picture greatly.

Table 3.2 Median ages and potential ageing support ratios, low fertility countries of Asia, 1980–2050

Country	1980	1990	2000	2010	2020	2030	2040	2050
Potential ageing support ratio (population aged 20–64/65+)								
Japan	6.67	5.15	3.62	2.61	1.91	1.74	1.45	1.31
South Korea	13.18	11.85	8.68	5.86	4.15	2.48	1.76	1.50
Singapore	11.93	11.52	8.78	7.37	4.28	2.47	1.78	1.58
China	9.54	9.30	8.48	7.88	5.44	3.84	2.50	2.20
Thailand	12.51	11.77	8.77	7.09	5.18	3.51	2.63	2.21
Median age								
Japan	32.6	37.4	41.4	44.7	48.2	51.4	52.6	52.3
South Korea	22.2	27.0	32.1	37.9	43.0	47.0	49.7	51.8
Singapore	24.5	29.3	34.5	37.6	42.7	46.5	48.9	51.4
China	22.1	25.0	29.7	34.5	38.1	42.5	46.4	48.7
Thailand	19.5	24.6	30.2	34.2	38.2	41.8	44.8	46.8

Source: Computed from UN World Population Prospects – the 2010 Revision (medium projection).

As shown in Table 3.2, the median ages of all the populations we are considering have risen sharply since 1980, and the ageing support ratios have fallen sharply. Both these trends are expected to continue until 2050. The decline in ageing support ratios will be particularly sharp over the coming decade – from 2010 to 2020 – in Japan and Singapore, whereas in South Korea, China and Thailand, the decade of the 2020s will see the sharpest fall in the ageing support ratios. In the 40 years between 2010 and 2050, the ageing support ratio will halve in Japan, and will fall by much more than this in the other countries. Such declines will require major adjustments of policies with regard to income support programmes, orientation of health services to give much more weight to gerontology, and labour market policy, including retirement ages. It will also require a re-thinking of the underlying rationale for policies throughout the region, which is that families should be responsible for the care of dependant elderly.

The ageing support ratio, as a macro-level indicator, is replicated, with considerable variation in particular cases, at the individual family level. For example, while in Thailand, most of the older elderly have many surviving children because they built their families during the high-fertility era, sharp declines are projected in the number of living children for those who will be in their 60s by 2015, because these cohorts were building their families in the era of declining fertility.

Table 3.3 Percentage distribution of the population aged 60 years or over, according to household composition

Country	Date	Living independently of others			With child or grandchild	With other relative	With non-relative
		Total	Alone	Couple			
Japan	2000	47.2	12.7	34.5	48.3	4.4	0.2
South Korea	2000	46.0	16.8	29.2	49.1	4.9[a]	
Malaysia	1983/85	16.7	5.8	10.9	79.8	3.1	0.4
Thailand	2002	20.6	6.5	14.0	65.7[b]	n.a.	n.a.
Singapore	1995	9.1	3.3	5.8	85.0	6.0[c]	
France	1994	82.1	28.7	53.4	15.3		2.6[d]
Italy	1994	62.9	22.6	40.4	34.6		2.4[d]
United States	2000	74.6	25.9	48.7	17.8	4.6	3.0

[a]Includes living with non-relatives.
[b]Does not include living with grandchild.
[c]Other living arrangements.
[d]Living with other adults, but not with partner or children.
Source: United Nations (2005, Table II.4); Kim (2004, Table 7.7); MCYS (1995, Table 4.1); Knodel and Chayovan (2008, Table 5.1).

It should be noted that living arrangements of the elderly do differ considerably in Asia from those in Western countries, with a much higher proportion living with a child or grandchild (see Table 3.3). Although the per cent of elderly Japanese and Koreans living with a child or grandchild has been gradually declining, it does not appear likely to reach levels as low as in France or the United States.

Demographic trends do, however, raise many issues about whether the family can be relied on as in the past to provide care for the needy elderly. There are a number of aspects to the problem. The first is the sharply declining ratio of potential carers to the numbers of elderly, as indicated by the potential support ratio in the figure above. The number of living children of older persons has been declining through movement of smaller birth cohorts into the main 'caring ages'. The second is that a high proportion of the potential carers (usually women) are now drawn into the paid workforce (consistent with government policy in these countries), and are therefore not available for full-time caring work. The third is that, despite the general improvement in the health status of the elderly at any given age (Crimmins 2004), the rising proportion of the elderly and the rising proportion of the elderly who are 'old-old' (i.e. 75+) will inevitably mean a rising load of frail and disabled elderly, who need full-time care. The ratio of the elderly population who suffer from senile dementia to non-working women at various ages is projected to rise substantially over the coming two decades in Japan (Ogawa 2006, Figure 11). This suggests that Japan will not be able to rely on the traditional family support network to care for the infirm elderly; the rise in the burden placed on middle-aged Japanese women providing in-home nursing care will simply be too dramatic.

Another trend at the family level is migration of adult children away from their parents' locality. This differs by country and region. In Thailand, particularly in rural areas, there is a tendency for children of the elderly to have migrated to the city. While they typically contribute financial support where necessary, and keep in frequent contact with parents through cell phones, etc.,[5] thus presumably providing emotional support, they are not available for day-to-day care (Knodel and Chayovan 2008).

Thus, it will be less possible for the family to provide intensive care for the disabled or frail elderly for the following three reasons: (1) the lowered proportion of children per elderly person, (2) the increased labour force participation of women (the traditional carers), and (3) the movement of children of the elderly to other localities. These trends have major implications for policy on elder care. Despite the tradition in Asian families of caring for family members in various kinds of need, and the official rhetoric about the key support role of the Asian family as an underlying (and by implication, unchanging) characteristic of East Asian societies, this traditional reliance on family will be subjected to intensive pressures. Governments will almost inevitably be forced to step in.

Divorce

Divorce rates in Western countries rose very substantially – with more than a doubling of the general divorce rate – in the two decades between 1960 and 1980. Since then, these rates have shown little change, although with the rise in cohabitation, divorce trends in these countries are becoming less meaningful as an indicator of dissolution of long-term relationships. In East Asian countries, though, divorce rates have been rising steadily since 1980, particularly in the period since 1990 in the case of Japan, South Korea and Hong Kong (see Table 3.4). The rise in South Korea was particularly sharp between 1995 and 2000 – the period in which the Asian financial crisis occurred. The usual risk factors explain only a small part of the rise in Korean divorce rates over

Table 3.4 General divorce rates (number of divorces per 1000 population aged 15+), OECD and East Asian countries, 1980–2005

	1980	1985	1990	1995	2000	2005
OECD countries						
Australia	3.6	3.3	3.2	3.5	3.3	3.2
France	2.0	2.5	2.3	2.5	2.4	3.1
Germany	1.9	2.5	2.0	2.5	2.8	2.8
United Kingdom	3.8	4.0	3.6	3.6	3.2	3.4
United States	6.7	6.3	5.9	5.6	n.a.	n.a.
Russian Federation	4.7	4.5	4.9	5.7	5.2	4.9
East Asian countries						
Hong Kong	n.a.	1.0	1.2	1.9	2.4	2.5
Japan	1.6	1.8	1.6	1.9	2.4	2.4
South Korea	0.9	1.3	1.3	1.6	3.2	3.3
China	n.a.	n.a.	1.0[a]	1.3[b]	1.3	1.7
Thailand	0.8	0.9	1.2	1.3	n.a.	n.a.
Singapore	1.0	1.0	1.6	1.5	1.6	1.9

[a]1992
[b]1997
Source: Calculated from data on numbers of divorces and on age structure from United Nations Demographic Yearbooks.

this period, implying 'transformations in normative regimes regarding divorce, which may have accelerated after the economic recession in the late 1990s (Lee 2006, p. 127).[6] In China, freeing up of divorce regulations in 2001 and 2003 may have contributed to the sharp rise in divorce rates in the 2000–05 period. In Taiwan, as in other East Asian societies, increase in divorce has taken place in a context of decreased prevalence of marriage. The chance of re-marriage after divorce has declined (Yang and Tsai 2009), indicating a growing acceptance of and perhaps preference for singlehood.

Divorce rates in Japan have risen to such an extent that Japan can no longer be considered as a society characterized by low levels of marital dissolution. Synthetic cohort estimates indicate that about one-third of marriages in Japan are likely to end in divorce (Raymo et al. 2004). It has been argued that traditional marriage stability in Japan, while it did not necessarily have much to do with whether a marriage was happy, at least gave some assurance that children would be cared for, and that wives could expect economic security. With the awareness of the increasing fragility of marriage, decisions about whether to marry and about whether to raise children when single motherhood is a possibility come more into play (Bumpass et al. 2009, p. 223).

Trends in divorce in East Asia appear, then, to be going the way of the West, and partly for the same reasons (Dommaraju and Jones, 2011). Substantial increases in divorce rates in East Asian countries signify a significant change in circumstances and attitudes to divorce, because in the past divorce carried a considerable stigma, and the pressure to remain in a disharmonious marriage for 'the sake of the children' and also for the sake of appearances and family honour, was very strong. It would appear that factors such as increasing economic independence of women and the pressures (and widened range of contacts) in the big city environments, in which an increasing proportion of East Asians live, are influencing divorce trends. More controversial is the issue of whether East Asian societies are becoming more individualistic and less governed by Confucianist norms. As noted earlier, there is considerable evidence that this is the case (Lesthaeghe 2010).

Policy implications

A few policy implications will be summarized, under three heads: those related to influencing fertility, those related to elder care, and those related to the role of singles.

With regard to the first of these, the East Asian countries have all been strengthening pro-natalist policies in recent years. In the cases of South Korea and Taiwan, adoption of pro-natalist measures has been quite recent, and only undertaken after fertility had fallen to such low levels that the need for action could no longer be ignored.[7] However, these policies are not as comprehensive as those in many European countries (Frejka et al. 2010). Even an increase in monetary incentives beyond the rather modest incentives currently offered cannot be expected to have much effect unless policies are in place to address the 'work-life balance' issues that appear to lie at the source of current low fertility levels. Addressing these issues effectively would require multiple interventions, such as handling maternity (and paternity) leave, child-care leave and child minding arrangements and relieving the pressures parents face in raising 'quality children'. In East Asian societies, there is still a long way to go in modifying gender relations, both in the household and the workplace, to relieve the pressures of the 'double shift' faced by working mothers.

With regard to the care of the elderly, as already noted, the characteristics and circumstances of families are changing in ways that will make it increasingly harder for them to deal with the strain of caring for the aged. For example, in Singapore, the percentage of elderly people is expected to treble in 25 years after 2010. The policy emphasis must be on active ageing, financial independence and a positive attitude towards the contribution by the elderly within families. Nonetheless, an increasing role of the government in elder care cannot be avoided.

On the role of singles in family and society, there is perhaps little that government policy can or should do. The modifications will work themselves out over time, and this process already appears to be evident in aspects such as lessened pressures on singles to marry (see Jones et al. 2012, for a discussion on Singapore). However, widening of the options available to singles through housing policies and aspects of labour legislation should certainly be considered to ensure that singles are not unduly disadvantaged by policies designed to encourage childbearing. There is need for more research into the changing roles of singles in society and the pressures they face.

Some broader issues

The economic success enjoyed by East Asian countries is exemplified by Singapore. Economic growth has been seen as the Holy Grail in a tiny country with almost non-existent natural resources. That growth has been seen as dependent on rising levels of human capital, and the heavy involvement of (increasingly better-educated) women in the workforce. Lee Kuan Yew famously lamented that educating women and giving them opportunities in the labour force had affected their traditional role as mothers. Educated women were having far fewer children than the less educated. As he put it – 'It is too late for us to reverse our policies.... Our women will not stand for it. And anyway, they have already become too important a factor in the economy' (Saw 2005, p. 248). Not only in Singapore, but elsewhere in East Asia the result has been increasingly low fertility and consequently the need to import human capital from abroad in order to maintain the high economic growth. But this is creating social tensions and fissures. Japan and South Korea are reluctant to accept permanent immigrants, but the pressure to do so will inevitably increase.

Aside from involving women more in the labour force, the economic success achieved by these countries has been heavily dependent on raising the quality of human capital through an 'education-oriented' society, attuned to pushing children to high educational performance. The dilemma is that the pressure this places on parents and potential parents is a factor contributing to the unsustainably low levels of fertility. The economic prosperity achieved will be enjoyed by fewer and fewer citizens and may itself be placed at risk by the downward spiral in the labour force and (with some delay) in the population size. There is a great irony here. The very pressures to prioritize economic growth and the factors that can contribute to it – long hours of work, involvement of women in the workforce on much the same terms as men, strong pressure on children to perform outstandingly in school, and the extra tuition and coaching that is considered indispensible for reaching this goal – contain the seeds of an inability of the population to replace itself.[8] Thus the successful East Asian economies are placed at risk by a shortage of people to continue to power the economies and enjoy their fruits, generated by the very factors that have resulted in the growth of these economies in the first place.

Kingsley Davis noted that 'replacement fertility is incompatible with advanced industrial society'. We might add – *particularly* when that society holds to Confucianist norms and is marked by fierce competition to drive children to better performance. Perhaps the basic model of East Asian economic growth needs to be modified to allow for adjustment to the forces that are undermining the traditional role of family, and making it impossible for the population to reproduce itself. If that means slower economic growth, this is perhaps a trade-off that must be accepted in the interests of avoiding either a downward spiral of population or a very substantial modification of the ethnic and cultural characteristics of East Asian societies implicit in relying on immigration to avoid substantial population decline.

Notes

1. Latest estimates for Thailand, based on registration data, suggest that TFR may now have fallen to 1.5.
2. The figure for South Korea is clearly much lower than in the other countries, but sharply increasing percentages single at younger age groups in South Korea (even higher than in Japan) strongly suggest that as these cohorts grow older, percentages single at ages in the 30th will rise sharply.
3. For example, in Singapore, 2010 census data show that 9.3 per cent of ever married women aged 40–44 were childless, a proportion that had been rising over time. It has been observed from survey data that in West Germany, there is a tendency for women either not to want any children, or to want (and have) two or more children, it seems because once having had a child, the problems this raises for working women are not greatly increased by having a second child. One-child families seem to be a smaller proportion than before (personal communication with Mandy Boehlke).
4. In the example given by Le Bras, 80 per cent of children are born into families of two or more children, but mothers of such families make up only 43 per cent of the cohort of women. Preston (1976, p. 105) also notes that the

transformation of all one-child women to childless women will always reduce average family size for women but will always raise average family size for children.

5. In Thailand, there has been an extraordinary rise in the proportion of the elderly living in houses with a telephone – from 15 per cent in 1994 to 76 per cent in 2007 (Knodel and Chayovan 2008, p. 41).
6. South Korean divorce rates appear to have levelled off since 2003 and to have fallen since the introduction in 2008 of a mandatory deliberation period before a couple could end their marriage (Junghyan 2009). Interestingly, divorce rates in Taiwan also peaked in 2003.
7. In all East Asian countries, there were long delays (measured in decades rather than in years) in modifying population policy after fertility fell below replacement level. For further discussion, see Jones et al. (2009, pp. 4–7).
8. Dalla Zuana's comment on the 'Phyrric victory' of the strong family system in Southern Europe – paradoxically, the family will eventually disappear for lack of adaptive capacity and absence of children (Lesthaeghe, 2010, p. 224). Similar comment may be appropriate for the East Asian countries.

References

Arifin, E. and Ananta, A. (eds), (2008) *Older Persons in Southeast Asia: An Emerging Asset* (Singapore: Institute of Southeast Asian Studies).

Atoh, M. (2001) 'Very low fertility in Japan and value change hypotheses', *Review of Population and Social Policy*, 10: 1–21.

Bumpass, L. L., Rindfuss, R. R., Choe, M. K. and Tsuya, N. O. (2009) 'The institutional context of low fertility: the case of Japan', *Asian Population Studies*, 5(3): 215–35.

Crimmins, E. M. (2004) 'Trends in the health of the elderly', *Annual Review of Public Health*, 25: 79–98.

Dalla Zuanna, G. (2002) 'The banquet of Aeolus: a familistic interpretation of Italy's lowest-low fertility', *Demographic Research*, 4(5): 133–61.

Dommaraju, P. and Jones, G. (2011) 'Divorce trends in Asia', *Asian Journal of Social Science*, 39(2011): 725–50.

Douglass, M. (2011) 'Global householding and international migration research – paradigms, emerging dynamics and public policy in East and Southeast Asia', paper presented in the conference 'Householding in Transition: Emerging Dynamics in "Developing" East and Southeast Asia', National University of Singapore, 25–26 July.

Eun, K.-S. (2007) 'Lowest-low fertility in the Republic of Korea: causes, consequences and policy responses', *Asia-Pacific Population Journal*, 22(2): 51–72.

Fan, C. C. (2011) 'Rural-urban migration, split households, and the left-behind in China', paper presented in the conference 'Householding in Transition: Emerging Dynamics in "Developing" East and Southeast Asia', National University of Singapore, 25–26 July.

Frejka, T., Jones, G. W. and Sardon, J.-P. (2010) 'East Asia childbearing patterns and policy developments', *Population and Development Review*, 36(3): 579–606.

Hirao, K. (2007) 'Contradictions in maternal roles in contemporary Japan', in T. Devasahayan and B. S. A. Yeoh (eds) *Working and Mothering in Asia: Images, Ideologies and Identities* (Singapore: NUS Press).

Hull, T. H. (2003) 'Demographic perspectives on the future of the Indonesian family', *Journal of Population Research*, 20(1): 51–66.

Jones, G., Straughan, P. T. and Chan, A. (2009) *Ultra-Low Fertility in Pacific Asia: Trends, Causes and Policy Issues* (London: Routledge).

Jones, G. W. (2002) 'The changing Indonesian household', in K. Robinson and S. Bessell (eds) *Women in Indonesia: Gender, Equity and Development* (Singapore: Institute of Southeast Asian Studies).

Jones, G. W. (2007) 'Fertility decline in Asia: the role of marriage change', *Asia Pacific Population Journal*, 22(2): 13–32.

Jones, G. W., Yanxia, Z. and Zhi, P. C. P. (2012) 'Trends and implications of rising singlehood in East and Southeast Asia: a Singapore case study', *Journal of Comparative Family Studies*, XXXX111(5): 731–50.

Junghyun, K. (2009) 'South Korea cools off on hot-headed, speedy divorce', *Reuters*, Tuesday, January 13.

Knodel, J. and Chayovan, N. (2008) 'Population Ageing and the well-being of older persons in Thailand: past trends, current situation and future challenges', *Papers in Population Ageing No. 5*, Bangkok: UNFPA Thailand and Asia Pacific Regional Office.

Lam, D. and Marteleto, L. (2008) 'Stages of the demographic transition from a child's perspective: family size, cohort size, and children's resources', *Population and Development Review*, 34(2): 225–52.

Lee, S.-S. (2009) 'Low fertility and policy responses in Korea', *The Japanese Journal of Population*, 7(1): 57–70.

Lee, Y.-J. (2006) 'Risk factors in the rapidly rising incidence of divorce in Korea', *Asian Population Studies*, 2(2): 113–32.

Lesthaeghe, R. (2010) 'The Unfolding Story of the Second Demographic Transition', *Population and Development Review*, 36(2): 211–51.

Mason, A., Phananiramai, M. and Poapongsakorn, N. (1993) 'Households and their characteristics', in B. O. Campbell, A. Mason and E. M. Pernia (eds) *The Economic Impact of Demographic Change in Thailand, 1980–2015* (Honolulu: University of Hawaii Press).

Montgomery, M. R., Arends-Kuenning, M. and Mete, C. (2000) 'The quantity-quality transition in Asia', *Population and Development Review*, Supplement to Volume 26: 223–56.

Ochiai, E. and Molony, B. (2008) *Asia's New Mothers: Crafting Gender Roles and Childcare Networks in East and Southeast Asian Societies* (Kent, UK: Global Oriental).

Ogawa, N. (2003) 'Japan's changing fertility mechanisms and its policy responses', *Journal of Population Research*, 20(1): 89–106.

Ogawa, N. (2006) 'Population aging and policy options for a sustainable future: the case of Japan', *Genus*, LXI(3–4): 369–410.

Preston, S. H. (1976) 'Family sizes of children and family sizes of women', *Demography*, 13(1): 105–14.

Raymo, J., Iwasawa, M. and Bumpass, L. (2004) 'Marital dissolution in Japan: recent trends and differentials', *Demographic Research*, 11(14): 395–419.

Retherford, R. and Ogawa, N. (2006) 'Japan's baby bust: causes, implications and policy responses', in F. R. Harris (ed.) *The Baby Bust: Who Will Do the Work? Who Will Pay the Taxes?* (Lanham, MD: Rowman and Littlefield Publishers).

Rindfuss, R. R., Choe, M. K., Bumpass, L. L. and Tsuya, N. O. (2004) 'Social networks and family change in Japan', *American Sociological Review*, 69(6): 838–61.

Straughan, P. T., Chan, A. and Jones, G. (2009) 'From population control to fertility promotion: a case study of family policies and fertility trends in Singapore', in G. Jones, P. T. Straughan and A. Chan (eds) *Ultra-low Fertility in Pacific Asia: Trends, Causes and Policy Issues* (London: Routledge).

Yi, C.-C., Wu, C.-I., Chang, Y.-H. and Chang, M.-Y. (2009) 'The psychological well-being of Taiwanese youth: school versus family context from early to late adolescence', *International Sociology*, 24(3): 397–429.

Xin, Y. (2004) 'The impact of the one-child family on China', *Innovation: The Magazine of Research and Technology*, 5(1): 58–9.

Zhou, W. (2010) 'Support network of the rural elderly in post-reform China: an illustration from Jiangsu Province', PhD thesis, Department of Sociology, National University of Singapore.

4
Childlessness: Choice and Circumstances

John Haskey

> Laws to encourage marriage and increase fertility ... designed to promote population growth ... were enacted by Augustus Caesar nearly 2000 years ago ... (but) there is no evidence that these measures had any effect on fertility. According to Tacitus, who like many of the eminent Romans of his time, was a childless man, the legislation of Augustus failed to achieve its object, 'so powerful were the attractions of childlessness'.
>
> (McCleary 1941)

> It is evidently necessary, in order to prevent the society from starving, that the rate at which the population increases should be retarded. But who are the persons that are to exercise the restraint thus called for, and either to marry late, or not at all?.
>
> (Malthus 1817, p. 282)

Introduction

Increasing the population has exercised nations throughout history; a large population was deemed desirable for military and economic purposes, and perhaps also for prestige. In England, though, once the population began to grow at such a fast rate, in the late 1700s, there was greater awareness of its increase and size, and its adverse consequences – that of poverty and starvation – were increasingly recognized as obvious evils. Marriage was seen as the key factor in population growth; when Malthus wrote his 'Essay on the Principle of Population', marriage was pursued by the aspiring classes (vide Jane Austen's novels) and widely recognized as the central pillar of family building, support and stability in society; however, family planning was probably negligible; and sexual activity naturally, and almost inevitably, led to children.

When Malthus wrote his 'Essay', he was primarily interested in arresting the rate of increase of the population via marital fertility; since then, the demographic landscape has changed out of all recognition; a profound transition. In the late twentieth and early twenty-first centuries, not only has marriage declined considerably as the sole form of partnership, but the advent of other demographic factors, such as divorce, cohabitation and lone parenthood have inevitably weakened the historic role of marriage as the vehicle by which children are born and reared. Also, a much greater diversity of family forms and of couples' and individuals' living arrangements, including living alone, has developed. Perhaps, most importantly, the advent of modern contraception has, for the first time in human history, allowed sexual relationships to be decoupled from reproduction.

As a result, the whole pattern of European fertility and especially childlessness has, *in theory*, over the recent decades been determined by individuals' conscious choices, except of course, in cases of infertility. Besides such incapacity, childlessness may be due to: the lack of an available partner; a situation judged unsuitable for child-rearing; women leaving it too late to start having children; or a deliberate choice not to have children. The analysis of fertility and childlessness is therefore a particular challenge in which economic factors, housing, labour force participation and unemployment, education, career choices, childcare availability, attitudes, individualism, gender roles, partnership history and cultural, societal and sexual norms have all been invoked as contributory explanatory mechanisms to the decision processes. Quality-of-life issues and the desire for self-fulfilment have been cited as key new factors influencing fertility in a 'post-modernist' world of demographic change (van de Kaa 2001). It has also been suggested that experts from other disciplines such as biology, genetics and political science might also be able to provide useful insights (Coleman 1998). In addition, due to the capricious nature of humankind, there is undoubtedly lack of planning, or conscious decision making, either to have or not to have children.

With relatively high levels of fertility pertaining for over two decades after the Second World War, demographic interest was primarily focused upon the factors encouraging fertility, especially economic factors. Subsequently, with fertility universally declining, interest turned to trying to identify the factors *discouraging* childbearing, and, especially, of bolstering childlessness. There has been a steady growth in the number of papers that have addressed the issue of childlessness; this chapter reviews and comments upon their findings, after first tracing the changes in fertility patterns in Europe to place childlessness in a broader context.

Data considerations

Data on childlessness are not quite so directly acquired as those on fertility; the main sources use birth registrations and population estimates, as well as results from censuses and surveys. Population estimates of the numbers of women can be used to derive estimates of the total number of women born in a given year, from which the numbers having had one or more births – derived from birth registration data – can be subtracted to give the numbers that are childless. In general, it is inadvisable to estimate any group as a 'remainder category', but if birth registration is virtually 100 per cent complete, and population estimates of those 'at risk' of giving birth are reliable, then the resulting proportion estimated to be childless should be dependable. Checking the consistency of the results against those derived from other sources is always advisable.

In recent decades, censuses and surveys have rarely asked questions on children that have been born to the respondent; usually questions refer only to children present in the household. Other difficulties can occur with survey data, usually involving the under-reporting of children by mothers at older ages, even of children living in the same household (Bhrolchain et al. 2011). It has long been known that there is a tendency to omit babies from the list of residents in the household in census returns. Specialized surveys on family intentions usually concentrate on women's attitudes to childbearing, although corresponding questions are also posed to their husbands and partners. Overall, though, there is a paucity of data on men's fertility and childlessness (Coleman 2000, pp. 29–60).

Historical trends in fertility

Fertility, as measured by the Total Period Fertility Rate (TPFR), which is the average number of children a group of women would have, were they to experience the set of age-specific fertility rates measured in a given year throughout their entire childbearing years, has declined considerably in most European countries (Frejka and Sobotka 2008; Sardon 2006). This substantial decrease, which has been well documented, is apparent from Figures 4.1 and 4.2, which trace the TPFRs for two different groups of European countries since 1950. Figure 4.1 gives the TPFRs for some of the Western and Northern European countries, whereas

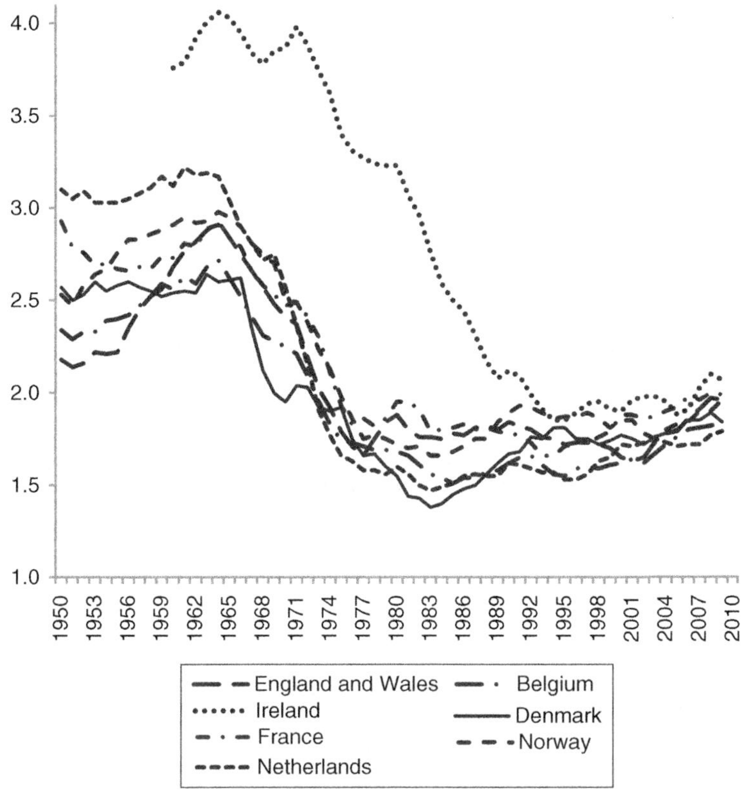

Figure 4.1 Total period fertility rates, selected European countries, 1950–2009

those in Figure 4.2 are for those from some Central and Southern European countries.

The turning point, marking the start of the decline in European fertility, occurred during the first half of the 1960s for most countries, although, for a few countries, such as Ireland, it was up to a decade later. Part of the reason for the decline lay in a sustained trend towards older age at childbearing, especially at the birth of the first child. Delaying the start of childbearing not only reduced the fertility rate, but also had repercussions on the timing of second and subsequent births, and, in many countries of Central, Eastern and Southern Europe, the proportions of women going on to have a second, third and fourth child consistently fell, which also depressed the fertility rate still further (Frejka and Sardon 2006b). Accompanying the

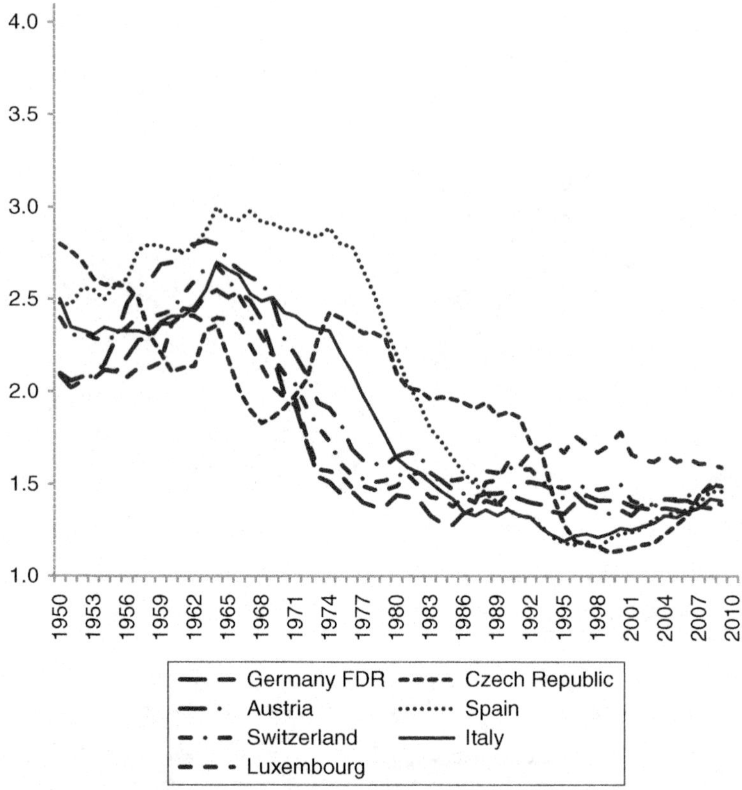

Figure 4.2 Total period fertility rates, selected European countries, 1950–2009

overall delay in childbearing has been the establishment of a new profile of smaller family size, and, as part of that picture, an increase in childlessness.

After reaching the low point of fertility during the 1970s, there was some form of plateauing, albeit with countries experiencing a wide spectrum of fertility levels, varying from about 1.2 to 1.9, but virtually all lower than the theoretical 'replacement value' of the population of 2.1. In the most recent few years, there has been a modest reversal – more apparent for the countries depicted in Figure 4.1 than those in Figure 4.2 (particularly the German-speaking countries) – marking the end, or temporary end, of delaying births, but fertility is still at its lowest level for many decades. Indeed, for many countries such as Germany (the former FDR), Austria and Italy, the most recent values, shown in Figure 4.2, are around 1.4, which is only some 70 per cent of replacement level. In contrast, for Western and Northern European countries, such as those shown in Figure 4.1, fertility is only slightly below replacement level.

Fertility by birth cohort

Fertility, as measured by the TPFR, tends to be particularly sensitive to changes in the *timing* of childbearing, that is, the delaying or indeed any bringing forward of births, and can fluctuate considerably. It is usefully supplemented by considering the average number of children a group of women, *born in a given year*, have *actually had* by the time they have reached the end of their childbearing years, which is usually taken as age 45. Comparing the trend in this 'birth cohort' measure of completed fertility, that is, for women born in successive years, allows the tempo of childbearing to be seen in its proper, overall, completed perspective. However, since any birth cohort of women need to reach age 45 for their childbearing to be complete, the *latest* birth cohort of women whose finished fertility can be confirmed is for those born 45 years earlier. Whilst such analyses inevitably cannot take into account fertility rates for younger women, as they have not yet reached age 45, they do allow the calculation of definitive proportions of all earlier birth cohorts of women who were childless, and trends to be discerned.

On this basis, cohort fertility increased in most European countries for women born in successive years of the 1920s, and generally peaked for those born around the mid-1930s, varying from an average of about 2.1 children to around 2.6 children per woman (Frejka and Sobotka 2008). Cohort fertility then declined for women born in the subsequent years of the late 1930s and 1940s and continued falling for most European countries for those born during the 1950s and 1960s, so that the most recent values are almost invariably lower than 2.1, the population replacement level.

Analysis of fertility on a cohort basis has also shown that the average age at first birth for women born in successive five-year periods since the end of the War has risen steadily, from the early 20s to the late 20s (see Figure 4.3). It has also indicated that, for most European countries, the postponement of first births is continuing, and will continue (Frejka and Sardon 2006a). They also found that, only for a very few countries, mostly in Northern Europe, the progress towards an older age at first birth has halted, and the proportions of women having their first child have stabilized. It follows that, with the persistent trend of relatively

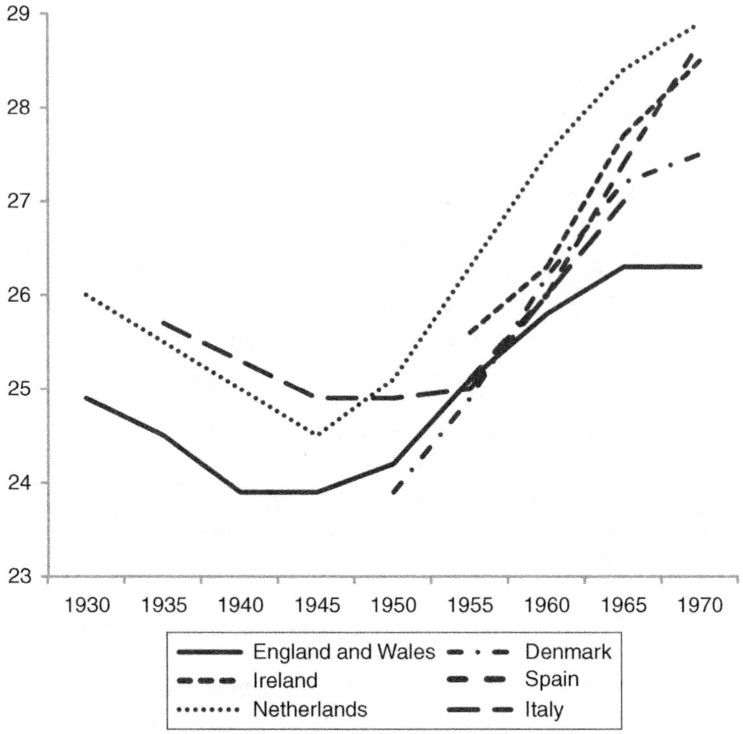

Figure 4.3 Average age at first birth, by birth cohort of women, 1930–70
Source: Sardon, 2006.

fewer women having had a first child, the proportions of women who are childless has been gradually increasing.

Childlessness by birth cohort

The trend towards increasing proportions of women remaining childless may be seen in Figure 4.4. For many countries, the proportions childless generally reached a minimum for women born in the years just after the Second World War. For subsequent birth cohorts, however, the proportions childless rose substantially from about one in eight to one in five for more recent birth cohorts around 1970.

This trend occurred in most countries, including, besides those shown in Figure 4.4, the former East Germany and Sweden. By the beginning of the 1960s, the 'relationship revolution' had begun, with divorce,

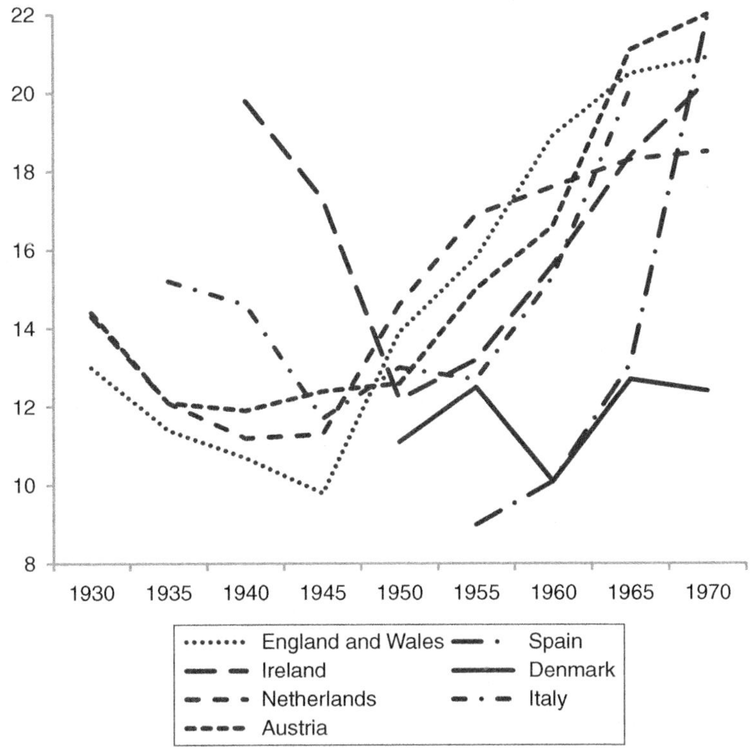

Figure 4.4 Percentage childless, by birth cohort of women, 1930–70
Source: Sardon, 2006.

cohabitation and births outside marriage all starting to increase. It is difficult to disentangle the effects of these different factors upon the overall growing extent of childlessness amongst women who grew up with these rapid changes. They would have reached the start of their childbearing years in the 1980s, when the 'tsunami' of the raft of changing social and demographic norms, summarized by the postulated 'Second Demographic Transition', struck Western society (Van de Kaa 1987). Whatever the influences and mechanisms, the proportion of women who were still childless grew yet further and, generally, at a faster pace.

Whilst there has been a sea change in childlessness for the successive groups of women born since 1940, childlessness actually *declined* amongst women born in the years leading up to 1940, that is, from around 1900 to 1940, having previously peaked amongst women born from 1880 to 1910 (Rowland 2007). Demographic estimates for France, Germany, the Netherlands and Finland suggest that between one-fifth and one-quarter of women born in 1900 remained childless (Rowland 2007). This reminder that childlessness has historically always been present in Europe, influenced by the postponement of marriage and economic circumstances, has been fully documented (Kreager 2004, pp. 1–45). Certainly, those born around the turn of the twentieth century, between about 1890 and 1910, would have been ready for parenthood just when The Depression struck, and, for slightly later cohorts, the Second World War would have interfered with the timing of their parenthood.

Indeed, in many European countries, the War resulted in many couples delaying having a family or not having a family at all – the involuntary choice that was the outcome of external events. In contrast, for women born in 1940, who reached childbearing ages in the more affluent and optimistic 1960s, when marriage and youthful marriage especially was still very prevalent, the number of births peaked, and the corresponding proportion childless was much smaller at between one-tenth and one-sixth. For the 1965 cohort whose childbearing years have just ended and who experienced fewer and later marriages, more cohabitation and below-replacement fertility, the proportion childless has risen to between one-eighth and one-fifth.

Hence, although the proportions of women who are childless have risen since the birth cohort of 1940, in general they have not (yet) returned to those of the 1900 birth cohort. Nevertheless, some authors consider the current situation to be one of a slight delay in a revival of historic levels of childlessness, and most demographic analysts incorporate an assumption of a further small increase in childlessness in their projections. Some researchers have suggested that up to one-quarter of women could remain childless, although it is certain that the proportion will be one in five in Austria, Finland, and possibly also in Ireland, the Netherlands and the western part of Germany (Sardon 2006).

Possible reasons for the changing prevalence of childlessness

Fertility intentions

Various surveys have been carried out over the years on the birth intentions of women, with women generally tending to overestimate their eventual completed family size. Inevitably, women at different ages, and therefore at different points in their childbearing years, express different intentions, and different degrees of uncertainty, with older women being more likely to express a definite intention, and also to expect slightly smaller numbers of children, on average, than younger women. However, in England and Wales, around 2000, women of most ages intended to have 2.1 children, on average, but those who in their late 30s – who were born between 1960 and 1965 – reported having an intended smaller average of just over 1.9 children (Smallwood and Jefferies 2003).

Of particular interest, in the present context, was the fact that, amongst this group of women in their late 30s who stated an intention on family size – whether with certainty or uncertainty – only 15 per cent around 2000 said that they intended to remain childless, although 20 per cent of them were still childless at that time. Hence for actuality to match intentions, three-quarters of the childless women would have had to remain childless, and the remaining quarter would have had to have a child during the next seven to nine years. Of note, too, is the fact that, amongst those women in their late 30s around 2000, only 14 per cent of those who were *certain* of their birth intentions said that they intended to have no children, whereas, of those who were *uncertain,* the corresponding proportion was almost double, at 25 per cent. (Women who were certain of their intentions formed 77 per cent, and those who were uncertain 23 per cent, of the sample of women in their late 30s around 2000.) As women whose birth intentions are uncertain tend to have fewer children than those who are certain, it is likely that the eventual proportion childless amongst this overall group of women – who were born between 1960 and 1965 – will be slightly under 20 per cent. Also, estimates from birth registration data on true birth order give this proportion amongst all women in their late 30s in 2001 as 22 per cent (Smallwood and Jefferies 2003).

In a later paper, using a time-series of data up to the more recent year of 2007, from the same survey, the General Household Survey for Great Britain, the proportion of childless women in their mid-30s who did not intend to have a child was shown to have declined fairly consistently between 1991–92 and 2005–07; from around 44 per cent to 25 per cent. However, the same survey showed that the proportions of women in their mid-30s who were actually childless rose consistently between 1991–94 and 2005–07, from 18 to 26 per cent (Bhrolchain et al. 2010). Further analysing this dataset, the authors found that, for each separate age group of women, the proportion of childless women in each survey year who expected to have at least one child was linearly related to the proportion of women who were childless in that year. The correlation was large, and the relationship suggests that birth intentions may be reflecting a response to the current *general* situation, rather than the future situation of the *individual respondent*, especially so as the direct link was present for each age group of women. Overall, the authors concluded that, throughout the 1990s, although women were anticipating a growing postponement of childbearing, their predictions were inaccurate on the eventual proportion who would have children, and the timing of their first births.

Postponement

The decline in fertility and increase in childlessness have been attributed to women's growing educational attainment and participation in the labour force. It has been argued that an increasing proportion of women have wanted to postpone having children until not only their education is complete, but also until they are established in their careers. Both these considerations tend to postpone the starting of a family; furthermore, women, once they have begun to advance in their profession, may wish to continue delaying having a child. Hence postponement is an important aspect of childlessness, since it determines whether progressively more women will be childless, or whether the ages of women having their first child will shift to an (even) older profile. And, of course, both tendencies can operate simultaneously. Making assumptions over how the fertility pattern of women who have not reached the end of their childbearing years will be completed is all the more difficult because of these two kinds of uncertainty. As a result, there have been few studies in which there has been an attempt to project the eventual proportion childless amongst those not yet around age 45.

One such study has, however, explored British data for both men and women from two birth cohort (sample survey) studies, one for those born in 1958 and the other for those born in 1970 (Kneale and Joshi 2010). The former, older cohort was last interviewed when aged 46, the younger cohort when 34. The idea was to use the information on childlessness from the older cohort, in which the women had just finished their child bearing, to make alternative assumptions on how the younger cohort would finish theirs. Amongst the older cohort of women, 18 per cent were childless by age 45 and about 23 per cent had been childless at age 34 – a smaller proportion than the 29 per cent at age 34 amongst the younger cohort. The first assumption was that the faster entrance to parenthood amongst the older cohort would be replicated for those aged over 34 in the younger cohort, on a constant proportional basis; that is, the ratio of propensities to enter parenthood in the younger years between the two cohorts would also apply at each older age too. The second assumption was that those still childless at age 34 in the younger cohort would experience exactly the same rates of first birth at future, older, ages as had those in the older cohort.

Calculations on the implied proportions childless were carried out on these two assumptions, separately for men and women, and separately according to their level of educational attainment. Inevitably, the set of proportions childless under the first assumption were uniformly larger than those for the 1958 birth cohort, as also were those under the second assumption, because at age 34 the proportion childless was already larger in the younger cohort than in the older cohort. Furthermore, understandably, the first 'ratio of propensities' assumption produced slightly larger proportions childless than the second 'same rates' assumption. For graduate women, the proportion projected to be childless amongst the 1970 birth cohort was found to be 31 per cent under the first 'ratio of propensities' assumption and 28 per cent under the second 'same rates' assumption. The corresponding proportions for graduate men were 40 and 31 per cent, respectively. The results from the first 'ratio of propensities' assumption are quite close to those derived next by the authors using a model taking both partnership characteristics and family formation intentions into account; 35 per cent, rather than 31 per cent, for graduate women, and 41 per cent, rather than 40 per cent, for graduate men.

However, the authors concluded that, for both methodological and computational reasons, a simpler model was to be preferred, one which included only fertility intentions, on the basis of which 25 per cent of graduate women and 27 per cent of graduate men (around one-quarter) were projected to be childless. This method, unlike the earlier methods, incorporated information on postponement expressed in respondents' own fertility intentions in the 1970 birth cohort sample survey, and takes into account evidence that later cohorts are postponing, as opposed to avoiding, parenthood. One important conclusion is that men's as well as women's views and characteristics should be taken into account, as witnessed by larger proportions of graduate men than graduate women delaying parenthood, with postponement not being solely due to the career choices of women, but probably reached by the joint decisions of both partners.

The fertility intentions of both partners, and the issue of postponement, were also the subject of another research project, using data from the British Household Panel Survey, which investigated differences and agreements in couples' intentions and their possible influence on their subsequent child-bearing (Berrington et al. 2004). Amongst women aged under 40 in 1992 who were childless and wanted a child, 95 per cent of their partners also expressed the same wish, but amongst the corresponding group of childless women who did *not* intend to have a child, a smaller proportion, around three-quarters, 76 per cent, of their partners also did not want to have a child. In general, there was a high degree of agreement between partners in their intentions, but it was very slightly lower when the two partners were not interviewed together.

The chance of a 35-year-old childless women actually having a child within six years – estimated from fitting a logistic regression model which incorporated besides other variables the woman's educational level and her partnership status – was found to vary considerably by a factor of around 7, according to the degree of coincidence of her intentions and those of her partner (if she had one) (Berrington 2004). Where both partners intended to have a child, the chance was estimated as 36 per cent; where the woman intended to have a child but her partner did not, it was 29 per cent, and where the woman had no partner and did not intend to have a child, it was 4 per cent. (Apart from the variability in these and other estimated chances, it is evident that the woman's intention is more important in her subsequent fertility than that of her partner's.) Overall, it was estimated that around one half of women who had postponed having their first child into their 30s would actually have a child within the next six years and the remainder could well, for one reason or another, become what the author terms 'perpetual postponers'.

Factors associated with childlessness

A variety of characteristics were compared between a sample of women who were still childless in 2005 when they were aged 45–49 and a corresponding sample of women who had had children, thus providing some key findings (Portanti and Whitworth 2009). The results were derived from a representative sample of over 12,000 women living in England and Wales who were born in the second half of the 1950s; the sample was drawn from the ONS Longitudinal Study, which has captured census and birth registration data from 1971 onwards. About one in six of the entire sample remained childless throughout, and, examining the women's legal marital status in 2001, a much larger proportion of childless women than of mothers were single (never married): 40 per cent and 8 per cent, respectively.

Being single, that is, never-married, however, does not necessarily mean that a woman is not, or has not been, in a union; in fact, when the two groups of women were in their early 30s, when childbearing might be expected to be high, almost one in four childless women was cohabiting, whilst the corresponding proportion of mothers was only about one in 12. Women who had been cohabiting in their early 30s were found to be more likely to remain childless than those who had been cohabiting at any other age; cohabiting is relatively (and consistently) more common amongst childless women than mothers. Taking both cohabitation and marriage into account, 53 per cent of childless women, when in their early 30s, had been living with either a cohabitant or a husband, whilst the corresponding proportion of mothers was 87 per cent, and these proportions were roughly similar to those which applied when the two groups of women had reached their early 40s. The study also found that at least 68 per cent of childless women had been living with a partner, either cohabiting or married, for at least one period during their childbearing years, whereas the corresponding proportion for mothers was 95 per cent. Consequently, although childless women were less likely to have had a partner, a sizeable proportion had, but yet they remained childless.

Women who had never married were consistently found to be more likely to remain childless, even if they were cohabiting. In addition, having one's marriage interrupted – either by divorce or being widowed – was found to be associated with childlessness, even if the woman remarried. One possibility (untested and not addressed by the authors) is that disruptions, breakdowns or, particularly, *changes* of partnerships, whether of informal unions or marriages, lead to durations of time when it is understandable that women do not want to contemplate having a baby; the after-effects of such events might be prolonged.

The study provided other important results: some new and some substantiating evidence from other studies. Childless women were found to be more likely to have a degree than mothers, and had a slightly higher social and economic status and were more often employed in professional, managerial and technical occupations. Childless women had a greater participation in the labour market than mothers, particularly for those in their early 30s, and childless women were more likely to own their own homes outright. Women with no siblings were found to be more likely to remain childless than those with siblings; possibly the absence of children at home when in childhood results in establishing a norm of no children in the home when in adulthood. In addition, amongst women in their 30s who were living with a partner or husband, significantly more childless women than mothers had a wider age difference with their partner, that is, relatively more were over five years older or younger than their partner. Childlessness was found to be more frequent amongst women whose educational level was higher than their partner's.

Priorities and preferences

The subject of childlessness in Europe, including attitudes to having children and priorities, was examined in a study using data from the Family and Fertility Surveys (FFSs) for up to 18 countries plus two British birth cohort studies (Hakim 2003a). The survey questions allowed voluntary childlessness to be divided into two groups: those who could be termed 'voluntary childfree' – who definitely did not want children, and those who were 'uncertain childless' – who answered 'Don't know' to at least one question on whether they wanted children. Hakim found that, for men and women aged under 40, in the majority of countries, fewer than one in ten expressed voluntary childlessness, whilst the proportions who were 'uncertain childless' were much more variable, ranging from 0 to 19 per cent. It was expected that the childless, and especially the voluntary childfree, would be distinctive in terms of values and attitudes, and this was found to be the case, albeit with not as great a difference as expected.

Hakim has emphasized the historical importance of contraceptives by which *women* can control their fertility, and this when coupled with equal opportunities for women have ensured that women's intentions and attitudes are key to understanding their fertility (Hakim 2003b). Recognizing the heterogeneity of women's preferences with regard to family building and work, she has advocated a new 'Preference Theory', for understanding and explaining fertility choices, concluding that women choose a lifestyle which is home- or family-centred, work-centred or adaptive (where work and family are combined). Consequently, questions on such lifestyle choices and preferences would usefully be included in fertility surveys as causal factors central to explaining fertility, and childlessness.

Many women decide, or discover, that it is impossible to combine raising a family with a demanding job, and choose, deliberately, to be childless. Many couples in this situation, prefer to describe themselves as 'child free' rather than 'childless' since the latter implies a loss or an unfulfilled need. Similarly, others decide not to have children for religious or ideological reasons, or just do not want them, or do not think they would make good parents.

In an earlier small-scale study, voluntary childlessness was found, for some, to be linked to the perceived attractions and advantages of a childless lifestyle, whilst for others, the choice of remaining childless was possibly due to a more fundamental rejection of motherhood, which was seen as distinct from feminine identity (Gillespie 1999). As well as active decisions not to have children, 'drifting' into childlessness was reported, as well as childlessness following on from compromises and partial choices.

In another study in the United States, factors concerning changes and persistence in the decision to remain childless were examined (Heaton et al. 1999). The researchers used a US national longitudinal survey, and two groups of Wave I respondents aged between 19 and 39 who had not had any children by the start of the study: women, and men who were either married or cohabiting. Respondents were asked at Wave I (1988) whether they intended to have a child, and, again at Wave II (1994) whether they intended to have a child (or another child). They were also asked about any births between Waves. Five types of respondents were identified: 'postponers'; 'switchers' to childless; 'intenders'; 'switchers' to wanting a child (or having become a parent); or consistently childless. Besides collecting a range of demographic, and partnership details at Wave I, questions were asked about the reasons for having children, attitudes to non-family lifestyles and views on the importance of various family relationships.

Older people were found to be more likely to be consistently childless, but also to be more likely to switch and decide to have children. Higher levels of education were found to reduce the likelihood of switching from childlessness to wanting children, but also to increase the chance of postponing having children. Not surprisingly, the respondents who expressed concern that children would adversely affect their leisure and social activities were unlikely to want children, and be more likely to be consistently childless, and, so too, were those who were concerned about the stability of their marriage. Respondents who voiced strong personal motivations for having children were least likely to postpone having children, as also were those who were married. Amongst those who were cohabiting, women were found to be more likely than men to postpone or decide against having children.

An alternative way of analysing the numbers of children women have had (their parities) has been developed over the last 20 years, by considering the 'Concentration of Reproduction' or CR. This index is similar in construction to that of the Gini coefficient based on the Lorenz curve of income, used to describe and measure income disparity. The present case quantifies the extent to which relatively few women have the majority of children and conversely, as part of the same story, the extent to which relatively many women have very few children between them. Amongst this latter group, of course, childless women figure prominently, and the CR is highly correlated with childlessness.

In a recent study, methods for decomposing changes in the CR into components, including one due to the proportion of women who were childless, have been derived and applied to a number of historic birth cohort datasets (Shkolnikov et al. 2007). Amongst other analyses affording new insights, the authors compared the change in the CR between the birth cohort of the early 1950s and that of the early 1960s for each of the 14 countries and decomposed the increase in the CR, which occurred in 11 of the countries, into the contributions for the different parities. They were able to *quantify* the contribution childlessness made to the change, and additionally measure it *comparatively* with the change in each parity group, hence placing it in complete context. For example, in England and Wales, the increase in CR was decomposed into a relatively large component due to childlessness, the relatively small components due to the decreases in the proportion of women with one child and the proportion of women with two children, and a microscopic increase in the proportion of women with three or more children. As in England and Wales, growing childlessness produced the greatest contributions to the total increases in CR in Ireland, Italy, Sweden, Denmark, Greece and Bulgaria.

Overall, the authors conclude that decomposition of the recent increases in CR suggests a particularly important role of growing childlessness, which, with other changes in parity distributions, suggests a further narrowing of the population base of reproduction and an increase in the CR.

Conclusions

One conclusion is certain from all the evidence and research described in this chapter and elsewhere – that projecting childlessness, either as part of a more complete picture on fertility or in its own right, is an inexact science. Fertility, and non-fertility, intentions are often not realized, and understandably, changing circumstances (both personal and general), greater experience, a more mature outlook and a realization of a finite or shorter time within which to have children can lead to altered wishes and goals at subsequent times. One possible solution for the researcher might be to try to adjust the results of currently expressed intentions with auxiliary information to derive better overall predictions, but it is none too clear what those other variables might be, and how they might be used. The problem is essentially that the respondent's future fertility is unclear to them, as well as to the demographic analyst.

Yet intentions, declared as far as they can, by the players themselves, seem to be the essential starting point as well as the most obvious predictor to employ. Improvements to questions have probably gone as far as they can; respondents are asked what they think they themselves will have regarding having or not having children, rather than a generalized ideal; they are also asked whether they are certain or uncertain concerning their intentions, or plainly do not know, so that each respondent's position is recorded as honestly and thoroughly as possible. In light of the research outlined previously, such intentions might usefully be supplemented by women's aspirations and attitudes on work, careers, home-making and partnerships – both informal unions and marriage – not only on their own *individual* hopes on these matters (such as I hope to marry my partner) but also their values and attitudes to issues on these topics *for society as a whole.*

In addition to individuals' own aspirations, wider societal norms and trends inevitably influence decisions. The first stage of the 'wider society' might well be the (male) partner, who, it has been seen, can shape or modify intentions, although perhaps only marginally. (Past partnership history, and especially periods of cohabitation may, however, according to studies described above, be more important, especially as cohabiting women have increased considerably in number and now represent almost one-third of all women in couples. Also, never-married women have been found to be more likely to remain childless, and with first marriage rates declining, another trend appears to favour increased childlessness.) Broader still, changing general attitudes to childlessness and large families can influence individuals' own ideas and views. A range of other factors too, such as overall unemployment, economic retrenchment and optimism or pessimism about the future in general, can influence decisions on childbearing.

Rather than trying to interpret developments in terms of women's choices and preferences, a more powerful explanation might well lie in women's desire for 'achievement', fuelled by the opening up of equal opportunities for women in all spheres, which is the key to understanding fertility and childlessness. Whether a woman can achieve a certain goal in either the employment context or in another field may depend upon whether the total resources available to her are sufficient to fulfil all goals, particularly the resources of *time* for having children and raising a family, *in addition* to realizing the other ambitions. To some extent, this is borne out by childless women being found relatively more frequently amongst professional and managerial occupations, and amongst those more highly educated, who undoubtedly have more and wider opportunities open to them. An increasingly competitive and individualistic society encourages a wide range of aims and targets and applauds their attainment; perhaps, amongst a minority, albeit a slowly increasing minority, the goal of having children has been pushed down the agenda.

References

Berrington, A. (2004) Perpetual postponers? Women's, men's and couples' fertility intentions and subsequent fertility behaviour, *Population Trends,* 117: 9–19.

Bhrolchain, M. N., Beaujouan, E. and Berrington, A. (2010) Stability and change in fertility intentions in Britain, 1991–2007, *Population Trends,* 141: 13–35.

Bhrolchain, M. N., Beaujouan, E. and Murphy, M. (2011) *Reported Childlessness: A Further Look at Cohort Estimates Based on Survey Time-Series Data,* ESRC Centre for Population Change Working Paper Number 11: 1–19, University of Southampton.

Coleman, D. A. (1998) *Reproduction and Survival in an Unknown World: What Drives Today's Industrial Populations, and to What Future?* Lecture presented in the NIDI Hofstee Lecture Series, 5, Amsterdam, (NIDI, The Hague).

Coleman D. A. (2000) Male fertility trends in industrial countries: theories in search of some evidence, in C. Bledsoe, S. Lerner and J. Guyer (eds) *Fertility and the Male Life-Cycle in the Era of Fertility Decline* (New York: Oxford University Press), pp. 29–60.

Frejka, T. and Sardon, J.-P. (2006a) First birth trends in developed countries: persisting parenthood postponement, *Demographic Research,* 15 (article 6): 147–80 (Max Planck Institute for Demographic Research).

Frejka, T. and Sardon, J.-P. (2006b) Cohort birth order, parity progression ratio and parity distribution trends in developed countries. *MPIDR Working Paper WP 2006–045*: 1–40, November 2006 (Max Planck Institute for Demographic Research).

Frejka, T. and Sobotka, T. (2008) Overall chapter 1: fertility in Europe: diverse, delayed and below replacement, *Demographic Research,* 19 (article 3): 15–46 (Max Planck Institute for Demographic Research).

Hakim, C. (2003a) *Childlessness in Europe.* Research Report to the ESRC on the funded project running December 2002–July 2003.

Hakim, C. (2003b) A new approach to explaining fertility patterns: preference theory, *Population and Development Review,* 29(3): 349–74.

Heaton, T. B., Jacobson, C. K. and Holland, K. (1999) Persistence and change in decisions to remain childless, *Journal of Marriage and the Family,* 61(2): 531–9.

Gillespie, R. (1999) Voluntary childlessness in the United Kingdom, *Reproductive Health Matters,* 7(13): 43–53.

Kneale, D. and Joshi, H. (2010) Postponement and childlessness – evidence from two British cohorts, *Demographic Research,* 19: 1935–68.

Kreager, P. (2004) Where are the children? in P. Kreager and E. Schröder-Butterfill (eds) *Ageing without children: European and Asian perspectives* (Oxford and New York: Berghahn Books).

McCleary, G. F. (1941) Pre-war European population policies, *Millbank Memorial Fund Quarterly*, 19(2): 105–20 (Blackwell).

Malthus, T. R. (1817) *An Essay on the Principle of Population; or a View of Its Past and Present Effects on Human Happiness with an Inquiry into Our Prospects Respecting the Future Removal or Mitigation of the Evils Which It Occasions.* The fifth edition with important additions. Volume II, Book III, Chapter III: Of systems of equality (continued) 1817 (London: John Murray).

Also appeared in: Additions to the fourth and former editions of: *An Essay on the Principle of Population; or a View of Its Past and Present Effets on Human Happiness with an Inquiry into Our Prospects Respecting the Future Removal or Mitigation of the Evils Which It Occasions.* Book III Chapter III: Of systems of equality (continued) 1817, p. 48. (London: John Murray).

Portanti, M. and Whitworth, S. (2009) A comparison of the characteristics of childless women and mothers in the ONS Longitudinal Study, *Population Trends,* 136: 10–20.

Rowland, D. T. (2007) Historical trends in childlessness, *Journal of Family Issues,* 28: 1311–37.

Sardon, J.-P. (2006) Recent demographic trends in the developed countries, *Population,* 61(3): 197–266.

Shkolnikov, V. M., Andreev, E. M., Houle, R. and Vaupel, J. W. (2007) The concentration of reproduction in cohorts of women in Europe and the United States, *Population and Development Review,* 33 (1): 66–99.

Smallwood, S. and Jefferies, J. (2003) Family building intentions in England and Wales: trends, outcomes and interpretations, *Population Trends,* 112: 15–28.

Van de Kaa, D. J. (1987) Europe's second demographic transition, *Population Bulletin,* 42: 1–47.

Van de Kaa, D. J. (2001) Postmodern fertility preferences: from changing value orientation to new behaviour, *Population and Development Review,* 27: 290–331.

5
Population Decline – Facing an Inevitable Destiny?

David Coleman and Bob Rowthorn

> in the multitude of people is the king's honour; but in the want of people is the destruction of the prince.
>
> (Proverbs 14: 28)

> the most decisive mark of the prosperity of any country is the increase in the number of its inhabitants.
>
> (Adam Smith 1776, *An Enquiry into the Nature and Causes of the Wealth of Nations*, p. 55)

Introduction

Birth rates have fallen below the level required to replace the population in almost all the populations of the developed world. Population decline already confronts almost all the countries of Central and Eastern Europe and many Asian countries. Total world population may be declining before the end of this century. Despite that, it is a neglected topic in demography – its analysis and its consequences overshadowed by the problem of population ageing. This chapter shows that population decline is a diverse phenomenon. The process of decline and its end-product of a smaller population size have different consequences. Modest rates of decline may be manageable and scarcely perceptible. Smaller population size may be irrelevant to most aspects of political,

---

A longer version of this paper: Coleman, D. and Rowthorn, R. (2011) 'Who's afraid of population decline? A critical examination of its consequences', in Ronald D. Lee and David S. Reher (eds) *Demographic Transition and Its Consequences* (Supplement to Volume 37 of *Population and Development Review*) pp. 217–48.

social and economic welfare and beneficial for environment and sustainability. In the future, adaptation to it may in any case become unavoidable.

Background

Fear of population decline, censuses to warn of it and pro-natalist and other policies to avert it, are almost as old as states themselves (Glass 1940; Teitelbaum and Winter 1985). Rulers and states in the past and present as well as state-less tribal societies found affirmation, strength and protection in population growth and cause for alarm in population decline, as the latter was considered a symptom and cause of failure and weakness. Where increases in productivity are difficult and where international trade is a zero-sum game, population becomes with land the chief factor of production, its increase to be encouraged by any means including conquest, prohibition of emigration and enslavement; its diminution to be avoided at all costs. Mercantilist thinking considered the global economy to be a zero-sum game and, with the difficulties of raising individual productivity, regarded population as a prime factor to be increased irrespective of the effect on individual standards of living.

Between the two World Wars, birth rates in many Western European countries and in the United States fell below the level of replacement (van Bavel 2010). The prospect of population decline implicit in those rates, formalized into alarming population projections (e.g. Charles 1938, pp. 73–105), prompted several governments to adopt pro-natalist policies to avert the 'twilight of parenthood' and 'race suicide'. The recovery of the birth rate and the 'baby boom' blew away those fears in most Western countries, at least for a while. Instead the world concerned itself with overpopulation. But since the end of the twentieth century, the demographic, political and business worlds have rediscovered population decline. For the latter, at least, this prospect is unappealing (see Longman 2004).

Until the 1980s, demographic transition theory took for granted that populations emerging from the transition would resume the previous pattern of maintenance of numbers sustained by approximately replacement-level fertility. That assumption was convenient, reasonable but evidence-free (Demeny 1997, pp. 94–110; United Nations 2002). Fertility in much of the developed world, except for Central and Eastern Europe, remained resolutely below the level of replacement from the 1970s onwards, and this trend was emulated by a growing number of developing countries, thus reviving the concerns of the 1930s (Chesnais 1996).

The era of rapid and sustained population increase was a short one in the broad sweep of human history. It dates back for little more than two centuries and is now drawing to a close in the West, with profound political and strategic implications. Before that 'great population spike', population decline was a constant preoccupation and a not-infrequent experience (Biraben 2004, pp. 9–31; Glass 1973).

Population decline – the current reality

Today, after the unlooked-for irruption of the baby boom, all its birth rates, with the exception of those in New Zealand, Iceland and (almost) France, have returned to below the level required to maintain the population. Without migration, the Western world faces population decline in the short or medium term, given the current levels of fertility. Many developing countries are likely to follow that example within a few decades. Natural increase remains positive in parts of north-west Europe and, thanks to recent increases in fertility, in the Czech Republic, Poland and Slovakia. Elsewhere, deaths exceeded births especially where chronic low birth rates have exhausted positive demographic momentum and turned it negative (Birg 2002; Ogawa et al. 2005; Schwartz 1998). The last generations completely to replace themselves in Western Europe were born in the 1950s (Sobotka 2008).

Japan's population tipped over the edge into decline in 2006. Official projections in Japan, gloomily assuming a future total fertility of a perpetual 1.3, project the population falling from 127.8 million in 2007 to 95.1 million in 2050, by which time natural decline would have reached 1.16 per cent per year (Government of Japan 2009, tables 1.4, 1.6). In China, Hong Kong, Korea, Taiwan and Singapore, despite very low total fertility, demographic momentum still keeps births ahead of deaths (Table 5.1).

The exciting 'decline' in Europe's population, both current and projected, of which the media are so fond, arises mostly because of the lumping together of Eastern Europe (including the European former Soviet Union) with all the other regions of Europe (Figure 5.1). The most severe decline is projected for Eastern Europe, with more modest declines in the longer term for Western Europe, and growth, not decline, for Northern Europe.

Taking all this together, the expectation for the future of the developed world is a picture of expanding diversity, not a collective descent into oblivion.

Table 5.1 Natural and total population change in selected European countries, 2011 (rates per 1000 total population)

States with increasing population 2011 (first 21)				**States with declining population 2011 (all)**			
Natural change		**Total increase**		**Natural change**		**Total decline**	
10.0	Ireland	Norway	13.2	−0.3	Greece	Moldova	−0.2
6.3	Albania	Kosovo	12.8	−0.4	Estonia	Estonia	−0.4
4.2	France	Switzerland	10.7	−0.6	Portugal	Belarus	−1.7
4.1	UK	UK	7.8	−0.8	Moldova	Greece	−1.8
3.8	Norway	Italy	7.3	−2.0	Germany	Germany	−2.0
2.7	Netherlands	Sweden	7.1	−2.2	Lithuania	Romania	−2.7
2.4	Switzerland	France	5.3	−2.2	Croatia	Hungary	−2.8
2.3	Sweden	Finland	4.8	−2.6	Romania	Portugal	−2.9
2.3	Belgium	Austria	4.6	−2.7	Belarus	Croatia	−3.2
1.9	Macedonia	Netherlands	4.5	−3.6	Ukraine	Ukraine	−3.2
1.9	Spain	Belgium	3.7	−4.1	Hungary	Serbia	−4.8
1.7	Finland	Denmark	3.6	−4.7	Latvia	Bulgaria	−5.7
1.7	Slovakia	Italy	3.2	−5.1	Bulgaria	Lithuania	−14.8
1.6	Slovenia	Ireland	2.8	−5.1	Serbia	Latvia	−16.0
1.2	Denmark	Slovenia	2.6				
0.3	Poland	Slovakia	2.2				
0.2	Austria	Czech Rep	1.8				
0.2	Czech Rep.	Russia	1.4				
−0.8	Italy	Germany	1.1				
−0.9	Russian Fed.	Spain	0.9				
−2.3	Germany	Poland	0.2				

Note: 'Natural change' is the difference between births and deaths, per thousand population; States below 1 million population excluded.
Source: Eurostat (2009).

Population decline and population ageing – divergent sisters

Population decline is often treated as a subtext of population ageing, which has received greater attention. In some aspects, these processes proceed in parallel, while in others they diverge. Decline and ageing may share a common cause in low birth rates, but one does not cause the other. Any reduction in birth rates promotes population ageing, even in youthful societies. Decline only follows (excepting the effects of migration) when the birth rate falls below the death rate. Inward migration (in the youthful pattern usually experienced in developed countries) acts similarly upon both, tending to reduce population ageing and decline, and preventing or reversing decline altogether if it is on a large enough scale. A reduction in mortality has opposite effects – tending to increase

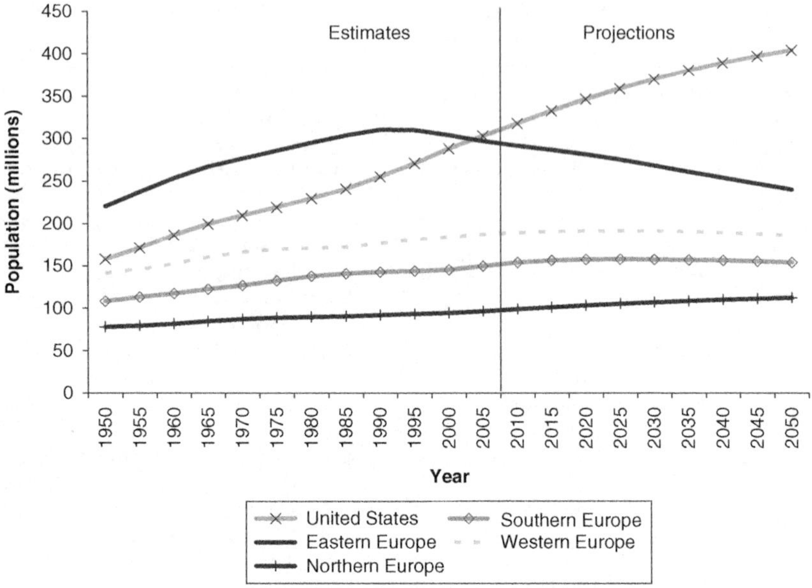

Figure 5.1 Population estimates and projections, USA and major European regions, 1950–2050 (millions)

population, or at least to moderate decline, while (in modern societies) also exacerbating population ageing.

Sub-replacement fertility, continued for many years in the absence of migration, has divergent effects on age structure and population size. Ignoring migration and mortality, it makes the population older for about two generations before the age structure comes to rest upon a new, older but stable distribution. Population size follows a different path, which continues downwards at an eventually constant rate. In the medium to long run, the effects on age structure are modest, whereas on population size the effects are eventually highly significant, tending towards extinction.

Reasons for fearing population decline

When considering the objections to population decline, and its possible benefits, it is important to make a distinction between the prospect and process of decline, and the fact of having a small population, or a smaller one than hitherto. A distinction must also be made between absolute and relative decline. A relative decline in population may still be a cause of concern if population growth falls behind that of political or economic rivals. Finally, the pace of decline matters. A given reduction in population will have different implications depending on whether it occurs gradually through the course of centuries or is compressed into a few decades.

Economic growth

As labour (equivalent to population) is one of the key inputs to production, it is axiomatic that population growth increases total output (or Gross Domestic Productivity, GDP) as long as additional workers can be employed. Conversely, declining population implies slower output growth, unless it is compensated by acceleration in productivity. Confidence in growth in numbers may underpin confidence among investors and inventors that their products and services will be launched onto a growing market that will sustain demand, and that a growing labour force can match demand with the required output. In theory, a larger population size permits greater economies of scale and division of labour, thus improving productivity. Manufactured products with high development costs come within the reach of growing capital markets.

In a closed economy, population decline, or even the end of population growth, pulls the rug from under these advantages and reverses them. It is accompanied by a greater degree of population ageing with all its costs. With the given productivity, GDP declines *pro rata* with numbers of people. Economies of scale may diminish. Shrinking markets and a diminished workforce could squeeze profitability – declining domestic demand, accompanied later as the workforce contracts, by rising wage pressures from an increasingly scarce labour supply. Weaker investment – discouraged by the prospect of declining markets – would mean that plants age and are less competitive. The psychology of the market becomes defensive, pessimistic and risk-averse when the cushion of population growth is no longer there, according to Jackson and Howe (2008, p. 113).

In a closed economy, declining population thus puts the spotlight on increasing standards of individual productivity and consumption to maintain the level of investment and confidence. Vulnerability to slumps may be higher without the prospect of long-term growth in demand to buoy up confidence. Products with high research and development costs can no longer be contemplated solely from the resources of the national economy. Ireland was a unique example of population decline in Europe from the 1840s to the 1950s, although only a nation-state from 1922. Official reports drew attention to high overhead costs in the provision of services, the limited domestic market, the discouragement of risk-taking and the lack of optimism about prospects (Walsh 1974, pp. 8–41).

Military security

Other things being equal, big countries have more political and military power than small ones (Kagan 2003; Kennedy 1988, pp. 158–84; McNicoll 1999). Population decline *ipso facto* reduces the potential size of armed forces. GDP, smaller than hitherto, can no longer support the domestic development of expensive equipment, and countries must either import it at a cost to the balance of payments or forgo it. The mechanization of warfare and the advent of nuclear weapons have not eliminated the importance of the balance of numbers between powers at similar levels of development. A classic example is the failure of the French population to grow in the nineteenth century, following its very early fertility transition. France began the nineteenth century as Europe's demographic, military and economic superpower. It ended it on par with the United Kingdom and Germany, to which it lost two provinces in 1871. Near-defeat in the First World War reinforced fears of population decline, confirmed by the final catastrophe of 1940 among other reverses (see Sauvy 1987, ch. 8, pp. 125–36; Teitelbaum and Winter 1985).

More recently, the power residing in the Kremlin has diminished with the diminution of population, space and economy under its control. After the loss of its satellites in 1989 (total population including the Soviet Union was 385 million) and the break-up of the Soviet Union itself in 1991, Russia will face an even further loss of capacity if its population declines as projected from 148 million in 1990 to 126 million by mid-century (Balzer 2005, p. 38; United Nations 2011). The relative decline of the Western powers projected for the twenty-first century, compared with the population increases of third-world countries, magnified by their economic growth, promises a radical shift in the strategic balance (e.g. Jackson and Howe 2008).

Civil political power

Numbers also matter in the peaceful exercise of power. Population determines representation in many international bodies (although not the United Nations) and is correlated with economic power. Representation in the European Commission and the European Parliament is directly related to population, although with a favourable weighting for small countries. G8 membership depends on GDP, closely related to population within today's developed realm. The UN 2008-based projections suggest that Germany's population will be eclipsed by that of the United Kingdom by 2050, with France not far behind – a development of considerable symbolic power, if nothing else. Smaller countries such as Bulgaria (Sugareva et al. 2006) and Hungary fear damaging de-population.

Is population decline really such a problem?

Population decline, therefore, is seen as bringing some disadvantages to any society.

So far we lack much empirical evidence that modern population decline will depress innovation, investment or individual wealth – the process has scarcely begun. Population in all the major West European countries, including the United Kingdom, had almost ceased to grow from the 1970s until the 1980s, until the revival of immigration from the mid-1980s. In Germany (Federal Republic) numbers fell slightly from 1973 to 1985. Despite that, German GDP continued to grow substantially, by 26 per cent over the period when compared with 29 per cent for 13 countries of Western Europe (United Nations Economic Commission for Europe's Economic Survey of Europe 1989–90, table A.1). No crisis of business confidence ensued, or was even discussed, or is now. However, the mood in Japan is more despondent (Akihiko 2006; Chapple 2004; Coulmas 2007). Economic pessimism about Japanese prospects is not universal. Over the decade of 1995–2005, Japanese GDP rose by 11.9 per cent and the population by 1.8 per cent. The IMF forecasts that in the following decade, 2005–15, population will fall slightly by 1.2 per cent, but GDP will rise by a further 10.6 per cent (IMF WEO database).

On closer scrutiny, some of the problems listed earlier lack substance, or may be advantageous. Current recession apart, the practical concern most often voiced is not unemployed resources and unemployment, as feared by Keynes (1936), but a shortage of labour hampering output and inflationary wage pressures. Concern about GDP can only be justified if national power, defence and international influence are given a greater weight than individual welfare. Naturally, total GDP tends to expand with total population size, but this has no necessary bearing upon individual welfare. As Sauvy (1969, ch. 6) pointed out, the 'power optimum' that gives greatest comfort to strategists and to rulers may be quite different from (usually bigger than) the population size that optimizes individual welfare. The interest of the poor might quite be otherwise. Those who sell their labour do better by making themselves scarce, not abundant.

On a global scale, there is no evidence of a positive relationship between population size and GDP per head, or between the growth rates of these variables. The same is true amongst the industrial countries (not shown separately) and also over a much longer time period. Using data from Maddison (2007), we computed growth rates over the twentieth century as a whole for a sample of 12 major west European economies, together with Canada, the USA, Australia, New Zealand and Japan. A regression of growth of GDP per head on population growth yielded a correlation coefficient equal to −0.12. With Japan excluded, the correlation was −0.25, indicating that, in the developed world, countries with lower rates of population growth tended to have higher rates of increase of GDP per head. Moreover, small industrial countries are just as rich as large ones (Barro and Sala-i-Martin 2003; Sheehey 1996).

While a large domestic market is obviously an advantage, as the US example shows, equivalent advantage may also arise from the adoption of free trade or membership of a trading block such as the European single market. The same principle applies to military and political affairs, where countries too small to have much influence on their own can increase their leverage by joining alliances. However, as the European Union and North Atlantic Treaty Organization (NATO) illustrate, alliances can be fraught with problems and can rarely mobilize their combined diplomatic or military resources as effectively as a large centralized state (Figures 5.2 and 5.3).

Small countries within a peaceful international order can have influence out of proportion to their size, such as the Irish Republic and Iceland (Krebs and Levy 2001; Weiner and Teitelbaum 2001, Ch. 3, pp. 21–37). Their impotence makes them convenient as neutrals. Some smaller states earn part of their living as uncontroversial hosts to international bodies. Small nations, with the same vote as the biggest, are thereby disproportionately influential in the UN General Assembly and are overrepresented among the institutions of the European Union. For the most part, it would be vain for countries locked into modern low-fertility demographic regimes to seek to change radically their position in the international league table of population size. And to try to do so through mass immigration would risk a serious breakdown of cohesion.

On the question of economies of scale, the significance of this factor depends on the extent to which overseas markets can compensate

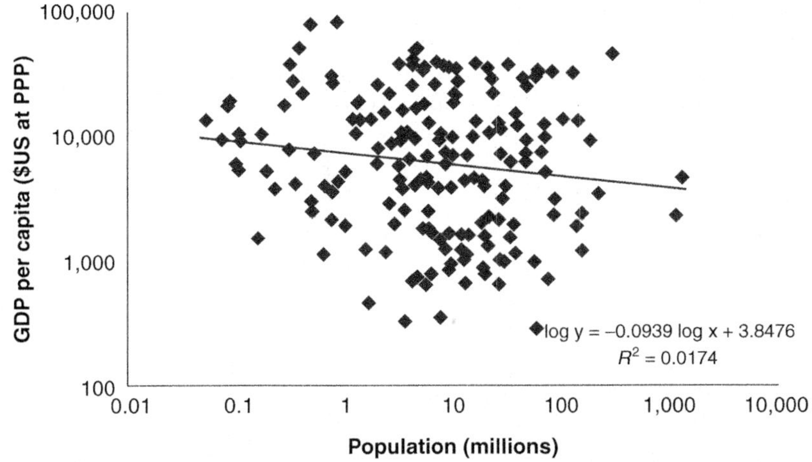

Figure 5.2 GDP per capita and population, 180 countries, 2006
Source: IMF, WEO data bases. All countries for which data are available are shown.

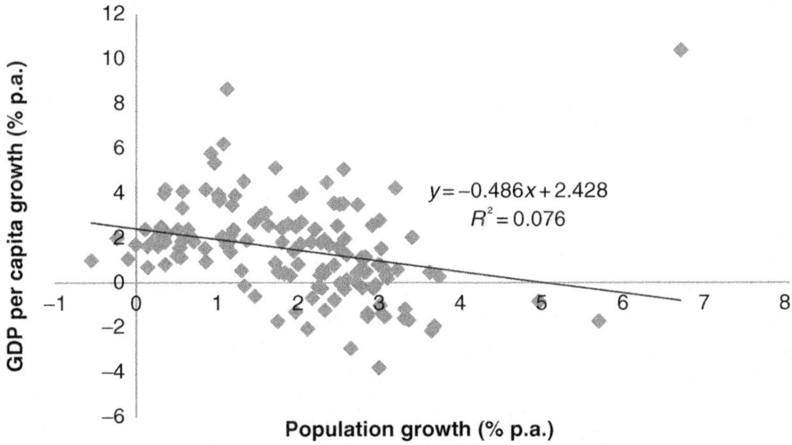

Figure 5.3 Growth rates of GDP per capita and population: 147 countries, 1980–2006
Source: IMF, WEO data bases. All countries for which data are available are shown.

for the diminution of domestic ones. Free trade makes national-level population decline less important because it increases the proportion of output that is exported. Countries with a small population typically export far more than large countries at the same stage of development. For example, in 2008, total US exports of goods and services were equal to 5.9 thousand dollars per capita. The corresponding figures for Finland and the Netherlands were 24.1 and 44.3, respectively (WTO database). Smaller economies, however, may lack the resources to invest in new highly competitive products requiring expensive research and development. But that can also apply to very large countries – there may be room in the world only for two major manufacturers of civil aircraft, and two or three of aero-engines, and a diminishing number of volume car manufacturers, for example.

As regards demand, some earlier worries have lost impact. Consumer demand for ever-cheaper goods appears to be insatiable – contrary to what Keynes (1936) and Reddaway (1939, 1977) – and before them Malthus (1803) – had feared. Superior macro- and micro-economic policies have developed in the Post-War years, with floating exchange rates, more open international trade, better management of inflation and a less regulated labour market and price mechanism. Consumer demand has been fuelled by the accelerating inventiveness of consumer products promoted by advertising in ways unheard of in earlier times, the outsourcing of manufacturing and borrowing. The recent economic crisis had nothing to do with population decline but was provoked by high consumption fuelled by excessive debt and failings in the financial sector.

Some claim that declining numbers, or small size, deprive countries of critical mass for research and development, driving specialists abroad. But between the prosperous countries of Western Europe there is no brain-drain from small to larger populations. Scholarship has always been mobile and international, and technical innovations in small countries (e.g. Nokia, and nuclear power, in Finland; advanced jet fighters and other weapons in Sweden) do not support such fears. The related notion advanced by Simon (1981), that population size and growth is essential because it produces more geniuses, to the general good, seems *a priori* absurd. The briefest refection upon the intellectual output of fifth century Greece, and of renaissance Florence, with the stagnation that followed, or the relative intellectual sterility of much larger populations then and today, allow us to dismiss it. There is no significant association between population size and the number of Nobel Prizes awarded per million of population. The smaller populations do better – first in rank is Iceland, the first eight (mostly Nordic) all have populations under ten million except for the United Kingdom.

The other side of the argument: the merits of population stabilization and decline

Long ago, the end of population growth was seen by the Royal Commission on Population (1949) as a relief from the balance of payments problems that have plagued many developed countries for most of the twentieth century, as competitive advantage in manufacturing was lost. Some imports of food, fuel and raw materials are unavoidable. With fixed land area, there are limits to sustainable food output; with fewer people self-sufficiency is easier and with it some relief from balance of payment costs. With food cheap on the international market, and wartime threats long forgotten, concern about food security has waned. But this concern is re-emerging as the era of abundant global food surpluses appears to be drawing to an end (Roberts 2008), a crisis hastened by global climate change and population increase.

As population diminishes and the stock of capital goods does not, the ratio of capital to population improves and the average person should therefore be wealthier. Resources can be directed to improve standards, not to make wider provision for a growing population. However, the capital stock needs eventually to be renewed and the annual cost of maintaining the complete transport network and other infrastructure may be unchanged, so that with a much smaller population the cost per head would be greater. Over the long run, a much smaller population also benefits from inheriting a capital stock designed for its more numerous ancestors.

Lower levels of usage in fixed distribution systems of drinking water and sewage disposal, for example, arising from population decline and other factors in Eastern Germany, can cause technical problems potentially affecting health (Hummel and Lux 2007). But in the shorter term, a modest reduction in size would take population back to a more comfortable stage, reducing congestion on transport networks and pressure on housing, for example. In many countries infrastructure provision – notably in transport – has badly lagged behind population growth and other factors of demand. London is already under serious water stress as a consequence of rapid population growth, among other factors (Environment Agency 2010).

The scarcity of labour in a declining population will inconvenience employers. But there are two important compensations. Employers will be obliged to review the efficiency of their operations and introduce equipment and techniques to increase productivity, substituting capital for labour and creating demand for higher technology products. Governments would be obliged to accelerate overdue reforms of raising retirement age. Much greater efforts would have to be made to mobilize the substantial population of unemployed youth, the 'NEETS' – Not in Education, Employment or Training, and the 'Underclass' – into the workforce. With abundant labour, immigrant or otherwise, this part of the population can be ignored, remaining in its marginalized and often criminalized state. Mobilizing this population would improve average income, cut crime and reduce inequality.

Costs of congestion and crowding should decline with smaller population, and journey to work times fall. Traffic could decline *pro rata* with population. With fewer people, fewer resources need to be devoted to new dwellings and their associated infrastructure once household formation had also ceased to grow. Housing could be built at a somewhat lower density as in the earlier twentieth century, with gardens free from the threat, or the temptation, of infill. Unsatisfactory housing, especially in peripheral social housing estates requiring apparently perpetual refurbishment, would be demolished and returned to open land. Costs of housing and of land would eventually fall with a stable or declining population. That might encourage family formation.

Environmental aspects of decline

The environmental consequences of lower population density could be considerable, and mostly favourable. Human population growth has been the biggest threat to wildlife (Hambler 2004, ch. 2). Most encroachment on the countryside would cease. With a relaxation of pressures, the intensification of agriculture, which makes much of the countryside a wildlife desert, would be relaxed. Some marginal land could revert to wilderness, as in previous eras of population decline (e.g. sixth century and late fourteenth century Europe). Expensive sea defences protecting low-lying coastal land no longer needed for agriculture could be abandoned, enabling land to be reclaimed by sea and salt marsh. In Western Europe, especially the United Kingdom, most 'nature' is man-made. The climatic climax vegetation (the stable natural state without human interference) over most of Europe is forest, to which untended land would revert within a century or so, after an un-aesthetic interval of scrub. Succession from agriculture back to forest brings a greater richness of species (Hambler 2004, ch. 7), and trees are effective carbon sinks.

Emissions and pollution of all kinds would be moderated (Costello et al. 2009). However, the number of households, not just people, is a most important component of environmental problems (Liu et al. 2003) and household numbers typically increase faster than population and could continue to grow even when population had started to decline. The environmental effects of the combination of economic growth with the relatively fast population growth in the United States, Canada and Australia (O'Connor et al. 2008) are correspondingly more potent, with US oil use projected to increase by 43 per cent by 2025 (Markham and Steinzor 2006). The projected diminution of Japanese, Russian and eventually Chinese populations may have corresponding environmental benefits.

The inevitable end of growth

The final argument is that population growth, and economic growth measured as GDP, must come to an end. Evidence for unavoidable shortage of fresh water in many parts of the world, even more than projections of food shortage, is mounting. Growth in population and economy together are bringing about their own limitation, if forecasts of the climate change that they provoke have any validity. The demographic consequences of climate change are even more difficult to project than climate change itself: uncertainty piled upon uncertainty. If the populations of the world do not reverse their growth, then negative feedback from our previous activities may force us to do so, in disagreeable ways.

Conclusions

Low fertility rates have focused attention on population decline, which is already under way in a number of countries. Some think it will become universal. Population decline and population ageing in modern societies share a common cause in low fertility. But one does not cause the other.

The process of population decline inevitably brings problems, although rates of decline might hardly be perceptible to contemporary observers. A smaller, stable population, once achieved, could have advantages. A smaller population size might of itself arrest further decline and permit the resumption of growth. The notion of homeostatic feedback between population size and family building was the foundation of Malthusian population theory and its existence is well documented for earlier centuries. Those processes have been neglected in much recent population thinking. The advent of population decline suggests that reconsideration is overdue.

Negative feedback in modern societies may have been underestimated. Populations may have 'overshot' their sustainable or comfortable limits. Inevitably, there are lags, protracted by the inertia of culture and tradition, between the beginning of negative effects upon family welfare of larger family size and larger population, and the responses of individuals to it (Ehrlich and Kim 2005). Demographic momentum exacerbates the delay. Fertility at or below replacement level was reached in most countries of Western European by the 1930s. But their populations have since increased by between 20 and 80 per cent, thanks partly to the transient baby boom and to migration but mostly as a consequence of demographic momentum. Recent studies in European countries have shown a negative relationship between population density and fertility (Kulu et al. 2009; Lutz and Quiang 2002; Lutz et al. 2006).

Negative feedback can be important at the national policy level as well. In some counties of the rich world, political pressure is growing for an explicit recognition of the need for measures to increase the birth rate, however ideologically unacceptable pro-natalist policies may have been regarded in even the recent past.

Defining optimum population for modern societies is difficult if not impossible. While it is clear that the process of decline has numerous drawbacks, these are only important if the decline is fast and protracted. Smaller population size, however, has social, economic and environmental advantages. And it may be forced on us, as a requirement for our survival, if the ultimate feedbacks from our growth arising from climate change come to pass.

References

Akihiko, M. (2006) *Shrinking-Population Economics: Lessons from Japan,* trans. Brian Miller (Tokyo: International House of Japan).

Balzer, H. (2005) *The Implications of Demographic Change for Russian Politics and Security*. Weatherhead Center for International Affairs Conference, Harvard University, Health and Demography in the States of the Former Soviet Union, 29–30 April 2005.

Barro, R. J. and Sala-i-Martin, X. (2003) *Economic Growth* (Cambridge, MA: MIT Press).

Biraben, J.-N. (2004) 'L'histoire du peuplement humain des origines à nos jours', *Démographie: anayse et synthèse V. Histoire du Peuplement et Prévisions,* in G. Caselli, J. Vallin and G. Wunsch (eds) (Paris: Institut National d'Etudes Démographiques), pp. 9–31.

Birg, H. (2002) 'Demographic ageing and population decline in twenty-first-century – Germany: consequences for the systems of social insurance', *Population Bulletin of the United Nations,* Policy Responses to Population Decline and Ageing, 44(45): 103–34.

Boardman, B. (2005) *The 40% House* (Oxford: Environmental Change Institute).

Boko, M., Niang, I., Nyong, A. and Vogel, C. (2007) *Africa, Intergovernmental Panel on Climate Change (IPCC) Working Group II Climate Change Impacts, Adaptation and Vulnerability. Working Group II Contribution to the IPCC Fourth Assessment Report. Intergovernmental Panel on Climate Change* (IPCC), World Meteorological Association/United Nations Environment Programme (WMO/UNEP) 36.

Breton, D., Condon, S., Marie, C.-V. and Temporal, F. (2009) 'Les départements d'Outre-Mer face aux defies du vieillissement démographique et des migrations', *Populations et Sociétés,* 460(October 2009): 4.

Champion, A. (ed.) (1989) *Counterurbanisation: The Changing Pace and Nature of Population Deconcentration* (London: Edward Arnold).

Champion, T. (2000) 'Flight from the cities?', in R. Bate (ed.) *On the Move: The Housing Consequences of Migration* (York: Joseph Rowntree Foundation), 10–19.

Chapple, J. (2004) 'The dilemma posed by Japan's population decline', *Electronic Journal of Contemporary Japanese Studies,* 2004 (Discussion Paper 5).

Charles, E. (1938) 'The effects of present trends in fertility and mortality upon the future population of Great Britain and upon its age-composition', in L. Hogben (ed.) *Political Arithmetic: A Symposium of Population Studies* (London: Allen and Unwin), 72–105.

Chawla, M., Betcherman, G. and Mukerji, A. (2007) *From Red to Gray: The 'Third Transition' of Aging Populations in Eastern Europe and the Former Soviet Union (overview)* (Washington, DC: The World Bank).

Chesnais, J.-C. (1996) *La crepuscule de l'occident* (Paris: Robert Laffont).

Clark, G. (2007) *A Farewell to Alms: A Brief Economic History of the World* (Princeton: Princeton University Press).

Costello, A., Abbas, M., Allen, A., Ball, S. et al. (2009). 'Managing the health effects of climate change', *The Lancet,* 373(16 May 2009): 1693–733.

Coulmas, F. (2007) *Population Decline and Ageing in Japan – The Social Consequences* (London: Routledge).

Dalla Zuanna, G. and Micheli, G. A. (eds) (2004) *Strong Family and Low Fertility: A Paradox? New Perspectives in Interpreting Contemporary Family and Reproductive Behaviour* (Dordrecht: Kluwer).

Daly, M. E. (2006) *The Slow Failure: Population Decline and Independent Ireland, 1922–1973* (Madison, Wisconsin: University of Wisconsin Press).

DaVanzo, J. and Grammich, C. (2001) *Dire Demographics. Population Trends in the Russian Federation* (Santa Monica: Rand).

Demeny, P. (1997) 'Replacement-level fertility: the implausible endpoint of the demographic transition', in G. W. Jones, R. M. Douglas, J. C. Caldwell and R. M. D'Souza. (eds) *The Continuing Demographic Transition* (Oxford: Clarendon Press), 94–110.

Dyson, T. (2005) 'On development, demography and climate change: the end of the world as we know it?', *Population and Environment,* 27(2): 117–49.

The Economist (2006) 'Incredible shrinking countries', 5 January 2006: 12.

Environment Agency (2010) *London State of the Environment Report 2010* (London: Environment Agency).

Ehrlich, I. and Kim, J. (2005) 'Endogenous fertility, mortality and economic growth: can a Malthusian framework account for the conflicting historical trends in population?', *Journal of Asian Economics,* 16: 789–806.

Eurostat (2009) *Data in Focus,* 31/2009.

Feser, E. and Sweeney, S. (2003) 'Out-migration, depopulation and the geography of US economic distress', *International Regional Science Review,* 26(1): 38–67.

Financial Times (2006) 'A labour shortage can be a blessing' by M. Lind, 8 June 2006.

Frejka, T. and Sardon, J.-P. (2004) *Childbearing Trends and Prospects in Low-Fertility Countries. A Cohort Analysis* (Dordrecht: Kluwer).

Glass, D. V. (1936) *The Struggle for Population* (Oxford: Oxford University Press).

Glass, D. V. (1940) *Population Policies and Movements in Europe* (London: Oxford University Press).

Glass, D. V. (1973) *Numbering the People* (Farnborough: Saxon House).

Hambler, C. (2004) *Conservation* (Cambridge: Cambridge University Press).

Haug, W. (2005) Policy challenges for emigration countries. Presentation to UNFPA/UNECE/NIDI Training Programme on International Migration, Geneva, 24–28 January 2005, http://www.unece.org/stats/documents/2005/01/migration/17.e.ppt

House of Lords Select Committee on Economic Affairs (2008) *1st Report of Session 2007–08: The Economic Impact of Immigration. Volume 1: Report HL Paper 82–1,* p. 84. *Volume II: Evidence. HL Paper 82-II,* p. 514 (London: The Stationery Office).

Hummel, D. and Lux, A. (2007) 'Population decline and infrastructure: the case of the German water supply system', *Vienna Yearbook of Population Research* 2007: 167–91.

Jackson, R. and Howe, N. (2008) *The Graying of the Great Powers* (Washington, DC: Center for Strategic and International Studies (CSIS)).

Kagan, R. (2003) *Of Paradise and Power. America and Europe in the New World Order* (New York: Alfred A. Knopf).

Kennedy, L. and Clarkson, L. A. (1993) 'Birth, death and exile: Irish population history 1700–1921', in B. J. Graham and L. J. Proudfoot (eds) *An Historical Geography of Ireland* (London: Academic Press), 158–184.

Kennedy, P. (1988) *The Rise and Fall of the Great Powers: Economic Change and Military Conflict from 1500 to 2000* (London: Unwin Hyman).

Keynes, J. M. (1936) 'The economic consequences of a declining population', *Eugenics Review,* 29: 13–17.

Krebs, R. R. and Levy, J. S. (2001) 'Demographic change and the sources of international conflict', in M. Weiner and S. S. Russell (eds) *Demography and National Security* (New York, Oxford: Berghahn), 62–105.

Kulu, H., Boyle, P. J. and Andersson, G. (2009) 'High suburban fertility: evidence from four Northern European countries', *Demographic Research,* 21(31): 915–44.

Laqueur, W. (2007) *The Last Days of Europe: Epitaph for an Old Continent* (New York: Thomas Dunne Books).

Lee, R. D. (1985) 'Population homoeostasis and English demographic history', *Journal of Interdisciplinary History,* 15(4): 635–60.

Lee, R. D. (1987) 'Population dynamics of humans and other animals', *Demography,* 24(4): 443–65.

Lesthaeghe, R. and Willems, P. (1999) 'Is low fertility a temporary phenomenon in the European Union?', *Population and Development Review,* 25(2): 211–28.

Liu, J., Daily, G. C., Ehlich, P. R. and Luck, G. W. (2003) 'Effects of household dynamics on resource consumption and biodiversity', *Nature*, 421(6922): 530–3.

Longman, P. (2004) *The Empty Cradle: How Falling Birthrates Threaten World Prosperity and What to Do about It* (New York: Basic Books).

Lutz, W. and Quiang, R. (2002) 'Determinants of human population growth', *Philosophical Transactions of the Royal Society B*, 357: 1197–210.

Lutz, W., Skirbekk, V. and Testa, M. R. (2006) 'The low fertility trap hypothesis: forces that may lead to further postponement and fewer births in Europe', *Vienna Yearbook of Population Research*, 2006: 167–92.

McDonald, P. (2006) 'Low fertility and the state: the efficacy of policy', *Population and Development Review*, 32(3): 485–510.

McMorrow, K. and Roeger, W. (2004) *The Economic and Financial Market Consequences of Global Ageing* (Berlin: Springer).

McNicoll, G. (1999) 'Population weights in the international order', *Population and Development Review*, 25(3): 411–42.

Maddison, A. (2007) *Contours of the World Economy, 1–2030 AD: Essays in Macroeconomic History* (Oxford: Oxford University Press).

Malthus, T. R. (1803) *An Essay on the Principle of Population, or, A View of Its Past and Present Effects on Human Happiness: With an Inquiry into Our Prospects Respecting the Future Removal or Mitigation of the Evils Which It Occasions*, 2nd ed. (London: J. Johnson).

Markham, V. D. and Steinzor, N. (2006) *US National Report on Population and the Environment* (New Canaan, CT: Center for Environment and Population).

Meadows, D. H., Meadows, D. L. and Randers, J. (1992) *Beyond the Limits: Global Collapse or a Sustainable Future* (London: Earthscan).

Meadows, D. H., Meadows, D. L., Randers, J. and Behrens, W. W. (1972) *The Limits to Growth. A Report for the Club of Rome's Project on the Predicament of Mankind* (London: Earth Island).

Müller, B. and Siedentop, S. (2004) 'Growth and shrinkage in Germany – trends, perspectives and challenges for spatial planning and development', *German Journal of Urban Studies*, 44: 1.

Myrskylä, M., Kohler, H.-P. and Billari, F. (2009) 'Advances in development reverse fertility declines', *Nature*, 460 (6 August 2009): 741–3.

O'Connor, M. and Lines, W. J. (2008) *Overloading Australia: how governments and media dither and deny over population* (Canterbury, NSW: Envirobook).

Ogawa, N., Kondo, M. and Matsukura, R. (2005) 'Japan's transition from the demographic bonus to the demographic onus', *Asian Population Studies*, 1(2): 207–26.

Reddaway, W. B. (1939) *The Economics of a Declining Population* (London: Allen and Unwin).

Reddaway, W. B. (1977) 'The economic consequences of zero population growth', *Lloyd's Bank Review. Reprinted as Economics Reprint no 17, Department of Applied Economics, University of Cambridge* (April 1977).

Reher, D. S. (2007) 'Towards long-term population decline: a discussion of relevant issues', *European Journal of Population*, 23(2): 189–207.

Roberts, P. (2008) *The End of Food* (New York: Houghton Mifflin).

Rostow, W. W. (1998) *The Great Population Spike and After. Reflections on the 21st Century* (New York: Oxford University Press).

Royal Commission on Population (1949) *Report Cmd. 7695* (London: HMSO).

Rozendal, P. and Moors, H. (1983) 'Attitudes towards population trends and population policy in the Netherlands, compared with some data from other western European countries', *European Demographic Information Bulletin*, 14(4): 141–9.

Sauvy, A. (1969) *General Theory of Population*, trans. Campos, C. (London: Weidenfeld and Nicholson).

Sauvy, A. (1987) *L'Europe submergée: Sud-Nord dans trente ans. Ch. 8 Nos trois defaites demographiques* (Paris: Dunod).

Saville, J. (1957) *Rural Depopulation in England and Wales 1851–1951* (London: Routledge and Kegan Paul).

Schwartz, K. (1998) 'Gibt es Alternativen zu der für Deutschland erwarteten Bevölkerungsentwicklung?' (Are there alternatives to the expected population trends in Germany?), *Zeitschrift für Bevölkerungswissenschaft*, 23(3): 335–41.

Sheehey, E. J. (1996) 'The growing gap between rich and poor countries: a proposed explanation', *World Development*, 24(8): 1379–84.

Simon, J. (1981) *The Ultimate Resource* (Princeton: Princeton University Press).

Skirbekk, V. (2005) 'Population ageing negatively affects productivity', *Vienna Yearbook of Demography*, 2005: 5–6.

Sobotka, T. (2008) 'The diverse faces of the second demographic transition in Europe', *Demographic Research*, 19(8): 171–224.

Statistisches Bundesamt (2006) *Bevölkerung Deutschlands bis 2050. Übersicht der Ergebnisse der 11. koordinierten Bevölkerungsvorausberechnung -Varianten und zusätzliche Modellrechnungen* (Wiesbaden: Statistisches Bundesamt).

Sugareva, M., Tzekov, N., Donev, D. and Boshikyov, D. (2006) 'Le vieillissement demographique dans les regions de dépopulation en Bulgarie du Nord-Ouest' (Demographic ageing in depopulated areas of North-West Bulgaria), in G.-F. Dumont, D. Argoud, R. Belot and P. Boquet (eds) *Les territoires face au vieillissement en Europe – géographie, politique, prospective* (*Areas Facing Ageing in Europe: Geography, Politics, Outlook*) (Paris: Ellipses Marketing. Colection Carrefours).

Sutter, J. and Tabah, L. (1951) Le notion de l'isolat et du population minimum, *Population*, 6: 481.

Teitelbaum, M. S. (2001) 'International migration: predicting the unknowable', in M. Weiner and S. S. Russell (eds) *Demography and National Security* (New York: Berghahn).

Teitelbaum, M. S. and Winter, J. (1985) *Fear of Population Decline* (London: Academic Press).

Testa, M. R. and Grilli, L. (2006) 'The influence of childbearing regional contexts on ideal family size in Europe', *Population*, 61(1–2): 99–127.

United Nations (2002) *World Urbanization Prospects. The 2001 Revision. Data Tables and Highlights* (New York: United Nations).

United Nations (2011) *World Population Prospects: The 2010 Revision* (New York: United Nations).

van Bavel, J. (2010) 'Subreplacement fertility in the West before the baby boom: past and current perspectives', *Population Studies*, 64(1): 1–18.

van Dalen, H. P. and Henkens, K. (2007) 'Longing for the good life: understanding emigration from a high-income country', *Population and Development Review*, 33(1): 37–66.

Vladov, V. (ed.) (2007) *National Demographic Strategy of the Republic of Bulgaria 2006–2020* (Sofia: Bulgarian Ministry of Labour and Social Policy).
Walsh, B. M. (1974) 'Ireland', in B. Berelson (ed.) *Population Policy in Developed Countries* (New York: McGraw Hill for The Population Council).
Weiner, M. and Teitelbaum, M. S. (2001) *Political Demography, Demographic Engineering* (New York: Oxford: Berghahn).
Wilson, C. and Airey, P. (1999) 'How can a homoeostatic perspective enhance demographic transition theory?', *Population Studies,* 53(2): 117–28.
Wrigley, E. A. and Schofield, R. S. (1981) *The Population of England 1541–1871 – A Reconstruction* (London: Arnold).

Part II

What Are the Reasons for Women Having Fewer Children?

6
Why Are Women Having Fewer Babies? The Views of Mumsnet Users

Justine Roberts, Kate Williams and Ann Buchanan

> Why are women having fewer babies? *Three Cs – careers, contraception and choice basically!*

In the previous chapters, international scholars have given evidence that low fertility rates and childlessness are rising around the world. But how does this play out in real life, where young mothers are daily making decisions to have or not to have more children? What reasons do current mothers give for having fewer babies, and what do they see as the barriers to larger families? The two principal authors here agreed to use their Mumsnet website to elicit some views. Within four days, there were more than 100 'postings'. Kate Williams was responsible for setting up the questions on the website.

Justine Roberts was one of the founders of Mumsnet, which was conceived in early 2000. The idea was to create a website where parents 'could swap advice about holidays, pushchairs and last night's TV'. Eleven years later, the site gets nearly 4 million visits per month (Mumsnet website 2011).

Although the site is staunchly apolitical, the views of its members are regularly scrutinized by media and politicians, and it has been credited as one of the most influential forces in the United Kingdom.

Originally, it was felt that the site attracted mainly a middle-class membership, but postings – for example, on the Summer 2011 British Riots – suggested that members come from a wide range of backgrounds, many having been brought up in relative poverty and living in the inner city areas where the riots took place.

Why do you think women worldwide are having fewer babies?

KateMumsnet (MNHQ) Friday 12 August 2011 13:06:44

Hello all

We've been approached by an academic researcher at the Oxford Centre for Research into Parenting and Children who's working on a book called 'No Time for Children'. The book will explore why fertility rates – the number of babies being born per mother – are actually falling the world over, despite a widespread belief to the contrary.

In China, for example, the worried government is reversing its one-child policy – but many adult 'onelies' now believe that one child is 'about right'. The same is true in Japan and Singapore, and fertility rates are also falling in Africa, Europe, Latin America and all over Eastern Asia.

The book will contain chapters written by an impressive roster of academic contributors, but its authors would also like to hear what mothers themselves think is going on, and what, specifically, they consider to be the barriers to having more children. If you'd like to contribute, please do post your thoughts here.

The views given here are based on the responses received. Although the discussion had a logical flow, for the purposes of this chapter, the responses have been organized into broad themes. The first part of this chapter considers the mothers' views of why women are having fewer babies and the second part, what mothers consider are the barriers to having larger families. The final section brings some of the ideas expressed to a conclusion, and sets out the initiatives that Mumsnetters feel would reduce the burden of raising children.

Why are women having fewer babies?

Most Mumsnetters were aware that they were living in a very different world to that inhabited by their parents and grandparents. Key to the change was the availability of contraception. Almost every posting mentioned this.

> Historically there was no contraception; when contraception became available I think there was a huge outcry that 'women wouldn't

> want it', yet the sales of the pill went through the roof, particularly amongst married women.
>
> My grandma had nine (children). She also made bread and cheese and cycled into town to deliver them to a local deli. Ireland has gone from (a situation where) five to seven (children) was average I'd say, as a norm, to 'only children' being almost as common as a family of two or three children in a family. In only two generations!

Others made the point that the shift from rural to urban living encouraged women to have fewer children:

> Raising kids in a close-knit rural community was easier than today's urban living, where children need to be entertained all the time.
>
> Increased movement from country into cities, as well as falling infant mortality rates has meant that having a big family is no longer desirable or necessary.

With contraception had come changes in sexual mores. Women were freer to refuse sex and able to choose when they would have babies.

> (In the past) women were obliged to have sex with their husband and could not realistically divorce until the last century; coupled with no contraception, this inevitably meant becoming pregnant multiple times.
>
> Until quite recently, women were not given the choice. Marriage was the only real career open to them and many didn't realize they could say no to their husband's 'pestering'. Tolstoy's wife, Sophia Tolstoy, for example, had 14 children by him, even though she was a very talented writer herself, judging by her recently published diaries. If she was born today, her life would look quite different. She would be able to pursue a writing career and divorce old Tolstoy for expecting her to write out War and Peace umpteen times for free while raising their children.
>
> (Without) electricity... what could you do after sunset but have sex? Now you can watch TV, send emails or post Mumsnet!

Not only were societies changing but families were also changing:

> Family dynamics have also changed – half-siblings, step-children, elderly parents needing help, children staying longer at home (most

> of the previous generation were out the house and earning by 18). This all impacts on the choices made.

Mumsnetters were aware that because contraception was both easily accessible and reliable in the United Kingdom, they were, compared to other mothers in the world, a relatively privileged group.

> It's only in countries where contraception has been cheap, easily available, and not frowned upon for a while that you need to start looking for other reasons.
>
> If (fertility is reducing) all over the world then there are still plenty of countries where the answer could be 'better access to contraception'.

Better education or striving to get better education

The possibility of controlling their fertility appears to have encouraged women to strive harder to achieve a better education. The self-respect gained from a career was also important.

> (Why are women having fewer babies?) Better education and better access to higher education.
>
> Better education for women and work opportunities for women (rather than their only future being to get married and have babies).
>
> I've had my two DCs[1] whilst doing my PhD and trying to get my academic career started and it's been very tough. Sometimes I think I'd like one more child but I'm not sure I could go through the toil of having a small baby again and the interruption to my studies and research. I'm only in my early 30s and I hope to get a lecturing job within the next five years and, with that, the possibility of a proper maternity leave. Should I have a third child? It will be a tough decision.

Other mothers felt that, combined with availability of contraception, it was the opening out of educational opportunities that was responsible for the fall in the birth rate.

> I thought it was pretty widely accepted that wherever educational and employment opportunities for women open up. The birth rate falls? So I'd rather hope that it's following in the wake of a trend in favour of educating girls properly.

Women's employment

Next to contraception, the most frequently mentioned reason for falling fertility rates was the increasing number of women in the workforce and the economic freedom that came with it. It was recognized that poorer women would always have worked, but the difference today was that many twenty-first century women had expectations of careers. The downside to this was that the mother's income frequently became essential in maintaining the family lifestyle.

> (Falling fertility rates are due to) a combination of factors depending on the type of society; for Western societies it is due to women having a greater presence in the workforce and unfortunately that lifestyle is not fully compatible with children.
>
> Agree mainly with women's role changing from that of housewife and mother to having a presence in the workforce as the core factor. And I reckon women recognize the importance of economic freedom, something you often lose if you stay at home.
>
> Don't forget the working classes always worked, whether they had children or not. Those children also often worked.
>
> I think the rise in women having careers is a cause – I'm a feminist and am obviously happy that women have fulfilling careers; however, in a household relying on two incomes; it's very hard for the woman to be able to give up work to have children.

Changing values

Alongside changing societies, increased education and employment of women have come markedly changing values. Whereas in the past, a woman's worth was based on her ability to provide numerous children, today other factors, such as having a good education and a career as well as a family, are valued.

> In patriarchal societies, broadly, a woman's status is pretty closely linked to her fertility – the more children, the more 'dutiful' she is seen to be; infertility can lead to being an outcast
>
> I think that overpopulation is created by patriarchies. Now that women are gaining more power and status, have greater access to contraception and to real economic independence, they are naturally choosing to have less or no children.

> My feeling is that in the past large families were useful for working together, as many hands were more helpful even if there were more mouths to feed as success was often down to pure manual hard work. However, success in life today generally depends on getting ahead in education and after-school activities and the fewer children you have the more time and money you have to invest in helping your offspring be successful in life.

With the changing attitudes to women have come new 'norms' of what is the ideal size for a family.

> Both DH and I are from large families but neither of us would ever want more than two children.
>
> I think the idea of the 'ideal' family size is largely based on DH and my family growing up (what you're used to). It's interesting that the normalization of 'only children' (in China) may be making people choose this option, whereas in this country this is still a stigma.
>
> I have friends who have chosen not to have any children at all. Availability of contraception and society being more accepting of such a choice have doubtless played a part.

With the other changes have also come choices about when to have children and in some cases more respect for women if they have careers.

> If you're middle class and intelligent, it's not an acceptable option (or even one worthy of consideration) to start having children early. I think contraception has led to this being an easy choice for both men and women – men can still have sex, but not have to agree to the possible consequence of doing so. This has of course also given women freedom, but has made choosing to have children an increasingly illogical and expensive thing to do.
>
> (Today) men have more respect for women and do not see them as housekeeper or baby machines.
>
> Can I afford a career? Yes. Will people judge me positively for it? Yes. Can I afford a big family? No. Will people judge me positively for it? No.
>
> It is interesting that the majority of posters see (a declining fertility rate) as a positive. I mean it is obviously positive in the sense that

> women don't have to have lots of children, that they aren't expected to; that they have other choices in life.

It was also noted that society was less critical about those who indulged in sexual relations outside marriage.

> (There is the) freedom to be sexually active outside of marriage without society disapproving, so people no longer have to get married so they can have sex.

Having babies later in life

With increased educational opportunities, more rewarding careers and higher aspirations for family life, some women had left having babies until their mid-30s or 40s. Some were aware that their biological clock was running out, while others waited until they became suitably 'broody'. Some of these older women had difficulties in conceiving and/or suffered distressing miscarriages.

> In the educated West I think it is mainly the personal choice of women leaving it later to start having children – I had my two when I was 31 and 35. I had been with my DH for 10 years when our first was born, so it was not that I didn't meet anyone until I was in my 30s, I just wasn't remotely broody until that stage in my life.

> I am almost 40. I left having my children to the second half of my 30s, as I just didn't want to have them before then. I was way too busy doing other stuff (career, but also having fun) to want to interrupt it all to have babies.

> For me, because I started later in life, either I have them very close in age, or I have less children. Women are leaving it too late to start a family. I have four friends in this category. They looked up one day and realized that their chance had gone.

> DH and I waited until we were 'set up' (house, good jobs, financially secure) before we tried for kids. I was only 28 when we started, but it was still a bit late for me. After six years of fertility treatments, we finally had twins – I would have liked four DCs but now I am 37 and DH is 42 we feel it is a bit late.

> I also had a miscarriage in between DS1 and DS2 and it took a fair few years to have DS1, so starting later is probably a factor too.

Mumsnetters noted that men often had different agendas, which delayed having children. Others disagreed, feeling that it was women who did not want to settle down.

> Men don't want to commit until late 30s so women have less time before their fertility declines.
>
> I would say we are having children later because we are waiting for male partner to grow up.
>
> (I disagree) Men love marriage. They're obsessed with it. Its women who don't want to settle down.

Better quality of life

Overall, there was a strong recognition that fewer children equalled a better quality of life for all. Some felt that they had had opportunities in their lives because their parents had limited the size of their family. Others were slightly ashamed to admit that they were stopping at one so that they could still enjoy life. Others worried about the need for a larger house if they had more children.

> A lot of it relates to the expectations we have about the lifestyles we can provide for our children, as well as our expectations for ourselves. If you are hoping to help your children through education to third level, if you want them to have a wide range of enjoyable experiences through their childhood, without wholly sacrificing your own interests in favour of theirs, then you are automatically deciding to limit their number (unless you are extremely rich).
>
> But I will be brutally honest and say that, while having more children has crossed my mind more than once, there is something incredibly liberating about only having one child of my own (albeit a child who has siblings, so doesn't miss out) and I certainly don't live life full of regrets. I have much more time for myself and for my relationship with my DP than if I had more than one child.
>
> Economically, we are now told we need so many things to raise our child that they are very, very expensive and people do not want to live with 14 people in a two-bedroom house (as the Victorians often did) so, since they have the means to stop subsequent pregnancies with contraception, they do stop.

> Something I often see here is that children need a room each. Therefore people feel they need a bigger house after one or two children and can't afford the four-bed house. The same could be said about cars too.

A range of other issues were touched upon by the mothers, which they felt had influenced their decisions. Children were healthier and few children died in childhood; there was better health care and in the United Kingdom this was free; for some groups, the pressures to have a son were less.

Wider societal context

It was interesting that only 5 out of 107 mothers were concerned about overpopulation and the possibility of benefit to the world from a smaller population.

> I don't think an ever-rising population is ecologically sustainable and I would like my children to have a nice world to live in. For all the rabbiting on about how many children people have in the third world, if you look at per capita resource utilization you quickly realize that it is us, not them, that there's too many of.

> The world is overpopulated, so if it's true that we are having less children, then I think that's good news!

Barriers to having children

Change in lifestyle once women have children

A number of Mumsnetters mentioned the huge change in their lives once they had children. This was particularly hard for those who had a glamorous life pre-children.

> We did a lot of interesting things in our late teens and early 20s – travelling, social events, clubs, sports, etc.

> There's a huge change in lifestyle for a woman once she has children – perhaps this wasn't such a marked change before women had careers and money of their own?

> The lives women lead prior to children are too often incompatible with the lives they will have to lead once they have children.

Having children is hard work

Mumsnetters emphasized that, even in the modern world, raising children was extremely hard work. Mumsnet's website obviously provided a vital life line for some mothers.

> It is interesting that if you read accounts of poorer women with large families from 100 odd years ago, the overwhelming impression is how relentless it all was.
>
> (Raising children) It's bloody hard work. Few jobs are as relentless as being a full time SAHM[2] and no one gives you the praise and credit given to people who do other difficult jobs. It's seen as natural that a mother manages with small children when, in reality, it's a constant struggle.
>
> Because there is no help, it is relentless and very hard work. I was going to have three but stopped after two because we were older and knackered by the time we'd had two.

Having children is also a risk to your health

A few mothers remembered the stress of child birth and this had put them off having other children. Some were even considering adoption rather than go through a second birth.

> I had a terrible pregnancy and a nightmare C Section. I never want to go through that alone, I am happy to raise a single child. And although I am considering adoption, DH does not agree.
>
> Many women have been treated appallingly by misogynistic doctors during their first birth and decide after that they would never go back for number two. Even with the best births (and I had a great one) you feel you've been hit by a truck. Then there's the PAIN!!!! Women are human. Maybe some women just can't be arsed by the PAIN.

Lack of family support

With modern mobility, new mothers were often separated from the natural support of their own mothers and kin. Paid help was less available. Some mothers were crying out for some time off.

> The upper classes often had larger families but they had paid help.
>
> In my opinion another important reason for not having more is that families are not as close as they used to be. You cannot rely on your

> parents and other close relatives to help with children because either you live too far away from them, or you had your children so old that your own parents are too old to help.
>
> I could cope with more children if I had Mum across the road, aunty on the next street, and I could let them play out on the road with the other neighbourhood kids all day.
>
> Also agree with the comment about no family support. I would love 5 hours off with my husband say once a month. But it will never happen, and it's draining without it. Having an extra child makes it even more difficult and costly to get support.
>
> And last but not least I have not had an unbroken night's sleep in five years. The idea of starting again with another baby makes me shudder.

In addition, communities did not appear to offer the support they may have done in the past:

> The sense of community doesn't exist anymore. You are not allowed to let your children play freely outside anymore, due to all the dangers. This means that if you have children, your freedom is history. I am sure that was not the case some decades ago.

The cost of children

This was another key issue raised by Mumsnetters. There were large numbers of postings around the cost of raising children. They noted that, in the past, children were an economic positive – in that they would help with the farm, trade and family business. They grew up quicker and became self-supporting earlier than today. Financial issues were one of the main reasons for limiting the number of children Mumsnetters had. Many families were struggling to pay their house mortgage and needed mother's salary to fill the financial gap in the family finances.

> Certainly the economics of having children has changed and is changing dramatically. Children used to be an economic positive for the family. They became productive much younger and with much less investment. In the West, children have gone from being an economic positive for a family to becoming an economic negative (though a positive for the country).

> For what it's worth, I am the only one of my group of friends to have had even one child. They all say it's a decision based on financial issues.
>
> Cost is a big one here – I can't have it all. I will need to go back to work to meet the mortgage as we can't manage on one salary.
>
> To be fair, it's lucky we're happy as we are as there's no way we could afford another. The costs of childcare and a big-enough house are totally prohibitive. DH works full time and I work part-time out of the home and part-time from home, so between us we have three jobs, and it's still not enough. I sometimes look at large families and feel a little jealous, but it's mostly a 'how do they do it? Wish I was that sorted' feeling, rather than a 'quick, get me pregnant' one.
>
> Logistics – how many children fit in a car? If you have more, how will you transport them? Not a problem when families lived and worked close together and walked everywhere.

Some mothers noted that there was beginning to be a divide between the richer and poorer families and those in the middle. One mother felt she would like to have more children if she was richer.

> Economic factors in this country mean that large families are usually polarized at the extremes of the income spectrum. So if you have lots of kids you are likely to be either very rich or very poor.
>
> I think the fact that very wealthy women in the United Kingdom often choosing to have large families shows the flip side – given the choice, many will choose to have more children if they could afford it.
>
> But I would love a massive family, and couldn't possibly afford it and also DH wasn't ready until now (I'm 31). I'm bright enough to have carved out a decent career (which DH and everyone I know expects me to leap back into as soon as possible) but not bright enough to have planned how to achieve the dream of having a big family – that would have involved purposefully choosing a rich man early in my 20s, who wanted loads of kids with me. Or a life on benefits with someone who wanted a big family but didn't earn enough to support them. I think it's more difficult for middle-class educated women to make the choice to have big families in the current political and economic climate.

Interrupted careers – damage to careers

Many mothers had invested heavily in their education, employment and careers. Although they noted that much had been done to improve the situation for women returning to work after childbirth, careers were still at risk.

> There is also the sad truth that many of us know that, despite all rhetoric to the contrary, our careers will be put on hold (and may never recover) if/when we have children.
>
> My career is part-time/on hold until kids go to school.
>
> For me personally, in the West, it's cost and juggling work and children. If I'd loved my job and wanted to pursue further promotion, I'd have stopped at two (or possibly even one). Instead, I have had third DC and accepted that my career is pretty much hosed. And DH had moved back into being an employee rather than contracting so we were more financially secure and could (just about, although have had a few gibbering moments) afford a third.

Cost of childcare

There was a particularly strong stream of postings about the cost of childcare. Mothers were aware that the situation in some Baltic countries made it easier for women to return to work and in these countries the birth rate was more static. The cost of quality childcare could use up the equivalent of one salary. Some parents had the choice of returning home where domestic help was readily available, but they chose to stay in England because they could work shorter hours and see more of their children.

> I think there is a relationship between how easily women think they combine career and work – e.g. in Italy, Spain, Germany there are pretty low birth rates I think, and rubbish support for working women – e.g. part-time is difficult to do etc. United Kingdom is better than those countries but worse than Scandinavia, which I think has a higher birth rate
>
> Even as a professional earning a good salary childcare eats up the equivalent of one income.
>
> Now that I live in the United Kingdom, I have two DCs and have to work full time so that we can survive. This is a so-called professional couple family with many postgraduate degrees between them.

> I imagine that if we were living in Singapore, we'd be more than fine financially (based on equivalent jobs) but would have a worse work-life balance.... But would have paid domestic help. Much of a muchness. Do I work like mad here but kinda get to go off on time to pick kids up from nursery (which costs an average person's income) rush home to get dinner on for starving kids who've not seen me the whole day, bath then bedtime? Or do I go to Singapore where I have the money to pay for domestic help to clean, cook and watch the kids but not the time to play with said children because I'm expected to work till late, travel for my work, and devote my life to work?

Intensive parenting and the new parenting theology

Extra pressure is put on mothers with aspirations for their children by the new parenting theology whereby enough is never enough.

> I think maybe we put more into it these days than we used to – I know my mum, for example, wasn't obsessed with parenting books, etc., in the way my generation are.
>
> Also, I would like to add that, as today's parents, we all want more for our children than we had as kids, in every sense, whether its material terms, education-wise and general quality of life. Perhaps more is expected of us as parents now, there is more pressure to create that ideal life for your children. I'm not sure entirely, but whenever my mum sees what we do for our DC's she always comments (a little sadly) 'we just got by with the basics, and that's just the way it was then'.
>
> (There are high) expectations and responsibilities in parenting – it is no longer acceptable to turf your brood out of the house for the whole day to entertain themselves.
>
> PS: and you have to save for braces too now. It's not enough just to put two kids through college now, you're expected to send them out into the world with American teeth!

Conclusion

Many of the responses from Mumsnetters suggest that they were, in the main, new mothers, well educated with careers, struggling with children in the early years. It is possible a group of mothers with older children may have responded differently. The mothers in this Mumsnet sample wanted the best for their children and were prepared to work hard to achieve it, but in 'getting there' the pressures were great. We have to remember that these women are relatively privileged, both as a sample but also as a group of young mothers living in a society with easy access to contraception, education, employment and considerable maternity and family benefits. They may feel that more could be done to ease the costs of childcare and the pressures of raising children generally. However, if these women's views are predictive of those in other societies who have yet to gain such opportunities, it seems unlikely that women will willingly choose to increase the size of their families. Increasingly, women all over the world will gain the benefits of their Western sisters; increasingly, they too will have choices, but their main choice is likely to limit the size of their family to one or two children.

> Education, choice, the increasing elevation of women's position in society, are all contributing to women recognizing that having a child or children disadvantages them in various ways, ranging from more serious things like income, health and job prospects through to things that may seem more trivial like figure, sex and social life. These disadvantages are usually felt to be more than made up for by the positives of having children, but those positives are in different fields – the disadvantages are still there and when you don't have children in today's materialistic, selfish society, why would an intelligent, educated woman want to deliberately disadvantage herself in comparison to younger women, childless women and men? This leads to either remaining childless, having fewer children to limit the damage and/or later childbearing, so there is less opportunity to have more kids. That sounds negative, but it's pretty much what I thought before having kids in my late 30s. I guess it's basically the 'women can't have it all' argument.

Legislation and family policies can make a difference

But the picture was not all negative. One Mumsnetter reflected that until 1992, a man could legally rape his wife in the United Kingdom, and this remains the case in many parts of the world today. Where contraception or abortion is not available, women are forced to rear a child that they may not have wanted. Legislation to protect women from spousal rape has obviously helped women.

Others Mumsnetters were aware that the wide range of benefits available to a mother in the United Kingdom did encourage her to think she could *both* retain a career and have a family.

But policies can have *negative unintended consequences,* such as that in Japan where policies were apparently intended to increase the birth rate.

> Think about it. Until 1992 it was legal for a husband to rape his wife because according to patriarchal laws rape is defined as a property crime. In other words, it only counted if a man raped a woman who did not belong to him. In the United States until recently, and in many countries, not only was spousal rape legal but abortion was illegal. So men had literally created a situation whereby women were impregnated against their wills and then forced to go through the pregnancy, and this was all enshrined by law.
>
> In countries such as the United Kingdom, where there is good maternity leave and decent childcare, and less of a glass ceiling, women tend to have more children, because they can combine work and motherhood quite well, and are therefore not forced to choose.
>
> In Japan, (where I live) the reasons are a little different. The ageing male government created policies where it was difficult for women to work and raise children simultaneously. Their policies were similar to those in Italy. The thinking behind it was that if women were forced to choose between family and career, they would choose children. This was a huge mistake. Given the choice, women choose work. Now that women can support themselves by other means, they don't get married and have children – not to the extent they did in the past. This is precisely what is happening in Japan right now.

Finally Mumsnetters gave a list of support, services and changes to the labour market which would make their lives easier and perhaps encourage them to have more children:

> (What we need is…) Decent childcare; change to the overburdening of women from domestic labour and childcare; changes to a job market that penalizes women for taking time out to have children; changes to the job market whereby it's possible to combine motherhood and decently paid work.

Notes

1. *Mumsnet shorthand*: DC = Darling Child; DH = Darling Husband; DP = Darling Partner; DS = Darling son; DD = darling daughter
2. *Mumsnet shorthand*: SAHM = Stay at Home Mother

7

Young Women's Relationships, Contraception and Unintended Pregnancy in the United States

Jennifer S. Barber, Yasamin Kusunoki, Heather H. Gatny and Jennifer Yarger

It may seem as if, with modern contraception, all children born are planned and wanted. This chapter suggests that this may not be the case. If we want to understand why women are having or not having babies, we need to examine more closely the reasons why some women, even those who have ready access to contraception, still have unplanned pregnancies.

(Ann Buchanan)

Introduction

In this chapter, we describe new research to investigate relationships, contraception and unintended pregnancies during the transition to adulthood. The Relationship Dynamics and Social Life (RDSL) study began with a 60-minute in-person interview about family background and current relationship characteristics. At the conclusion of the interview, respondents were enrolled in the journal-based portion of the study, which consisted of a 5-minute survey via web or phone and occurred weekly for 2.5 years. We begin by describing the prevalence and significance of unintended pregnancy in the United States and the

The research is supported by funding from the Eunice Kennedy Shriver National Institute of Child Health and Human Development (RO1 HD050329, R01 HD050329-S1, R24 HD041028) and from the National Institute on Drug Abuse (R21 DA024186).

limitations of past research on unintended pregnancy as background for our study. Then we describe the specific aims of our study and its design strengths. Next we provide a description of the young women in our sample, their relationships and their pregnancy intentions as of the baseline interview, as well as a summary of any changes across the weekly journals. Finally, we provide a summary of study findings that provide new insights into the contexts producing unintended pregnancies among young women. The results presented throughout the chapter are preliminary as data collection only recently ended in January 2012.

Unintended pregnancy in the United States

Although the United States experienced declines in unintended childbearing in the 1970s and early 1980s, levels have recently risen, and the most recent national estimates indicate that approximately 35 per cent of live births from 1997–2002 were unintended at the time of conception (Chandra et al. 2005). Unintended childbearing is associated with a wide range of negative health statuses for children and mothers (Brown and Eisenberg 1995). In fact, the combination of these negative health statuses and rising levels of unintended childbearing led the US Department of Health and Human Services (in its National Health Promotion and Disease Prevention Objectives) to target a substantial reduction in unintended childbearing in its objectives for 2000 (formulated in 1990), 2010 (formulated in 2000) and 2020 (formulated in 2010). According to data available from the most recent national estimates of unintended childbearing, the goal for 2000 was not met, and the goal for 2010 likely was not met either. Research that has addressed the social consequences of unintended childbearing suggests that they may be severe, may permeate multiple aspects of social life and may persist for the very long term (Axinn et al. 1998; Barber et al. 1999; Baydar 1995; Brown and Eisenberg 1995).

The causal nature of the relationship between unintended childbearing and negative health statuses is the subject of some debate (Barber and East 2009, 2011; Barber et al. 2003; Brown and Eisenberg 1995; Joyce et al. 2000, 2002; Korenman et al. 2002). Unfortunately, without random assignment of unintended births (experimental designs), it is impossible to determine causation with great certainty. Unintended births are drawn disproportionately from lower income mothers with less education. Thus, it is unclear whether the children would suffer negative outcomes regardless of whether their births are unintended. Some analyses featuring fixed-effects models suggest that perhaps these relationships are not causal, because siblings within the same family experience similar outcomes regardless of the intention status of their birth (e.g. Joyce et al. 2000). Although it is impossible to completely rule out this unobserved heterogeneity hypothesis, new evidence suggests that many of the consequences of unintended childbearing are likely to apply equally to all children in the family, not just the child born from the unintended birth (Barber and East 2009, 2011; Barber et al. 2003). Thus, a family-level effect is to be expected – rather than an effect on only the child born from the unintended pregnancy. Unfortunately, as Joyce et al. (2000) suggest, the fixed-effects model strategy may not be an appropriate approach if the consequences of unintended childbearing that produce the relationship between unintended childbearing and child development are experienced by all of the children in a family. Thus, it seems likely that at least part of this negative association is causal.

While the debate continues to swirl around the consequences of unintended pregnancy, there is no debating the harmful health and social status consequences associated with it. Yet most scholars, caught up in the escalating discussion of cause and effect, have largely ignored a key question: why are unintended pregnancies so prevalent, and what, if anything, can social scientists do to better understand their occurrence? In fact, the high rates of unintended pregnancy are a major health and public policy concern, even if they have no causal consequences, because the occurrence of pregnancies to women who do not want them is itself a negative health outcome. For this reason, the United States' Office of Population Affairs operates the country's Title X family planning clinic programme with the main aim of offering services to ensure that women do not have pregnancies they do not want (Alan Guttmacher Institute 2002; Frost 1996, 2001; Mosher 1990). A more comprehensive scientific understanding of unintended pregnancy is essential to the formulation of programmes and related policies aimed at reducing unintended pregnancy.

Mismatches between intentions and behaviour – such as an unintended pregnancy – are also of great theoretical interest. A long-standing body of theory in the social sciences argues that individuals' beliefs, attitudes and intentions are an essential determinant of their behavioural choices (Ajzen 1988; Fishbein and Ajzen 1975; Mead 1934). On the other hand, the confrontation between these intentions and the physical, social or psychological constraints that prevent individuals from realizing their intentions is an equally long-standing topic of theoretical inquiry (Alexander 1989, 1990; Alexander et al. 1987; Coleman

1994; Giddens 1984). Clearly individuals do not always choose nor are they always able to act in ways that are consistent with their intentions (Bagozzi and Warshaw 1990; Grube and Morgan 1990; Liska 1984; Schoen et al. 1999; Wright 1998). Recent theoretical advances in the study of relationships among attitudes, intentions and behaviour explicitly recognize these constraints (Ajzen 1988, 1991; Ajzen and Madden 1986; Gibbons et al. 1995, 1998). Nevertheless, empirical evidence of the micro-dynamics connecting intentions, behavioural constraints and behaviour remains illusive. Investigation of unintended pregnancy has the potential to advance these theories because pregnancy-related attitudes and intentions must confront constraints related to relationships, sexuality, contraception, contraceptive failure and activities that compete with childbearing to determine actual pregnancy outcomes (Schoen et al. 1999). Investigating the detailed micro-dynamics of the social context of unintended pregnancy will provide significant new insight into these issues.

Limitations of past research on unintended pregnancy

One of the major obstacles to scientific research on unintended pregnancy is the measurement of unintended pregnancy. Most study designs, such as that used in the National Survey of Family Growth (NSFG), feature a single cross-sectional interview with lifetime retrospective reporting. As a result, all measures of unintended childbearing are based on retrospective reporting of intention, contraception, happiness and relationship status for pregnancies that occurred sometime before the interview, often years before the interview. Each of these important dimensions is subject to somewhat different levels of retrospective reporting error, but methodological research on surveys suggests that these errors will be substantial and significant (Groves et al. 2001; Schwarz and Sudman 1994; Sudman et al. 1996). Of greatest concern is that individuals alter their feelings to become more consistent with behaviour (Festinger 1957; Williams et al. 1999), which may produce substantial underestimates of the true level of unintended childbearing. A second, closely related concern is that retrospective reporting severely limits the extent to which these studies can measure temporal dynamics in intentions and attitudes, relationship characteristics or contraceptive use. In other words, existing measures of intentions, relationships and contraception are limited to a single referent time point per pregnancy and do not measure how behavioural, attitudinal and contextual aspects of relationships and contraceptive use may change directly before or after a pregnancy.

Longitudinal studies, which interview the same young women multiple times, address some potential shortcomings of the cross-sectional measures. The National Longitudinal Study of Adolescent Health (Add Health), the National Longitudinal Survey of Youth (NLSY) and the National Survey of Families and Households (NSFH) are all important alternatives to the cross-sectional measures of unintended pregnancy. Multiple interviews with the same young women at multiple times allow measurement of intentions, contraception, happiness about pregnancy and relationship characteristics at one time point, followed by subsequent measurement of pregnancy. This design greatly reduces the risk of retrospective reporting error. Unfortunately, even in these designs, lengthy gaps between interviews greatly increase the chance of changes in the immediate context of pregnancy and retrospective reporting errors about that context. Without very frequent re-interviews, it is impossible to fully capture the temporal dynamics in intentions, contraception, happiness towards pregnancy and relationship characteristics. The costs of face-to-face interviews prohibit frequent re-interviewing – an alternative strategy is a high scientific priority.

An innovative new approach to studying unintended pregnancy

To address the critical limitations in the existing measures of unintended pregnancy, the RDSL study intensively measured these key processes. Specifically, we collected weekly journal-based attitudinal and behavioural measures of pregnancy, relationships and contraceptive use, and are conducting semi-structured follow-up interviews with young women who avoid pregnancy as well as those who become pregnant. These measures reduce the retrospective reporting period to one week and capture the dynamics in attitudinal and behavioural aspects of relationships and contraceptive use during the early adult years, when both the instability and the risk of unintended pregnancy are at their peak. We believe that a weekly measurement strategy balances the need for a routine with the costs of minimizing measurement error while not being overly burdensome to respondents.

Our overarching question for this project asks how prevalent unintended pregnancy is during the transition to adulthood, and why. To advance our understanding of the processes leading to unintended pregnancy during the transition to adulthood, this project has four specific aims: (1) collect new detailed, dynamic measures of unintended pregnancy; (2) collect new detailed, dynamic measures of behavioural, attitudinal and community-context aspects of relationships (including sexual behaviour), contraceptive use, pregnancy and activities that compete with childbearing; (3) provide alternative estimates of the prevalence of unintended pregnancy based on new, prospective measurement strategies and directly compare these new prevalence estimates to those based on national studies; and (4) determine which attitudinal, behavioural and contextual aspects of relationships, contraceptive use and activities that compete with childbearing increase unintended pregnancy rates during the transition to adulthood.

Study design

Our study uses a population-based sample of 1003 young women, ages 18–19, residing in a Michigan county. A 60-minute face-to-face baseline survey interview was conducted between March 2008 and July 2009 to assess important aspects of family background; demographic information; key attitudes, values and beliefs; current and past friendship and romantic relationships; education; and career trajectories. At the conclusion of this baseline interview, all respondents were invited to participate in a weekly journal-based study – a mixed mode (Internet and phone) survey for 2.5 years. Each week respondents chose to complete the journal either by logging into the study's secure website or by calling a toll-free number and completing the journal with a live interviewer.

Respondents were paid $1 per weekly journal with $5 bonuses for on-time completion of five weekly journals in a row. Automated reminder email and/or text messages were sent to respondents weekly. If a respondent was late, study staff first attempted to contact her by phone and later by email and letter in attempt to regain her participation. Respondents who became 60 or more days late were offered an increased incentive for completing the next journal. Small gifts (e.g. pen, chap stick, compact, pencil) were also given to respondents to award continued participation.

Our incentive scheme, coupled with the cooperative nature of this age group and their interest in the subject matter, resulted in extremely high cooperation rates: an 83 per cent response rate and a 94 per cent cooperation rate for the baseline interviews. Over 99 per cent of respondents who completed a baseline interview enrolled in the weekly journal portion of the study (N = 992). Journal response rates are high. At the conclusion of the study, 84 per cent of baseline survey respondents had participated in the journal study for at least 6 months, 79 per cent for at least 12 months, and 75 per cent for at least 18 months. In total, respondents completed 58,594 weekly journals.

Characteristics of the young women in our study

Table 7.1 presents the percentage distribution of the socio-demographic characteristics among the 992 respondents enrolled in the journal portion of the study as of the baseline interview. Age is coded in years (mean = 18.7). Race is coded as white (64 per cent), African American (34 per cent), Native American (2 per cent) and Asian or Pacific Islander (1 per cent). Ethnicity is a dichotomous variable, coded 1 if the respondent is Latina (8 per cent) and 0 otherwise. Education is operationalized as the highest grade completed with those who completed 12th grade or less coded 1 (63 per cent) and those who completed more than 12th grade coded 0. School enrolment is created using information about the type of school in which the respondent is currently enrolled and highest grade completed and includes the following categories: (1) not enrolled and did not graduate high school (8 per cent), (2) not enrolled and did graduate high school (22 per cent), (3) high school (13 per cent), (4) two year college/vocational/technical/other (29 per cent) and (5) four year college (27 per cent). Employment status is a dichotomous measure, coded 1 if the respondent was employed at the time of the baseline interview (50 per cent) and 0 otherwise. A respondent is coded as receiving public assistance (27 per cent) if she identified receiving at least one of the following: (1) Special Supplemental Nutrition Program for Women, Infants and Children, (2) Family Independence Program (FIP), (3) cash welfare or (4) food stamps. Respondents were also asked whether they had enough money at the end of the month. Response categories include: (1) some money left over (48 per cent), (2) just enough money to make ends meet (34 per cent) and (3) not enough money to make ends meet (19 per cent). A dichotomous measure indicates whether the respondent was currently living with a parent or grandparent (69 per cent). Family structure is based on information about who the respondent lived with while growing up and includes the following four categories: (1) both biological parents (46 per cent), (2) biological parent and step-parent (6 per cent), (3) single biological parent only (40 per cent) and (4) other situations (8 per cent). Parental income is measured as a categorical variable: (1) $14,999 or less (14 per cent), (2) $15,000–44,999 (28 per cent), (3) $45,999–74,999 (19 per cent), (4) $75,000 or more (18 per cent) and (5) don't know/refused (20 per cent).

Table 7.1 Characteristics of respondents at baseline interview, RDSL, 2008–12

	Percentage or mean
Age	18.7
Race	
White	63.5
African American	33.6
Native American	2.1
Asian	0.8
Ethnicity	
Non-Latina	91.9
Latina	8.1
Highest grade completed	
12th grade or less	62.9
More than 12th grade	37.1
School enrolment and type	
Not enrolled and did not graduate	8.4
Not enrolled and did graduate	22.3
High school	13.3
Two year college/vocational/technical/other	28.7
Four year college	27.3
Employment status	
Not employed	49.8
Employed	50.2
Receiving public assistance	
No	73.2
Yes	26.8
Enough money at end of month	
Some money left over	47.8
Just enough money to make ends meet	33.7
Not enough money to make ends meet	18.5
Living with parents/grandparents	
No	30.6
Yes	69.4
Family structure	
Two biological parents	46.1
One biological parent/one step parent	6.1
One biological parent only	39.6
Other	8.2
Parent's income	
$14,999 or less	14.4
$15,000–44,999	28.0
$45,000–74,999	19.3
$75,000 or greater	18.0
Don't know/refused	20.3
N	992

Descriptive findings on young women's experiences with sex, contraception, relationships, pregnancy and pregnancy intentions

Next we describe the sample of young women, including their sex, contraception and pregnancy experiences, their relationships and their pregnancy intentions. The tables describe the 992 respondents enrolled in the study, as well as a summary of changes reported in the weekly journals by the 953 respondents who completed more than one weekly journal. Recall that all results are preliminary as data collection only recently ended in January 2012.

Table 7.2 presents the sex, contraception and pregnancy experiences of respondents as of the baseline interview. Over 76 per cent have ever had sex. The average age at first sexual intercourse was about 15 years. The median number of lifetime partners among those who had ever had sex was three. Almost two-thirds of the sexually experienced respondents reported ever having had sex without using birth control.

Table 7.2 Sex, contraception and pregnancy experiences of respondents at baseline interview, RDSL, 2008–12

	Percentage or mean (median)
Ever had sex	
No	23.1
Yes	76.9
Age at first sex[a]	15.66 (16)
Lifetime number of sexual partners[a]	4.42 (3)
Ever had sex without birth control[a]	
No	36.7
Yes	63.3
Number of prior pregnancies	
Zero	77.2
One	14.6
Two or more	8.2
Currently pregnant	
No	94.5
Yes	5.5
Probably pregnant	
No	98.6
Yes	1.4
N	992

[a]Among sexually experienced respondents ($N = 763$).

We operationalize a pregnancy as a report of a positive pregnancy test or a respondent reporting that she is 'probably pregnant'. Almost one-quarter of respondents reported at least one previous pregnancy. About 5 per cent were pregnant at the time of the baseline interview and about 1 per cent were probably pregnant.

Table 7.3 presents select characteristics of respondents' current relationship as of the baseline interview (over 73 per cent of the 992 respondents reported being in a relationship at the baseline interview). Approximately 2 per cent of respondents in a relationship were married to their partners, another 10 per cent were engaged, and about 14 per cent were living with their partners. The remaining 73 per cent were not married, engaged or cohabiting, but still reported a partner. About 20 per cent of respondents' relationships were with a partner who was the same age and over 30 per cent had a partner who was three or more years older. About 13 per cent of respondents reported that their partner was a different race than her own. Relationship length ranged from less than one month to over eight years with an average length of about 18 months. Over three-quarters of the relationships involved sexual activity, and 76 per cent had talked about birth control with their partner. About 12 per cent of respondents had at least one child with the partner. The majority of relationships were exclusive and both satisfaction with and commitment to partners was high (about 4 on a scale of 1 (not at all) to 5 (extremely)). Both the respondent and partner had equal power in the vast majority of relationships. About two-thirds of the respondents had ever fought with their partner and about 16 per cent reported that their partner had disrespected, threatened or hurt them.

One key strength of our project is a detailed, nuanced and prospective measure of pregnancy intentions. We measured future pregnancy intentions *weekly* using two questions, one about the positive desire to get pregnant and have a baby and one about the desire to *avoid* getting pregnant and having a baby. Respondents were asked, 'First, how much do you want to get pregnant during the next month? Please give me a number between 0 and 5, where 0 means you don't at all want to get pregnant and 5 means you really want to get pregnant.' They were then asked, 'And next, how much do you want to avoid getting pregnant during the next month? Please give me a number between 0 and 5, where 0 means you don't at all want to avoid getting pregnant and 5 means you really want to avoid getting pregnant.' Due to small cell sizes, 0–2 are collapsed into one category and 3–5 are collapsed into one category; the vast majority of young women answered 0 for 'want to get pregnant' and 5 for 'want to avoid getting pregnant'. Respondents were

Table 7.3 Characteristics of respondents' relationship at baseline interview, RDSL, 2008–12

	Percentage or mean (median)
Relationship type	
Married	2.3
Engaged	10.2
Cohabiting	14.2
Other relationship	73.3
Age difference between partners	
Partner 1–2 years younger	11.2
Partner same age	20.4
Partner 1–2 years older	37.6
Partner 3+ years older	30.8
Race difference between partners	
No	87.4
Yes	12.6
Length of relationship (months)	17.76 (11)
Ever had sex with partner	
No	21.5
Yes	78.5
Talked about birth control with partner	
No	24.4
Yes	75.6
Had a child with partner	
No	87.8
Yes	12.2
Spend a lot of time with partner	
No	15.6
Yes	84.4
Exclusive with partner	
No	11.5
Yes	88.5
Satisfaction with partner	4.14 (4)
Commitment to partner	4.50 (5)
Power in relationship	
Respondent	11.5
Partner	1.6
Both	86.9
Ever fight	
No	35.6
Yes	64.4
Partner ever disrespected/threatened/hurt respondent	
No	83.7
Yes	16.3
N	731

Table 7.4 General pregnancy intentions of respondents at baseline interview, RDSL, 2008–12

	No desire to avoid pregnancy	**Strong desire to avoid pregnancy**	**Total**
No desire to get pregnant	Indifferent 2.28%	Negative 95.33%	97.61%
Strong desire to get pregnant	Positive 1.41%	Ambivalent 0.98%	2.39%
Total	3.69%	96.31%	100%

Table 7.5 Partner-specific pregnancy intentions of respondents at baseline interview, RDSL, 2008–12

	No desire to avoid pregnancy	**Strong desire to avoid pregnancy**	**Total**
No desire to get pregnant	Indifferent 4.64%	Negative 88.92%	93.56%
Strong desire to get pregnant	Positive 3.74%	Ambivalent 2.70%	6.44%
Total	8.38%	91.62%	100%

first asked these questions without referencing a specific partner (general pregnancy intentions), and next in reference to the specific partner they reported that week (partner-specific pregnancy intentions).

Tables 7.4 and 7.5 present cross-tabulations of the positive and negative components of general and partner-specific pregnancy intentions. Table 7.4 shows that the majority (95 per cent) of young women reported no general desire to get pregnant and a strong desire to avoid pregnancy as of the baseline interview. About 1 per cent were positive (strong desire to get pregnant and no desire to avoid pregnancy), over 2 per cent were indifferent (no desire to get pregnant and no desire to avoid pregnancy) and less than 1 per cent were ambivalent (strong desire to get pregnant and strong desire to avoid pregnancy). Table 7.5 reveals similar overall patterns for partner-specific pregnancy; however, respondents are more positive about pregnancy when referring to a specific partner. This is largely because respondents who have a partner are more positive and less negative about pregnancy than respondents who do not report a partner. Note that the per cent of women who reported no desire to get pregnant and a strong desire to avoid pregnancy was

Table 7.6 Changes across journals among respondents who completed more than one weekly journal, RDSL, 2008–12

	Percentage
Any new partner	
No	36.0
Yes	64.0
Ever got back together with a partner after a break	
No	56.6
Yes	43.4
Ever forgot to use birth control	
No	75.5
Yes	24.5
Any change in pregnancy status	
No	69.8
Yes	30.2
Any reports of a pregnancy	
No	73.7
Yes	26.3
Any live birth	
No	83.4
Yes	16.6
Partner ever disrespected/threatened/hurt respondent	
No	54.6
Yes	45.4
N	953

lower when asked about pregnancy with their partner and the per cents of positive, indifferent and ambivalent intentions were each higher.

Respondents were repeatedly asked several of the same questions across the weekly journals in order to capture change. Table 7.6 presents preliminary descriptive results for respondent-level summary measures of some of the changes that are captured in the weekly journals for those respondents who completed more than one weekly journal (about 96 per cent of the 992 respondents). About 64 per cent of respondents had at least one new partner. The majority of these new relationships were changes in partners between weeks versus going from not having a partner in one week to having a partner in the next week (results not shown). Over 40 per cent of respondents got back together with a partner after a break in the relationship. Almost 25 per cent of respondents forgot to use birth control during the study as a reason for non-use in a previous week ('forgot' was one of the choices provided). About 30 per cent of respondents experienced at least one change in pregnancy status among the categories of not pregnant, probably pregnant and positive pregnancy test (e.g. not pregnant to probably pregnant). Among those who experienced such changes, the number of changes ranged from 1 to 17 with an average of 2.8 changes per respondent (results not shown). About 26 per cent of respondents reported a pregnancy and about 16 per cent of respondents had a baby during the study. About 45 per cent of respondents reported that their partner had ever disrespected, threatened or hurt them during the study period.

Multivariate findings on contexts producing unintended pregnancies

The study also examines which attitudinal, behavioural and contextual aspects of relationships, contraceptive use and other activities increase unintended pregnancy rates during the transition to adulthood. While it is not possible to describe all of our results in this area, here we highlight some key preliminary findings.

Relationship seriousness and instability

The formation, dissolution and character of heterosexual romantic relationships are key determinants of unintended childbearing that are understudied (Brown et al. 1999). Our data allow us to examine the types of relationships – particularly the dynamics of those relationships – that produce pregnancies among young women. First, we examine multiple relationship domains, both individually and in tandem. Specifically, we focus on multiple indicators of the seriousness of the relationship and also indicators of volatility in the relationship. Second, we examine these characteristics at multiple dynamic levels – the individual's current relationship, the history of that relationship and the individual's overall relationship history with all partners. Third, we use our fully dynamic, weekly measures of women's experiences to directly examine instability in their relationships.

The analyses suggest that both seriousness and instability are important. Time-intensive and exclusive relationships are particularly likely to produce pregnancies. Further, this effect does not appear to be due to the types of young women who enter these relationships – current involvement in a time-intensive or exclusive relationship increases pregnancy risk *net of* prior experiences with these types of relationships. These serious relationships appear to mainly increase pregnancy risk via increased sexual activity and less so via contraceptive behaviour. Finally, changes and instability in living arrangements are associated with increased risk of pregnancy, as well. Neither living with a partner in a particular week nor a history of living with a partner is strongly related to the risk of pregnancy. However, young women who move in with and away from their partners more frequently have a higher pregnancy risk than young women who *either* remain living with or apart from their partner continuously.

In addition, young women's relationship experiences affect their contraceptive behaviours. We investigate the effects of time-varying measures that capture the seriousness and instability of relationship experiences on imperfect contraceptive use, and we explore reported *reasons* for imperfect use among the imperfect users. The results suggest that both the seriousness (e.g. cohabitation, spending a lot of time together, exclusivity) and instability (e.g. concurrency, conflict and partner transitions, such as getting back together with a previous partner) of young women's relationship experiences increase the risk of imperfect contraceptive use. In addition, different relationship experiences are associated with different reported reasons for imperfect use. For instance, partner transitions, such as getting back together with a previous partner, are associated with a greater likelihood of reporting 'no method available', being engaged or cohabiting is associated with a greater likelihood of reporting 'not trying to avoid pregnancy', and conflict is associated with a greater likelihood of reporting 'partner did not want to use a method'.

Relationship conflict

We also investigate the role of relationship conflict in pregnancy. Experiences with conflict within a relationship have been shown to compromise the use of contraceptive methods (DiClemente et al. 2001; Wingood et al. 2001), so it is likely that conflict also increases the risk of pregnancy. First, we examine current conflict within a specific relationship at the approximate time the pregnancy occurred. Being in a relationship that includes arguing and fighting and/or unequal decision making is associated with early pregnancy net of socio-economic characteristics and prior experiences related to pregnancy that are highly predictive of pregnancy. Second, we examine history of conflict with the current partner. A history of arguing and fighting, swearing, threats/violence and unequal decision making with the current partner is associated with early pregnancy. Third, we examine young women's history of conflict with *any* partner. A history of arguing and fighting, swearing, threats/violence and unequal decision making with any partner is also associated with early pregnancy. We also confirm that the association between conflict and pregnancy is net of a three or more year age difference between the partners. These results suggest that the tendency to enter conflictual relationships, conflictual relationships themselves and current experiences with conflict are all associated with increased risk of early pregnancy.

Pregnancy scares

Our study also examines pregnancy scares as a possible predictor of unintended pregnancy. A pregnancy scare is when a woman who wants to avoid pregnancy believes she is pregnant, but later learns that she was not really pregnant. We find that a relatively large number of young women report pregnancy scares during the transition to adulthood, and that these pregnancy scares often precede the report of a confirmed pregnancy. However, there is little existing research on pregnancy scares, even though they are likely to be important to our understanding of unintended pregnancy among young women. Our preliminary results indicate that pregnancy scares are a strong predictor of unintended pregnancy, independent of socio-demographic characteristics and early pregnancy-related experiences. Nearly one-quarter of young women in our study who experienced an unintended pregnancy *first* experienced a pregnancy scare. This suggests that the experience of a pregnancy scare can be used to better define the population to which unintended pregnancy intervention efforts should be targeted.

Attitudes

Attitudes are another crucial aspect of the context of pregnancy. In our study, we assess the relationship between a very wide array of attitudinal measures and early pregnancy. We find that a range of attitudinal measures are related to pregnancy rates among young women. Particularly strong and consistent predictors include perceptions of friends' and parents' approval of pregnancy and related behaviours; positive perceptions of others who become pregnant and engage in related behaviours; desires, willingness and expectations to become pregnant and engage in related behaviours; general attitudes towards pregnancy and related behaviours, particularly feelings that the respondent is not ready for sex, birth control is a hassle, and pregnancy has negative consequences; positive attitudes towards caring for children; and the respondent's perception that she may be unable to become pregnant.

We also explore the proximate determinants that explain the relationship between attitudes and pregnancy. Overall, attitudinal measures that are related to sexual behaviour are explained by actual sexual behaviour, measures that are related to contraceptive use are explained by contraceptive behaviour, and attitudes that are not limited to sex or contraception tend to be explained by both behaviours. In general, we find support for two broad types of attitude-behaviour models described in the literature: rational models that posit a direct link between wanting to become pregnant (and have a baby) and actually becoming pregnant, and models that posit an irrational component to behaviour.

School enrolment

Finally, it is also important to consider the relationship between activities that compete with childbearing during the transition to adulthood, such as school enrolment, and unintended pregnancy. Past research has established a negative relationship between level of educational attainment and unintended pregnancy. Although educational attainment and enrolment are known to exert unique effects on family formation behaviour, relatively few studies have examined the influence of enrolment on the risk of unintended pregnancy. Our analyses indicate that the risk of unintended pregnancy is significantly lower among women enrolled in school than among those not enrolled. In addition, we examine factors that may mediate the relationship between school enrolment and pregnancy, including perceived norms, expectations, attitudes towards contraception, relationship characteristics and sex and contraception. Our results suggest that perceived norms surrounding college attendance and early parenthood help mediate the effects of enrolment on unintended pregnancy. However, the primary reason why women enrolled in school have a lower risk of unintended pregnancy than those not enrolled is because they use contraception more consistently.

Conclusion

This chapter presents the background and motivation for our study as well as a detailed description of the study design. We also provide a first look at the characteristics of the young women enrolled in our study and factors that increase their risk of pregnancy. The results presented here are preliminary and are just a preview of the rich information we are collecting. These young women represent a diverse set of circumstances and life experiences. Our findings indicate that attitudinal, behavioural and contextual aspects of relationships, contraceptive use and activities that compete with childbearing increase the risk of pregnancy during the transition to adulthood. Furthermore, a unique feature of our study is the ability to capture these dynamic experiences over time. The preliminary results presented in this chapter indicate that these young women experience many important life events and changes from week to week, which may have implications for unintended pregnancy. For example, we have found that moving in and out of cohabitations increases the risk of pregnancy above and beyond the dramatic increase associated with current cohabitation. In other words, the *instability* itself increases pregnancy risk. We have also found that a *history* of serious relationships, particularly at a young age, is associated with higher risk of early pregnancy – net of whether the young woman is *currently* in a serious relationship. And, the initial period after getting back together with a prior partner also seems to be a particularly fertile situation for an unintended pregnancy. These insights will inform future research on unintended pregnancy and may help inform the policies and programmes 'on the ground' which intervene to reduce the risk of unintended pregnancy.

References

Ajzen, I. (1988) *Attitudes, Personality, and Behavior* (Chicago: Dorsey).

Ajzen, I. (1991) 'The Theory of Planned Behavior', *Organizational Behavior and Human Decision Processes*, 50: 179–211.

Ajzen, I. and Madden, T. J. (1986) 'Prediction of Goal-Directed Behavior: Attitudes, Intentions, and Perceived Behavioral Control', *Journal of Experimental Social Psychology*, 22: 453–74.

Alan Guttmacher Institute (2002) *Family Planning Annual Report: 2001 Summary*. Submitted to the Office of Population Affairs, U.S. Department of Health and Human Services.

Alexander, J. C. (1989) *Structure and Meaning: Relinking Classical Sociology* (New York: Columbia University Press).

Alexander, J. C. (1990) *Action and Its Environments: Toward a New Synthesis* (New York: Columbia University Press).

Alexander, J. C., Smelser, N. J. and Munch, R. (eds) (1987) *The Micro-Macro Link* (Berkeley, CA: University of California Press).

Axinn, W. G., Barber, J. S. and Thornton, A. (1998) 'The Long-term Impact of Parents' Childbearing Decisions on Children's Self-Esteem', *Demography*, 35(4): 435–43.

Bagozzi, R. P. and Warshaw, P. R. (1990) 'Trying to Consume', *Journal of Consumer Research*, 17: 127–40.

Barber, J. S., Axinn, W. G. and Thornton, A. (1999) 'Unwanted Childbearing, Health and Mother–Child Relationships', *Journal of Health and Social Behavior*, 40(3): 231–57.

Barber, J. S., Cooksey, E., Young-DeMarco, L. and Hurst, D. (2003) 'Unintended Childbearing and Children's Cognitive Ability and Achievement'. Paper presented at the annual meetings of the Population Association of America, April 30–May 4, Minneapolis, MN.

Barber, J. S. and East, P. (2009) 'Home and Parenting Resources Available to Siblings Depending on Their Birth Intention Status', *Child Development*, 80(3): 921–39.

Barber, J. S. and East, P. (2011) 'Children's Experiences after the Unintended Birth of a Sibling', *Demography*, 48(1): 101–25.

Baydar, N. (1995) 'Consequences for Children of Their Birth Planning Status', *Family Planning Perspectives*, 27: 228–34, 245.

Brown, S. S. and Eisenberg, L. (1995) 'Demography of Unintended Pregnancy', in Sarah S. Brown and Leon Eisenberg (eds) *The Best Intentions: Unintended Pregnancy and the Well-Being of Children and Families* (Washington, DC: National Academy Press), pp. 21–49.

Brown, B. B., Feiring, C. and Furman, W. (1999) 'Missing the Love Boat: Why Researchers Have Shied Away from Adolescent Romance', in W. Furman, B. B. Brown and C. Feiring (eds) *The Development of Romantic Relationships in Adolescence* (New York: Cambridge University Press), pp. 1–16.

Chandra, A., Martinez, G. M., Mosher, W. D., Abma, J. C. and Jones, J. (2005) 'Fertility, Family Planning, and Reproductive Health of U.S. Women: Data from the 2002 National Survey of Family Growth', National Center for Health Statistics, *Vital Health Stat*, 23(25): 1–160.

Coleman, J. S. (1994) *Foundations of Social Theory* (Cambridge, MA: Belknap Press of Harvard University Press).

DiClemente, R. J., Wingood, G. M., Crosby, R. A., Sionean, C., Brown, L., Rothbaum B., et al. (2001). 'A Prospective Study of Psychological Distress and Sexual Risk Behavior among Black Adolescent Females', *Pediatrics*, 108: e85.

Festinger, L. (1957) *A Theory of Cognitive Dissonance* (Evanston, IL: Row-Peterson).

Fishbein, M. and Ajzen, I. (1975) *Belief, Attitude, Intention, and Behavior: An Introduction to Theory and Research* (Reading, MA: Addison-Wesley).

Frost, J. J. (1996) 'Family Planning Clinic Services in the United States, 1994', *Family Planning Perspectives*, 28(1): 92–100.

Frost, J. J. (2001) 'Public or Private Providers? U.S. Women's Use of Reproductive Health Services', *Family Planning Perspectives*, 33(1): 4–12.

Gibbons, F. X., Gerrard, M., Blanton, H. and Russell, D. W. (1998) 'Reasoned Action and Social Reaction: Willingness and Intention as Independent Predictors of Health Risk', *Journal of Personality and Social Psychology*, 74(5): 1164–80.

Gibbons, F. X., Gerrard, M. and Boney-McCoy, S. (1995) 'Prototype Perception Predicts (lack of) Pregnancy Prevention', *Personality and Social Psychology Bulletin*, 21: 85–93.

Giddens, A. (1984) *The Constitution of Society* (Los Angeles: University of California Press).

Groves, R. M., Biemer, P. P., Lyberg, L. E., Massey, J. T., Nicholls, W. L. and Waksberg, J. (eds) (2001) *Telephone Survey Methodology* (New York: John Wiley & Sons).

Grube, J. W. and Morgan, M. (1990) 'Attitude-Social Support Interactions: Contingent Consistency Effects in the Prediction of Adolescent Smoking, Drinking, and Drug Use', *Social Psychology Quarterly*, 53(4): 329–39.

Joyce, T., Kaestner, R. and Korenman, S. (2000) 'The Effect of Pregnancy Intention on Child Development', *Demography*, 37(1): 83–94.

Joyce, T., Kaestner, R. and Korenman, S. (2002) 'On the Validity of Retrospective Assessments of Pregnancy Intention', *Demography*, 39(1): 199–213.

Korenman, S., Kaestner, R. and Joyce, T. (2002) 'Consequences for Infants of Parental Disagreement in Pregnancy Intention', *Perspectives on Sexual and Reproductive Health*, 34: 198–205.

Liska, A. E. (1984) 'A Critical Examination of the Causal Structure of the Fishbein/Ajzen Attitude-Behavior Model', *Social Psychology Quarterly*, 47(1): 61–74.

Mead, G. H. (1934) *Mind, Self and Society: From the Standpoint of a Social Behaviorist* (Chicago: University of Chicago Press).

Mosher, W. D. (1990) 'Use of Family Planning Services in the United States: 1982 and 1988', in *Advance Data from Vital and Health Statistics*, no. 184 (Hyattsville, MD: National Center for Health Statistics).

Schoen, R., Astone, N. M., Kim, Y. J., Nathanson, C. A. and Fields, J. M. (1999) 'Do Fertility Intentions Affect Fertility Behavior?', *Journal of Marriage and the Family*, 61(3): 790–9.

Schwarz, N. and Sudman, S. (eds) (1994). *Autobiographical Memory and the Validity of Retrospective Reports* (New York: Springer Verlag).

Sudman, S., Bradburn, N. M. and Schwarz, N. (1996) *Thinking about Answers: The Application of Cognitive Processes to Survey Methodology* (San Francisco, CA: Jossey-Bass).

United States Department of Health and Human Services (1990) *Healthy People 2000 Objectives* (Washington, DC: United States Department of Health and Human Services).

United States Department of Health and Human Services (2000) *Healthy People 2010 Objectives* (Washington, DC: United States Department of Health and Human Services).

United States Department of Health and Human Services (2010) *Healthy People 2020 Objectives* (Washington, DC: United States Department of Health and Human Services).

Williams, L., Abma, J. and Piccinino, L. J. (1999) 'The Correspondence between Intention to Avoid Childbearing and Subsequent Fertility: A Prospective Analysis', *Family Planning Perspectives*, 31(5): 220–7.

Wingood, G. M., DiClemente, R. J., McCree, D. H., Harrington, K. and Davies, S. L. (2001) 'Dating Violence and the Sexual Health of Black Adolescent Females', *Pediatrics*, 107(5): e72.

Wright, B. R. E. (1998) 'Behavioral Intentions and Opportunities among Homeless Individuals: A Reinterpretation of the Theory of Reasoned Action', *Social Psychology Quarterly*, 61: 271–86.

8

Crisis and Control: Russia's Dramatic Fertility Decline and Efforts to Increase It

Brienna Perelli-Harris and Olga Isupova

Introduction

The breakup of the Soviet Union brought about one of the most unexpected economic and social upheavals of the twenty-first century. Nearly overnight, economic and political systems were demolished, leaving a population confused and uncertain. The crisis not only led to widespread unemployment, wage stagnation and inflation, it also created a demographic crisis, with substantial migration and increases in mortality. The changes also led to shifts in family formation behaviour. Marriage declined, divorce increased and births outside of marriage increased. Most notably, fertility rates plunged. During the last decade of the twentieth century, the largest former Soviet Republic – Russia – witnessed one of the lowest fertility rates in the world.

Russia and Eastern Europe were not alone in experiencing 'lowest low' fertility (Goldstein et al. 2009; Kohler et al. 2002); many parts of Southern Europe and sections of East Asia also achieved Total Fertility Rates (TFRs) below 1.3. However, the Eastern European countries had a unique pattern of fertility. While the decline in most of southern, and even central Europe, was due to a rapid postponement of first births, with women delaying childbearing into their late 20s and early 30s, Eastern Europeans continued to maintain an early pattern of fertility. The mean age at first birth in Russia remained relatively young for Europe, hovering around 22 until the late 1990s when the mean age at first birth started slowly to increase. Also unusual (compared to Western countries) was the near universality of first births – nearly all women had one child. Thus, Russia's very low fertility rate was a result of the vast majority of women having one birth at a young age and then stopping.

Russia represents a striking case of how massive social and economic change can collide with long-held cultural traditions, resulting in an unforeseen pattern of demographic behaviour. The decline to extremely low fertility with a preponderance of only children would not have been predicted by most demographers. During the post-Soviet period, the demographic situation became so acute that the government reacted by instituting one of the most ambitious pro-natalist policies the world has ever seen. These pro-natalist policies proposed an outlay of 'maternity capital' that would contribute funds towards housing, education for a child or retirement pension for the mother – a payment of about 250,000 rubles ($10,000) indexed to inflation. Although many are sceptical at the extent to which these policies raised or will raise fertility, the country did witness a shift in fertility patterns and a diversification of reproductive behaviour in the early 2000s. Thus, the massive changes at the turn of the century have led to changes in demographic behaviour, although with a Russian twist.

In this chapter, we explore the reasons and mechanisms that led to the changes in demographic behaviour. We first describe the entrenched norms and values that maintained the early pattern of childbearing at the beginning of the post-Soviet period. Next we turn to the social and economic crisis of the 1990s and discuss how a myriad of economic, psychological and ideational factors may have contributed to the decline in second and higher-order births. We then describe the government's reaction to the decline in fertility and the policies implemented to address the demographic crisis. Using survey and qualitative data, we demonstrate how the public responded to these policies and how the policies impacted fertility behaviour. Finally, we conclude with the most recent data on Russia, data which suggests a diversification in family forms. This leads us to speculate about Russia's future fertility. Two decades after the dissolution of the Soviet Union, Russia is still struggling with low fertility: will couples start to have more than one child, or are only children here to stay?

Entrenched patterns of early fertility

Russia's early age pattern of fertility dates back centuries, as in other countries east of 'Hajnal's line', which runs from Trieste to St Petersburg (Coale 1992). Historical patterns of household formation, which include multi-generational households and young brides, have resulted in entrenched norms about the ideal age of first birth. These norms of early childbearing have been pervasive throughout society and slow to change. For example, the mean age at first birth hovered around 22 or 23 throughout the 1980s and early 1990s, and only in 1998 did it rise above age 23 (Zakharov et al. 2010). The greatest per cent of all births continued to occur between ages 20 and 24 into the late 1990s and early 2000s (Zakharov et al. 2010).

Ethnographic studies in the early 2000s revealed several factors that continued to push women to have their first child relatively early. First, due to social norms, women felt pressure from peers and parents to marry and have at least one child early rather than risk becoming an 'old maid'. Once a couple moves in together, little planning occurs, and instead becoming a parent 'just happens' (Rotkirch 2012). Second, it was not uncommon for university students to have children while at school. One young student from this ethnographic study explains how she balanced caring for a baby and studying: 'You see, my mum helps me; my friends from my group at the University write two copies of the lecture down for me. When I am at University, I always run home for a while when there is time to breastfeed. It is so good that we live so close to University.... I know that it is important to breastfeed as long as possible. But I do not want to skip a year of study' (Ashwin et al. 2010). Thus, with the help of parents, who often provide childcare or even live with their married children, it is usually not as difficult to combine student and mother roles as in Western societies (Perelli-Harris 2005).

Third, in-depth studies show that the medical establishment has also encouraged women to give birth at relatively young ages. According to one study, Russian doctors have medically and socially defined the appropriate age range of giving birth to 18–28; these doctors even recommend abortions, or at the very least C-sections, for older women (Gabriel 2005). As one doctor in Gabriel's 2005 study said, 'There is a time when it is just better, physiologically, to have a baby. After 28, everything is less flexible. Things don't stretch the way they do when you're younger. You're just older and it's much, much harder' (Gabriel 2005, p. 77). In addition, modern forms of contraception such as oral contraceptives and Intrauterine Devices (IUDs) only became widely available in Russia in the 1990s; before then, Russian women relied primarily on abortion for unwanted pregnancy. The Soviet medical community had discouraged using modern contraceptives due to the high level of hormones and concerns about side effects, and abortion was seen as 'comparatively harmless and convenient' (Popov and David 1999). Nonetheless, women were unlikely to abort unintended first pregnancies, due to fears of post-abortion sterility or complications that would result in childlessness. Thus, the lack of efficient contraceptives to avoid unwanted pregnancies combined with the reluctance to abort first pregnancies contributed to maintaining the early age at first birth.

Explanations for the decline to very low fertility

With the breakup of the Soviet Union, fertility rates in Russia plummeted to a low of 1.16 in 1999 (Zakharov 2008). The reasons for the decline in fertility, particularly the curtailment or postponement of second births, have been widely debated in the literature. One of the most prominent explanations for the decline to very low fertility was the economic crisis that jarred the country during the transition from communism to capitalism (Kohler and Kohler 2002). During this period, Russia experienced a sharp increase in unemployment and social stratification (Gerber 2002), and poverty increased (Mroz et al. 1999). Proponents of the economic explanation argue that couples curtailed second births because of economic uncertainty and the rising costs of children (Kohler and Kohler 2002). Relying on economic theories of fertility, which posit that couples weigh the costs and benefits of childbearing (Becker 1991), this perspective argues that couples delay or postpone childbearing when experiencing involuntary job loss or a substantial decline in income and resources. Therefore, childbearing may have declined during the post-communist transition, because children simply became too expensive.

Although it may seem likely that couples would restrict their childbearing due to lack of resources or financial concerns, most micro-level studies examining the relationship between economic indicators (e.g. income and employment) and fertility have found few significant effects. In a study from the 1990s, income and fear of job loss had no effect on fertility in the post-communist period, or if anything, the effect was positive (Kohler and Kohler 2002). Other studies have also failed to find a relationship between income and fertility (Kharkova and Andreev 2000; Perelli-Harris 2006). Moreover, second birth rates differed little by education or occupation; instead, all women, regardless of strata, experienced a uniform decline in second births (Billingsley 2011). Another study, however, finds that intra-generational downward mobility is negatively related to second birth rates for men and women (Billingsley 2010). This finding suggests that individuals, especially men, who transitioned from a higher to lower occupational class had lower second birth rates than their counterparts who experienced no downward transition.

Men, and to some degree women, may have restricted their childbearing behaviour if they experienced a loss in status during the post-Soviet period. Finally, other studies found that Russians, again men in particular, who participated in extra-income generating activities, such as a second job, informal work, or agricultural production were also more likely to have and want a second child (Buhler 2004; Perelli-Harris 2006). Thus overall, the studies suggest that individuals who experienced substantial declines in occupational status may indeed have lower birth rates, but those who take on additional jobs may be better able at coping and having more children.

The economic consequences of the crisis clearly had a detrimental effect on families' finances, but the larger casualty might have been on families' functioning and psychological well-being. The breakdown in social norms and responsibility that occurred during this period can be considered a state of 'anomie', after Emile Durkheim's use of the word to describe a loss of moral standards (Durkheim 1984 [1893]; Perelli-Harris 2006; Philipov 2002). The social and political changes that swept across the country led many individuals to feel a loss of control, resulting in high levels of stress and anxiety (Leon and Shkolnikov 1998). Consequences of stress and anomie can be seen in the rapid rise in morbidity and mortality (Shkolnikov et al. 1998), especially due to alcohol, accidents and suicide (Gavrilova et al. 2001). In highly educated societies like Russia, where parents are more likely to invest in their children and desire high 'quality' children, this type of environment was not likely to be conducive to bringing another child into the world. Couples may have had the means to do so, but they might not have wanted to raise a child in such turbulent times.

Nonetheless, fertility did not fall to zero during this period, and indeed a substantial proportion of the population continued to have more than one child. One study has shown that subjective well-being, or life satisfaction, was positively related to wanting and having a second child in Russia, regardless of household income or other economic measures (Perelli-Harris 2006). Although it may seem rather intuitive that happier people would be more likely to have additional children, this finding is particularly interesting given the context of anomie, stress and general hardship. The finding suggests that people who are optimistic in times of trouble are more likely to have more children.

Despite the economic crisis and general turbulence, some have argued that declining fertility may have been less a consequence of financial hardship and anomie than the 'inevitable' process of modernization or 'Westernization' that has led to radical changes in the family in Western

Europe (Lesthaeghe and Surkyn 2002; Zakharov 2008). Changes in the family, including increases in cohabitation, nonmarital childbearing, divorce and delays in marriage and fertility, are considered to be a set of behaviours often called the 'Second Demographic Transition' (SDT). Proponents of the SDT attribute changes in family behaviour to shifts in attitudes and values that stem from the process of individualization that occurs as material needs are met (Lesthaeghe 2010). As women begin to favour education and career, and the opportunity costs of childbearing increase, they begin to delay entrance into parenthood and have fewer children. Although it is unlikely that the rapid decline in fertility in Russia began with the SDT, since first births only started to be postponed well into the economic crisis, the SDT may help to explain changes occurring later in the post-Soviet period, when the economic crisis was not as acute. As Western ideas about women's independence and employment possibilities have infiltrated into the country, women may have begun postponing marriage and childbearing to pursue other educational and career opportunities.

Despite changing attitudes and values that may seem to be pushing Russia closer to the West, however, the norms about having at least one child and preferably two have remained strong. Fertility rates over the past few decades may show women having only one child, but a two-child family has remained desirable for the vast majority of Russians. The 2009 survey 'Family and Fertility' conducted by the Russian State Statistics Committee indicated that the average desired number of children was 2.28 for women and 2.38 for men, although expected number of children was only 1.72 for women and 1.90 for men (Rosstat 2010). The two-child norm dates back politically to a push for two-child families in the 1960s. 'One child is good, two are better' stated a Soviet propaganda poster from 1968 (Rotkirch 2012). Qualitative research helps to explain these norms. When asked about the ideal number of children, one respondent from a study by Rotkirch (2012) answered, 'Without a doubt, I want two children. Having just one seems somehow incomplete and it is very sad to be the only child in a family.'

It is important to note that in Russia, the spacing between first and second children has been much longer than in other countries (Gerber and Perelli-Harris 2009; Zakharov 2008). Several studies have shown that the gap between first and second births is around five to six years (Rosstat 2010). Therefore, even though the time spent with only one child has increased – leading to very low fertility rates – it is possible that many couples will begin to have second births again, once economic and social conditions stabilize. Given the expressed desire to have more than one child, the decline to very low fertility may only be a temporary phenomenon, reversed relatively quickly. On the other hand, the norm for early births, at least before age 30, is still widespread, and women who gave birth in their early 20s in the 1990s will now be reaching their mid-30s. Women still in their reproductive ages express 'health concerns' as one of the main reasons for not having or delaying a second child (Rotkirch 2012). Thus, it is unclear what will win out in the end: the ideal two-child family model or the fear of being too old to have another child.

Political alarm and policy reaction

The state has long been concerned about declining fertility and fewer births in Russia. Part of the concern during the Soviet period was due to a labour force deficit stemming from male losses during the Second World War, but the Soviet Union also wanted to increase population size to establish its role as a world superpower. As a result, the Soviet state encouraged women to work and stay in the labour force after birth. The state passed measures expanding access to day care and allowing mothers to work shorter days with more flexible hours. Then, in 1981, Soviet Russia introduced maternity leave for all women regardless of occupational sector or type of job. This was combined with other child and welfare benefits, a special tax on childless men and women, and subsidies for 'mothers of many children' that included reduced time in housing queues and privileged access to everyday supplies (Zakharov 2008). Childcare in Russia at that time was so widespread that it resulted in the ideal model of 'every woman working, every woman having at least one child' (Tiomkina et al. 2002). Russians began to rely on the state to help them balance family and work.

Studies show that Soviet policies had mixed effects on overall fertility. On the one hand, the policies of the late 1980s did appear to have had a short-term impact on fertility rates, particularly by increasing second birth rates (Zakharov 2008). However, the fall in fertility in the 1990s suggests that the former Soviet policies had a much smaller impact in the long run. Nonetheless, Russian maternity leave policies in particular do seem to have had a positive effect on fertility and promoting women's attachment to the labour force. Gerber and Perelli-Harris (2009) show that women on maternity leave had higher rates of returning to work, lower rates of quitting or losing their jobs, and higher rates of changing employers than comparable women not on maternity leave. Despite anecdotal evidence that suggests that employers discriminated against mothers, the quantitative findings from this study show that maternity leave protected women, and even more so during the early post-Soviet period. In addition, women who took maternity leave and then returned to work had higher second birth rates, suggesting that maternity leave provided a positive experience for raising young children. Of course, mothers who were predisposed to having more children may have been more likely to take maternity leave – and despite a series of sensitivity analyses, the authors cannot rule out this option altogether – but the strength of the findings suggest that maternity leave policies can in fact work (Gerber and Perelli-Harris 2009).

Although Soviet and post-Soviet family policies may have been relatively generous compared to those in many Western countries, they did not prevent the rapid decline in fertility of the 1990s, as already discussed. At the turn of the century, the extreme lows in fertility coupled with rising mortality led to a 'demographic crisis' that caught the attention of the nation and the world. The population growth rate in Russia had not only begun to slow, it reversed, resulting in a loss of as many as 700,000 people per year (Editors 2006). The shrinking population was seen as a threat to the country's national supremacy and its ability to maintain power. Thus, in May 2006, Russia's president Vladimir Putin addressed the nation to discuss the demographic crisis, or 'the most acute problem facing our nation today'. Despite the startling decline in life expectancy and pertinent issues related to immigration, the main focus of Putin's speech was on fertility and how to raise the birth rate. Putin discussed his ideas for why women were not having children – primarily economic reasons – and extolled mothers' virtues. He called for the restoration of family values and emphasized the importance of family life. He also proposed one of the most ambitious family policy agendas ever aimed at increasing fertility.

Putin promised several measures to stimulate fertility, particularly intended to induce women to have second children. The state was to increase monthly maternity benefits for women with children under 18 months. Benefits were to be paid to all women regardless of previous work experience, although working women would receive higher payments. Additional allotments were to be paid out upon pregnancy and birth. In addition, the state was to subsidize day care facilities, as well as provide payments to families to help cover the costs of childcare. Finally, and most radically, the state was to provide 'maternity capital' to women who gave birth to (or adopted) a second or higher-order child (Zakharov et al. 2010). (Note that the Russian state almost exclusively provides benefits to mothers; a father can acquire maternity capital only if the mother is dead or considered legally incompetent.) This very large lump sum – on the order of 250,000 rubles and set to rise with inflation – could only be spent on the improvement of family housing, the child's education, or the mother's future pension, although minor adjustments were made later (e.g. a small amount of the money could be used immediately after childbirth, and the uses were expanded to include buying land).

The initial reaction to Putin's policies was mixed (Rotkirch et al. 2007). Many politicians saw Putin making a concerted effort to raise fertility in Russia, but academics were sceptical that it would achieve its stated goals. Liberals critiqued the plan as not being sufficient to stimulate fertility, or if it did, it would only encourage the low-income strata of the population, while feminists pointed out that it ignored men's responsibilities for care-giving (Rotkirch et al. 2007). But the real concern was whether women had heard about Putin's policies and whether the policies would encourage them to have another child. One representative survey of women aged 16–34 conducted by Gerber and Mendelson in 2008 asked women about their knowledge and opinion of maternity capital. The per cent of women who knew about maternity capital was encouraging: 52 per cent were able to state the exact amount of the plan, an additional 12 per cent were off by about 50,000 roubles and 24 per cent had heard of the plan, but were unable to state the amount. Only about 9 per cent had never heard of the plan at all. However, only 42 per cent understood that it would be paid out when the child turned three years old. And the per cent who thought it would influence them was very discouraging: only 4 per cent thought it would have a strong influence on their decision, 20 per cent said it would somewhat influence their decision, another 16 per cent said it would have a weak influence, while 44 per cent said it would have no influence at all. For women who already had one child (the target group), the responses were very similar, although even more (54 per cent) said it would have no influence at all on their decisions (Gerber and Mendelson 2008).

The qualitative research on this issue has also revealed a negative public reaction and exposed the inadequacies of the policies (Ashwin et al. 2010). When asked about maternity capital, one respondent answered,

> O.K., maternity capital. But what does it do for me? To me, it is of no help. I have a flat. Well, I can use it for child's education.... But anyway, the money is needed much more during the first 3 years of the child's life. I need to invest so much in a child, and a pregnant

> woman, she also needs a lot of things. And, second, when she is on maternity leave, where will she get her living from? Either her husband must earn a lot, or.... Therefore, now, women never have children until they have made some career, to be honest. Otherwise, what will I live on? These pitiful 6000 rubles per month? This is just crazy.
>
> (Ashwin et al. 2010)

Besides raising fertility, one of the main goals of maternity capital was to help young families acquire housing, in effect infusing Russia's fledgling mortgage market with government subsidies (Zavisca 2012). However, it turns out that the maternity capital is usually not sufficient for purchasing a house or placing a down payment on a mortgage. For example, as a proportion of housing costs, maternity capital is insufficient to make the minimum 30 per cent down payment on a conventional mortgage (Zavisca 2012). In addition, most families who could use maternity capital for a mortgage would have been rich enough to afford the mortgage anyhow; poorer couples would not have had a high enough income to qualify for a mortgage even with maternity capital (Zavisca 2012). Therefore, the policy falls short of assisting young couples with one of the most important requirements for having a second child: sufficient space. As another respondent from the Ashwin et al. research states: 'We have a child which requires A LOT of money – and this is our mortgage. It is good that we managed to improve our housing conditions. But we have to pay for that, and the idea of a second child does not come to our mind anymore...' (Ashwin et al. 2010).

Thus, according to public opinion polls and in-depth interviews, it is not clear that putting significant resources into 'maternity capital' is the best way to stimulate fertility. First, the options for using 'maternity capital' are limited, thereby alienating the majority of women who cannot decide how best to use the funds. In fact, three years after the policy was introduced, only 11 per cent of those eligible had used maternity capital (Zakharov et al. 2011). In addition, the maternity capital may be unintentionally exacerbating social inequality: providing the benefit in the form of housing assistance is only useful for those who have high incomes or pre-existing housing wealth (Zavisca 2012). Thus, many parents and potential parents need the financial support in more flexible forms, for example, as an increased benefit in the first years of the child's life or as a monthly payment during maternity leave at levels closer to the costs of living in the region. Alternatively, the support could be directed towards investments in childcare, which has been shown to be effective in other settings (Rindfuss et al. 2010).

Finally, these latest policies do not motivate couples to have a first child. Although aimed at supporting families with housing needs, the policies are not aimed at improving the quality of children's lives, but instead increasing the quantity of children (Zavisca 2012). According to the latest statistical data and research, encouraging couples to have their first child may become an issue for the first time in Russian history.

Recent trends in childbearing behaviour

During the first years of the post-communist period, when Russia was faced with massive economic and social change, Russians tenaciously maintained historical and cultural patterns of fertility. The most recent years, however, have brought about an unravelling of these deeply entrenched patterns. Recent statistics now show signs of increasing diversification of reproductive behaviour, particularly in the age at first birth and the probability of having a first birth at all (Zakharov 2011). The probability of having a first birth in 2009 was lower than in the 1990s, indicating that women are postponing childbearing more than ever before (Zakharov 2011). In fact, the mean age at first birth for all Russian women in 2009 was 24.4, suggesting a steady increase since its low in the mid-1990s. Note that due to limited data, this figure was calculated using only half of the Russian regions and not St Petersburg or Moscow, where mean age at first birth (MAFB) is likely to be much higher. The higher MAFB suggests that social change, accompanied by shifting values, attitudes and economic pursuits, has produced a fundamental shift in childbearing behaviour. This quote from research by Ashwin et al. (2010) reflects the shifting priorities of the new generation, 'I married 10 years ago, while still studying at the University, but nothing has changed in my family since then. I mean, we have no children. Well, this is just temporary. We simply have no time, we are working, always on business trips, always doing other things.'

In addition, for the first time, childlessness appears to be increasing, and some Russian women are indicating that they want to remain 'childfree'. Although cohort fertility rates for the youngest cohorts are still not available, the predicted per cent of women remaining permanently childless is as high as 17 per cent, up from 6 to 7 per cent in the 1980s and 1990s (Zakharov 2011). Given that infertility treatments are now widely available, leaving only a small percentage of couples truly unable to have children (Zakharov et al. 2011), a large proportion of the newly childless do not have children due to the inability to find a partner, other constraints or because they simply prefer not to have children. Survey responses still suggest that desired childlessness is still extremely low – only 0.2 per cent of those surveyed in the 2009 Russian Statistical survey (mentioned above) wanted 0 children and 0.6 per cent expected to remain childless. Qualitative research, however, suggests that the 'childfree' are now gaining in numbers and no longer feel social pressure to conform to norms about childbearing. For example, participants in the Internet website *ru_childfree in Livejournal* differ from women of previous generations when they write about their reasons for not having children. As one participant writes, 'Does anyone have problem with parents, these people of Soviet times, wanting grand-children? Or, is this only my problem? They simply cannot understand that I am never, ever going to have any' (Childfree Ru 2011). Given the social pressure that created nearly universal childbearing, the ability to express such opinions – and carry them out – is remarkable.

The fertility pattern is also diversifying in terms of parity. After the introduction of Putin's pro-natalist policies, the number of births at all parities except first did increase slightly, especially second-order births. But, according to Zakharov (2011), the increase in the number of births may be partly due to age structure, since women born in response to the 1980s' policies are now reaching reproductive age. And even though there has been an increase in the number of second births, the probability of having a second child still remains lower than in the 1980s. The probability of having a third or fourth birth, on the other hand, has almost returned to 1980s levels, although the probability is very low in absolute terms. Thus, the group of women with one child, which was growing proportionally faster than any other parity in the 1990s, has now become smaller, not only because of the growing number of women with two and more children, but because of increasing childlessness. This means that the distribution of fertility is now no longer as concentrated among women with one child but has begun to spread out among women with different numbers of children.

The increase in births has resulted in a rise in the Russian TFR to 1.54 in 2009. Although women are steadily postponing first births, the increase in higher parity births is offsetting this trend. Note, however, that the major cities of Moscow and St Petersburg have not seen as much of an increase in TFR, that is, 1.41 and 1.40, respectively, most likely due to the even steeper increase in the mean age at first birth (Zakharov 2011). These cities have experienced greater economic development than other parts of Russia, thus alleviating some of the pressures of the post-Soviet economic crisis, but nonetheless, the challenge of balancing two careers in a large city may outweigh the economic advantages and lead couples to postpone parenthood until their lives are more stable. In addition, these cities have better access to contraceptive technology (Sakevich 2010), assisting women in avoiding unintended pregnancies and facilitating the postponement of parenthood. Thus, even though the number of births may be increasing throughout Russia, the rest of the country may experience an even greater postponement of childbearing in the near future, thereby keeping the TFR low for many years to come.

Conclusion

Has the experiment in maternity capital worked, or would fertility rates have increased anyhow? The immediate increase in births, especially second births, since Putin's 2006 address does suggest that the policies are working, indicating that the stimulus probably influenced short-term period fertility rates. It is questionable, however, whether the policies will impact long-term cohort fertility – similar to what happened with the policies implemented in the 1980s (Sakevich et al. 2006). However, it is still unknown whether the policies motivated couples who were anticipating having another birth or convinced couples who would otherwise not have had another birth to do so. Also, given the lack of individual-level data, it is difficult to disentangle whether the rise was a direct result of the maternity capital policy. Many other factors may have led to the increase, for example, the improvement in economic circumstances, the fulfilment of the two-child norm, or the inevitable adjustment to life instability after a crisis.

It is also important to recognize that the increase in fertility, albeit slight, has led to unintended consequences. The Russian government should have predicted that the policy would increase the number of births, but it failed to predict a shortage of municipal day care facilities. Parents must now wait in long queues for slots in publicly funded childcare centres. The shortage has been so severe that parents have organized Internet social movements to demand an increase in facilities. The situation is especially tense in the poorer cities of Russia, where salaries are low, alternative family forms of care are not always available, and mothers' salaries are necessary for a decent standard of living. As stated by the activists of the movement detivsad.ru (assessed 20 March 2011): 'Many women must stop working or opt for jobs requiring lower qualifications, because of a shortage of day care. The current situation forces many current and potential moms to choose between motherhood and professional development.'

These new developments suggest that Russian women are now faced with many of the same challenges as their Western counterparts. During the Soviet period, 'essential' gender roles were deeply entrenched, resulting in greater occupational segregation and a distinct gender division of household duties. Soviet women struggled to balance the 'double-burden' of working inside and outside the family home (Tiomkina and Zdravomyslova 2004). But the work demands were often fewer and conditions more flexible, in recognition of women's important role in the home. Today, women not only struggle to balance work and family, they are more often struggling to balance *career* and family with limited support. The demands of a privatized labour market can be harsh for women with children. Perceptions about living standards and material achievement are also requiring women to contribute significant amounts to household income and take less time out of the labour force for childbearing and rearing. Unfortunately, for the most part, men's participation in household duties has not increased sufficiently to reduce demands on women. Compared to other countries, the gender distribution of housework in Russia is still very unequal and women must continue to shoulder the majority of housework (Tiomkina and Zdravomyslova 2004).

In conclusion, the future of Russian fertility is uncertain. Despite a pervasive two child norm, the obstacles to having two children may simply be too high. Women are now facing new pressures to balance career and work, with little support from their husbands. Due to their previous experience with socialist state support, Russians tend to rely heavily on the state to help them balance work and family. At the same time, there is little trust in the government to provide that support (Zavisca 2012). Although Putin's maternity capital may seem like a constructive way to help families, in reality it is less than ideal for helping Russians deal with some of their most significant concerns: housing, income and a stable society. Thus, even as conditions in Russia improve, it is not at all clear that fertility will rise to pre-crisis levels again.

References

Ashwin, S., Goncharova, N., Ilyina, M., Isupova, O., Kozina, I., Lytkina, T., Omelcheko, E., Popova, I., Semina, M., Tartakovskaya, I., Zhidkova, E. and Yaroshenko, S. (2010) 'Gender differences in employment strategies of Russian men and women', LSE Research Committee Seed Fund (RCSF).

Becker, G. (1991) *A Treatise on the Family* (Cambridge, Mass.: Harvard University Press).

Billingsley, S. (2010) 'Downward social mobility and fertility decline in Russia', *Stockholm Research Reports in Demography*, Stockholm.

Billingsley, S. (2011) 'Economic crisis and recovery: changes in second birth rates within occupational classes and educational groups', *Demographic Research,* 24: 375–406.

Buhler, C. (2004) 'Additional work, family agriculture, and the birth of a first or a second child in Russia at the beginning of the 1990s', *Population Research and Policy Review,* 23: 259–89.

Childfree Ru. (2011) *Soobshestvo russkoyazychnyh childfree* [Online]. Available: http://ru-childfree.livejournal.com/, date accessed 20 March 2011.

Coale, A. J. (1992) 'Age of entry into marriage and the date of the initiation of voluntary birth control', *Demography,* 29: 333–41.

Durkheim, E. (1984 [1893]) *The Division of Labour in Society* (London: Palgrave Macmillan).

Editors (2006) 'Vladimir Putin on raising Russia's birth rate', *Population and Development Review,* 32: 385–9.

Gabriel, C. (2005) 'Our nation is dying – interpreting patterns of childbearing in post-Soviet Russia', in C. B. Douglass (ed.) *Barren States* (Oxford, UK: Berg Publishers): 73–92.

Gavrilova, N. S., Evdokushkina, G. N., Semyonova, V. G. and Year, G. L. A. (2001) 'Economic crises, stress, and mortality in Russia', in *The Population Association of America Annual Meeting,* 28–31 March 2001, Washington, DC.

Gerber, T. (2002) 'Structural change and post-socialist stratification: labor market transitions in contemporary Russia', *American Sociological Review,* 67: 629–59.

Gerber, T. and Perelli-Harris, B. (2009) 'Maternity leave in turbulent times: effects on labor market transitions and fertility in Russia, 1985–2000', *MPIDR Working Paper,* Rostock.

Gerber, T. P. and Mendelson, S. (2008) *Young Russian Women on Procreation, Trafficking, and Prostitution: Myths, Reality, and Policy Implications* (Moscow: Carnegie Center).

Goldstein, J. R., Sobotka, T. and Jasilioniene, A. (2009) 'The end of "lowest-low" fertility?', *Population and Development Review,* 35: 663–99.

Kharkova, T. and Andreev, E. M. (2000) 'Did the economic crisis cause the fertility decline in Russia: evidence from the 1994 microcensus', *European Journal of Population,* 16: 211–33.

Kohler, H.-P., Billari, F. C. and Ortega, J. A. (2002) 'The emergence of lowest-low fertility in Europe during the 1990s', *Population and Development Review,* 28: 641–80.

Kohler, H.-P. and Kohler, I. (2002) 'Fertility decline in Russia after 1990: the role of economic uncertainty and labor market crises', *European Journal of Population,* 18: 233–62.

Leon, D. A. and Shkolnikov, V. M. (1998) 'Social stress and the Russian mortality crisis', *Journal of the American Medical Association,* 279: 790–1.

Lesthaeghe, R. (2010) 'The unfolding story of the second demographic transition', *Population and Development Review,* 36: 211–51.

Lesthaeghe, R. and Surkyn, J. (2002) *New Forms of Household Formation in Central and Eastern Europe: Are They Related to Newly Emerging Value Orientations?* (Brussels, Belgium: Interface Demography (SOCO) Vrije Universiteit Brussel).

Mroz, T., Mancini, D. and Popkin, B. (1999) *Monitoring Economic Conditions in the Russian Federation: The Russia Longitudinal Monitoring Survey 1992–98* (Chapel Hill, North Carolina: USAID, Carolina Population Center, University of North Carolina).

Perelli-Harris, B. (2005) 'The path to lowest-low fertility in Ukraine', *Population Studies,* 59: 55–70.

Perelli-Harris, B. (2006) 'The influence of informal work and subjective well-being on childbearing in post-Soviet Russia', *Population and Development Review,* 32: 729–53.

Philipov, D. (2002) 'Fertility in times of discontinuous societal change: the case of Central and Eastern Europe', *MPIDR Working Paper* (Rostock, Germany: Max Planck Institute for Demographic Research).

Popov, A. A. and David, H. P. (1999) 'Russian Federation and USSR successor states', in H. P. David (ed.) *From Abortion to Contraception* (Westport, Conn.: Greenwood Press).

Rosstat (2010) *Kratkie itogi vyborochnogo obsledovaniya 'Semya I rozhdaemost'* [Online], http://www.gks.ru/free_doc/2010/family.htm, date accessed 15 April 2011.

Rotkirch, A. (2012) *Two Children Is in the Zone of Social Misery: Childbearing and Risk Perception among Russian Women* (Stockholm: Sodertorn).

Rotkirch, A., Temkina, A. and Zdravomyslova, E. (2007) 'Who helps the degraded housewife?', *European Journal of Women's Studies,* 14: 349–57.

Sakevich, V. (2010) 'Planirovanie semyi v Rossii', *Demoscope Weekly,* February 8–21: 409–10.

Sakevich, V., Zakharov, S. and Vyshnevsky, A. (2006) 'Modernizatsiya rozhdaemosti', in A. G. Vyshnevsky (ed.) *Demographicheskaya modernizatsia Rossii 1900–2000* (Moscow: Novoe Izdatelstvo).

Shkolnikov, V., Cornia, G., Leon, D. and Mesle, F. (1998) 'Causes of the Russian mortality crisis: evidence and interpretations', *World Development,* 26: 1995–2011.

Tiomkina, A., Rotkirch, A. and Zdravomyslova, E. (2002) 'Sovetskie Gendernie Kontrakty i Ih Transformacia v Sovremennoy Rossii' [Soviet Gender Contracts and their Transformation in Contemporary Russia], *Sociological Studies,* 11: 4–15.

Tiomkina, A. and Zdravomyslova, E. (2004) 'Gosudarstvennoe konstruirovanie gendera v sovetskom obshestve', *Issledovaniya sotsialnoi politiki,* 1: 299–322.

Zakharov, S. V. (2008) 'Russian Federation: From the first to second demographic transition', *Demographic Research,* 19: 907–72.

Zakharov, S. V. (2011) 'Rost chisla rozhdeniy v Rossii zakonchilsia?' ['The End of Birth Numbers Increase in Russia?'], *Demoscope weekly,* NN, February 7–20, NN 453–4, http://demoscope.ru/weekly/2011/0453/demoscope0453.pdf, date accessed 4 November 2012.

Zakharov, S. V., Isupova, O. and Sakevich, V. (2010) 'Rozhdaemost i vosproizvodstvo naseleniya', in A. G. Vyshnevsky (ed.) *Naselenie Rossii 2008* (Moscow: State University High School of Economics): 77–185.

Zakharov, S. V., Isupova, O. and Sakevich, V. (2011) 'Rozhdaemost i vosproizvodstvo naseleniya 2009', in A. G. Vyshnevsky (ed.) *Naselenie Rossii* (Moscow: State University High School of Economics): 84–178.

Zavisca, J. (2012) *Housing the New Russia* (New York: Cornell University Press).

9

The Choice of Having a Second Child and Its Implication for Future Family Structure in China

Zhenzhen Zheng

Introduction

The number of one-child families has been increasing since the 1970s in China. This has been due to the promotion of family planning and the more strict birth policy which has become dominant in cities and in some rural areas. One of the consequences of the birth policy is the 'four-two-one' family structure (four grandparents, two parents, one child). It has raised concerns especially where elderly care is mainly dependent on the family.

Birth policy today, in most provinces, now allows couples to have two children if both of them have been an only child. In some provinces this also includes cases where one of the partners is an only child and has a rural *hukou* (a rural residential permit).

As more and more only children enter the age of marriage and childbearing, it was anticipated that the 'four-two-one' family structure would become less common as policy-makers assumed that most only child couples would have two children instead of one.

The real situation is, however, more complicated. It has been found, both in urban and some rural parts of China, that the proportion of couples having a second child is not large. Such only-child couples, however, are still young, and they have another 20 years during which they could have another child. This increases the uncertainty about future family structure. The big question is: How many of the young couples with one child will have two children? Since most married couples do have children in China, but families with more than two children are extremely rare, the major difference is between having one child only and having two. If couples who can have two children choose to just have one, the impact will be large enough to change the mid- to long-term population projection for China, especially in areas where the proportion of only-child couples is high.

The close connection between childbearing behaviour and fertility intentions has always been an important research topic. But before the twenty-first century in China, there were limited surveys on childbearing, let alone more specific surveys on fertility intention. More recently, regional and small scale surveys in China have included simple questions such as: 'What is your ideal number of children?' and 'Do you prefer to have a daughter or a son?'. However, even without these surveys, the changes over the last two decades of twentieth century are obvious. The ideal number of children has rapidly decreased to one or two, that is to below 2.1, the replacement level. In both rural and urban areas, the majority of people say they want to have two children, and most say that they would prefer to have one son and one daughter (Feng and Zhang 2002). The question about the ideal number of children parents would like to have was asked in 1997, 2001 and in the 2006 National Population and Family Planning Survey, with very similar results (averages of around 1.7 children in each survey). When only married women were asked about their preferences in 1997 and 2001, it is estimated by the author that the rate was slightly higher, 1.77 and 1.75, respectively. However, results from such a simple question are not particularly convincing. Almost all the surveys took place after the implementation of the provincial Family Planning Regulations (mostly in 1980s), which clearly defined the upper limit on the number of children a couple could have, usually one or two (for details about the birth policy, see Gu et al. 2007). Studies show that 'having less children' is often related to more internalized perceptions of the right size of a family, rather than to external policy pressure. Nevertheless, many Chinese policy-makers were concerned that the underlying fertility desire could be much higher than what people chose to report in surveys. With more choices about their fertility behaviour, and more couples eligible to have two children, there was likely to be more variability in family size. Thus, further studies of fertility intention were important for the development of population policy.

In recent years, most fertility intention surveys have taken place in urban China. This is because in cities dominated by the 'one-child policy', there are now more and more couples who are eligible to have two children. These recent surveys among urban youth found that: (1) the childbearing desires of youths who were an only child did not differ from those who had siblings; (2) about half or more urban youth who were an only child believed that one child per family was ideal, and they often did not have any preference for the gender of the child (such as Feng 2004; Ma 2007); (3) a survey in four cities found that only-child youth actually had fewer children than the number of children they had stated they wanted (Song and Chen 2010). The results of the fertility intention surveys and the above urban studies broadly correspond to the framework outlined by Miller and Pasta (1995). Miller and Pasta (1995) distinguished between questions of desire which refer to what people want to do and of intention which asks what people plan to do. In China as a result of all these studies, we currently have a much better understanding of fertility intentions. The only child has rooted itself as a social norm. This is the family's image a couple or single young person hold in their minds when thinking about how many children they will have. However, this image will possibly be adjusted according to their life experience and changes.

We have also learnt something about young couples' childbearing plans, that is, whether to have another child and when. It is found that there are gaps between ideal and desired family size with a small but significant decrease from ideal to desired size. It is also found that there are gaps between desired family size and childbearing plans, with an equally significant decrease. Although some youth reported two children per couple is ideal, and they are entitled to have two by the current birth policy, they stated that they had decided to stop at one. Since almost all the related surveys are cross-sectional, there is still one step missing to complete the pathway. If a woman originally said she want to have the second child, will she really do so? And who are more likely to have these second children?

The Choice of having second child: evidence from Jiangsu, China

An introduction to the Jiangsu Fertility Intention and Behaviour Study (JFIBS)

JFIBS is a collaborated longitudinal research designed to study about childbearing desire, intention and behaviour. The first wave of data collection took place in early 2007 and the second in early 2010 in six selected counties along the east coast of Jiangsu Province, with two counties each representing different economic levels in this part (south, middle and north, with the northern part being the least developed among the three). The six counties differ in population dynamics and economic development. However, they have converged to current low fertility and share much more similarities than before. The objective of the Jiangsu study was to find out and to analyse the link between birth policy and real fertility, and to look for possible childbearing responses to policy change.

The Jiangsu study was proposed to address research inquiries such as: (1) fertility desire, opinions, intention and plan about childbearing among young couples, especially when there are more choices; (2) the relationships between birth policy and ideal family size, childbearing attitude and intention, and childbearing practice; and (3) the role of policy, cultural, social-economic, familial and individual factors in childbearing decision. Childbearing behaviour is the main variable to be explained, while fertility desire and childbearing intention are intermediate variables which predict the outcome, and these are also variables of research interest. Institutional, cultural, social-economic and demographic factors play different roles in community, family and individual to affect individual's fertility desire and childbearing intention.

Jiangsu is one of the provinces with the lowest fertility in China, and the provincial natural increase rate has been lower than 3‰ since 2000. Although Jiangsu is a province in the post–population transition era already, the trajectory of fertility change in Jiangsu is very similar to that of China albeit with lower rates.

The study population covers women aged 18–40 and their household members in the six counties, utilizing a two-stage cluster sampling design. In the first stage, a village in rural areas or a neighbourhood in urban areas was used as the primary sampling unit. A weighted sampling scheme was used to randomly select 49 primary sampling units. In the second stage, an attempt was made to interview every woman aged 18–40 in each of the selected units. Trained interviewers (mainly community staff) carried out face-to-face interviews using a standardized survey questionnaire. The 2007 baseline survey has a sample of 18,513 women and the follow-up has 20,827 with 76 per cent had the baseline survey, and the follow-up rate is 86 per cent.

The survey asked questions about reproductive preferences and intentions, including a question on what the respondent's ideal family size would be in the absence of the one-child policy. To some respondents, these questions are hypothetical. To others, they are real, as some of the young respondents are allowed to have two children under the current policy. The survey also included questions aimed at collecting individual, household and community data on economic changes, such as non-farming activities, migration, income and cost of children's education. In addition, we also gathered data on individual value orientations, with some questions adopted from other surveys, such as in the International Social Survey Program (ISSP) and the World Values Survey (WVS).

Fertility intention: major findings from the baseline

The baseline survey of JFIBS found that despite policy allowance and while generally believing that having two children with a balanced sex composition was the ideal family formation, the majority of the survey respondents had no plan to have two children. Among couples who were eligible under the current policy to have two children, the majority said that they have voluntarily chosen to have only one child, and they cited economic considerations as the primary reasons for this choice.

The survey found that there was a considerable gap between ideal and reality regarding having one or two children. Maternity remains highly valued. Although almost all women agreed that to have children was necessary for married couples, mainly for personal satisfaction and family happiness, at the same time, a large majority also agreed that 'one is good enough'. Overall 57 per cent reported that one child was ideal. Further breaking down the respondents into two groups by birth policy, we found that the group that were entitled to have two children had a similar ideal number of children compared to the total sample: 55 per cent of them also believed one child was ideal. The rest thought two children was ideal for a family, only 21 per cent already had two children, and most of the others had no intention of having two (Zheng et al. 2009).

In fact, less than 10 per cent of women who were eligible to have two children already had two in the 2007 survey. Of these a major proportion consisted of remarried women or women with a first child who was disabled. The majority of women not wanting the second child selected reasons such as 'one is good enough' and 'children cost too much'.

We also performed a multivariate analysis of survey data and individual in-depth interviews. They indicated that economic transformation in this part of China had brought with it an increased sense of economic uncertainty. Young Chinese couples were concerned with their own economic conditions and the opportunities and risks their next generation might face. Economic conditions and concerns over economic cost stood out as the most important forces affecting fertility intention. Personal attitudes towards marriage and childbearing showed that the traditional large family ideal was giving way to a small family norm with only one or two children.

In sum, the reasons for favouring one child only appeared to be a combination of increased standards of living and economic uncertainty, a less traditional view on marriage and childbearing and a sustained government birth control programme implemented by social mobilization, public propaganda campaign and routine surveillance – this scenario forms the broad context of China's new reproductive regime. Economic conditions and concerns over economic cost stood out as the most important forces that affected fertility intention. Personal attitudes towards marriage and childbearing showed that the traditional large family ideal was giving way to a small family norm with only one or two children.

With findings from only one cross-sectional survey, we cannot know to what extent plans will translate into behaviour. The question remained unsolved about whether the respondents would really practice what they said. It was impossible to guess without at least one follow-up visit to check. Accordingly, the research team revisited the survey site early 2010.

Linkages from intention to practice: major findings from the JFIBS follow-up

In the follow-up survey questionnaire, there are two separate questions about ideal family size and personal preferred number of children: (1) What do you consider as the ideal number of children for a general family, not considering the government's birth control policy and other constrains? (2) How many children would you like to have? The average answer was 1.65 to the first question, and 1.42 to the second. Most of respondents gave a consistent report on the two questions, 35 per cent select 'one' for both, and 41 per cent selected 'two' for both. However, inconsistency was also present. Twenty-three per cent believed that two children per family were ideal, but actually they themselves preferred to have one. The opposite was quite rare; only 0.8 per cent reported their ideal number of children as one but had chosen to have two.

In the follow-up survey, 6 per cent of married woman with one child at the time of the baseline survey gave birth to a second child. Childbearing plans were associated with childbearing behaviour during the three-year period, but gaps were also found. Forty-four per cent (46/105) of women who were sure about having another child in the 2007 survey actually did give birth to the second child during 2007–10, while some

Table 9.1 Number of children from ideal to reality, married women eligible to have two children by birth policy ($N = 5705$)

By birth policy	Ideal	Preferred	Currently have	Currently have plus plan to have
2	1.7	1.5	1.1	1.3

Source: Follow-up survey of JFIBS (2010).

others had changed their decision to not wanting another child. Meanwhile, only 2 per cent (37/1878) of women who did not plan to have another child in 2007 gave birth to the second child by 2010. This shows an associated relationship between fertility intention and behaviour. It also implies a consistency of not wanting the second child but inconsistency of wanting the second child. Further examination found that women with more decisive childbearing ideas and clearer childbearing schedules were more likely to put their plan into action.

It is reasonable to say that the ideal number of children is an upper ceiling that may never be reached in contemporary China. The personal preference is closer, if yet a little higher, than actual behaviour. The number of children women currently have plus children they plan to have is probably the closest estimation of future fertility. Thus, by linking the baseline and follow-up surveys, a connection from birth policy to behaviour can be established as seen in the table (Table 9.1). This shows a clear decreasing fertility rate of almost 0.2 at each step. At most, we expect that 30 per cent of couples will have two children in the study sites. However, to complete the pathway, a second follow-up is needed to discover the total number of children born by the end of the reproductive life of the women. Our respondents in the surveys are still young.

Factors related to having a second child

In the 2010 follow-up survey, women who already had two children were asked about the main reason for having the second child. These were: one child is lonely (52 per cent); the birth policy allows a second child (52 per cent); we want to have both a son and a daughter (31 per cent); we want to satisfy the older generation's expectation (23 per cent). Similar reasons were found among those who planned to have a second child.

In our interview with women in the field, 'one child is lonely' was a common opinion of most women, with or without siblings. The birth policy was more of a condition than a reason: only 6 per cent said 'birth policy allows' was the only reason.

Were those who desired having both a son and a daughter mainly longing to have a son? This does appear to be the case. Although no one admitted to having a preference for a son during the interview, the result of multivariate analysis shows that only childbearing intention and gender of the first child were significant predictors for having the second child. No clear pattern was found on the effect of other demographic, social and economic factors (Cai et al. 2010).

Nearly a quarter of women had a second child in order 'to satisfy older generation's expectation', and a similar proportion said that parents or parent-in-laws had some influence on childbearing decisions. This influence was often indirect, for instance, such as the old generation offering considerable support or willingness to participate in childcare. A study on intergenerational ties and fertility preferences found that preference for a grandson and a granddaughter as well as a woman's willingness to take advice from the parental generation promoted fertility desire. In addition, potential childcare provision from grandparents boosted fertility preferences (Chen et al. 2011). In-depth interview with local women found that having the second child was often a very conscious decision of the couple, especially regarding the consideration of who would take care of the baby. From field visits we found that almost all women who had had a second child in the last three years had willing grandparents to help take care of their newborn baby. Most of the young mothers we visited returned to wage work soon after maternal leave. Having a second child, therefore, might reflect grandparents' desire to have more grandchildren.

Less than 5 per cent of women said that they had a second child because of contraceptive failure (i.e. an unplanned pregnancy). Their pregnancy histories showed that most of the live births were reported as planned pregnancies, and most induced abortions were due to unintended pregnancies.

Discussion and policy implication

The research indicates that the one child family is becoming a social norm in parts of China, regardless of whether the parents are themselves only children or not. Our surveys show that people's fertility intentions do not correspond closely to birth policy, but rather is more individualized. Birth policy is not the major and only determinant of childbearing decisions. One of the implications from our findings is that if the majority of only child couples have one child only of their own, a considerable fraction of families in China will end up with a 'four-two-one' pattern. This will mean we will have a very different society to that we have today.

China has experienced more than two decades of below replacement fertility. The surveys presented here and others reflect findings similar to the rest of the world: below replacement fertility with a slightly higher fertility intention compared to fertility outcome; the gaps between ideal family size, expected family size, fertility intention and childbearing practice; the reasons for not reaching reproductive goals; fertility intention as a 'moving and missing', that is, a changeable target over time; and so on. When fertility intention is very low, probably among the lowest in the world, this is a matter of concern. Such a low fertility intention and even lower real fertility may lead to a negative increase 'trap' in the future if it continues.

References

Cai, Y., Wang, F., Zheng, Z. and Gu, B. (2010) 'Fertility intention and fertility behavior: Why stop with one?' Paper presented at *'From Intentions to Behaviour: Reproductive Decision-making in a Macro-micro Perspective'*, Vienna, Austria, 2–3 December 2010.

Chen, F., Ji, Y., Cai, Y., Zheng, Z. and Gu, B. (2011) 'Do parents matter? Intergenerational ties and fertility preference in a low fertility context', paper presented at *2011 Annual Meeting of Population Association of America*, Washington, DC.

Feng, X. (2004) 'Fertility desire of urban youth – current status and comparative analysis', *Jiangsu Social Sciences*, 4: 175–81.

Feng, X. and Zhang, Q. (2002) 'Changes of urban and rural fertility desire over the two decades', *Market and Population Research*, 5: 21–31.

Gu, B., Wang, F., Guo, Z. and Zhang, E. (2007) 'China's local and national fertility policies at the end of the twentieth century', *Population and Development Review*, 33(1): 129–47.

Ma, X. (2007) 'Would you want to have the second child? – a study on one-child family in Beijing urban areas', *Almanac of China's Population*, 278–89.

Miller, W. and Pasta, D. (1995) 'Behavioral intentions: Which ones predict fertility behavior in married couples?', *Journal of Applied Social Psychology*, 25(6): 530–55.

Song, J. and Chen, F. (2010) 'Reproductive behaviors and preferences of China's urban youths: deviation and determinants', *Chinese Journal of Population Science*, 5: 103–10.

Zheng, Z., Cai, Y., Wang, F. and Gu, B. (2009) 'Below-replacement fertility and childbearing intention in Jiangsu Province, China', *Asian Population Studies*, 5: 3, 329–47.

10
Childbearing and the Impact of HIV: The South African Experience

Lorna Benton and Marie-Louise Newell

Introduction

A demographic transition of falling birth and death rates has been widely observed across much of Europe and the Western world in parallel with economic development. Yet there is conflicting evidence surrounding the much anticipated African transition (Zaba and Gregson 1998). In response to regional economic and political development, a limited number of sub-Saharan countries have observed declining birth rates in the past 20 years. Increased urbanization, improved education, health services, higher prevalence of contraceptives and access to reproductive health care has led to a swift reduction in fertility rates in Zimbabwe, Botswana, Nigeria, Kenya and South Africa (Kalipeni 1995). This effect is most pronounced in South Africa, where fertility rates of 2.4 births per woman in 2009 were exactly half those in 1980 and are now the lowest in sub-Saharan Africa (The World Bank 2008).

Meanwhile, in 2008, sub-Saharan Total Fertility Rates (TFRs) of 5.1 births per woman were almost double the global average of 2.54, although these had declined from 6.7 in 1980 (The World Bank 2008). Improved food access, sanitation and medical care have facilitated a reduction in mortality in countries such as Niger and Mali where fertility rates remain unchanged since the 1960s and are amongst the highest globally.

In parallel with economic growth and prosperity, the greatest declines in births per woman can be observed in the northern and southern regions of Africa (Kalipeni 1995), coinciding with the spread of major HIV epidemics across the continent (Terceira et al. 2003). Table 10.1

Table 10.1 Births per woman, 1989 and 2008, and Adult HIV prevalence (%)

Country	Births per woman (1980)	Births per woman (2008)	Adult HIV prevalence (%) 2007/2008
Highest TFR in Africa (2008)			
Chad	6.8	6.2	3.5
Mali	6.7	6.5	1.5
Niger	8.1	7.1	0.8
Somalia	6.8	6.3	0.5
Uganda	7.1	6.3	5.4
Lowest TFR in Africa (2008)			
Botswana	6.2	2.9	23.9
Kenya	7.5	4.9	7.4
Nigeria	6.9	5.7	3.1
South Africa	4.8	2.5	18.1
Zimbabwe	7.1	3.4	15.3

illustrates how the decline in fertility has been greatest in countries with some of the highest burdens of HIV.

In 1989, Caldwell speculated that HIV would be the catalyst for the onset of the sub-Saharan fertility transition (Caldwell et al. 1989), although a more recent revision of this view places a greater emphasis on economic and cultural determinants (Caldwell 2000; Cohen 1998). It is assumed that the epidemic could influence population fertility rates through (a) increased mortality amongst reproductive age groups, (b) reduced fecundity of HIV-infected women and men (c) changes in reproductive behaviour to avoid pregnancy and prevent the spread of the disease. More recently, it has been suggested that with the roll-out of the HIV treatment programmes, HIV effects on fertility, if any, would be altered by the impact of effective Antiretroviral Therapy (ART), reducing morbidity and mortality as well as preventing mother-to-child transmission of infection.

In addition to the burden placed on an individual's health, the cultural impact of HIV is multifaceted. The decision to have a child is shaped by a complex variety of economic and cultural factors, and the full extent to which the HIV epidemic interacts with these factors to determine fertility patterns in South Africa is also not well understood.

In South Africa, where 5.6 million people are currently living with HIV, the effects are likely to be most pronounced. The country has had one of the lowest birth rates on the continent since the 1980s, a decline that has occurred in parallel with strong socio-economic development and the emergence of one of the highest burdens of HIV in the world (WHO 2010; The World Bank 2008). This chapter will first address the unique political, cultural and economic context in which childbearing is determined in South Africa before discussing the possible contribution of HIV to the shape of this transition.

A South African transition

Population trends and HIV

Birth rates have fallen steadily under relative socio-economic development marking an early entry to demographic transition similar to countries such as Egypt, Tunisia and Lesotho (Kalipeni 1995; Moultrie and Timaeus 2002). Young estimated that population levels in South Africa should reach 110 million by 2050, instead they have remained below 50 million for almost 50 years under slowing rates of population growth attributed to falling fertility and HIV-associated mortality (Young 2005) (Figure 10.1).

South Africa faces one of the fastest growing and heaviest burdens of HIV in the world with an adult prevalence of 17.5 per cent resulting in more than 310,000 HIV-associated deaths each year (WHO 2010). The epidemic has placed a disproportionate burden on people of reproductive age with the highest national estimates amongst women aged 25–29 years (32.7 per cent) and men aged 30–34 years (25.8 per cent) (South African Department of Health 2003). HIV-associated death amongst these age groups effectively removes a cohort of potential childbearing adults from the population and limits the proportion of the population able to bear children (Gregson et al. 2009).

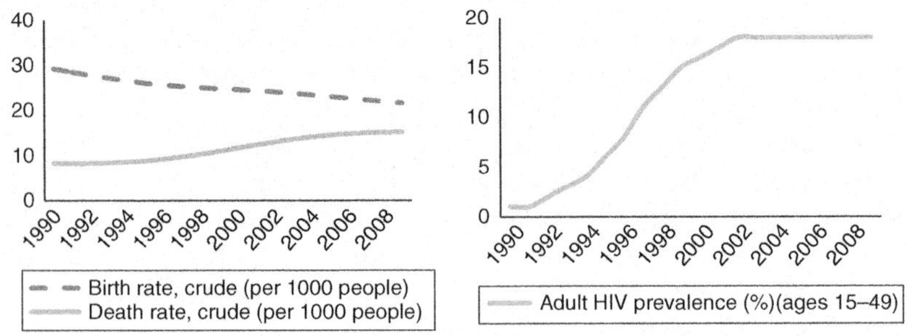

Figure 10.1 Birth and death rates and adult HIV prevalence in South Africa since 1990

Source: Data taken from World Bank (The World Bank 2008).

Improved survival of mothers and children living with HIV through access to ART could alleviate these changes to the age structure of the population that is attributable to HIV (Herbst et al. 2009; Ndirangu et al. 2010). European studies have demonstrated the efficacy of Highly Active Antiretroviral Treatment (HAART) in reducing mother-to-child transmission to rates as low as 0.1 per cent (Townsend et al. 2008). Since 2001, treatment has been made freely available for pregnant women through Prevention of Mother-to-Child Transmission (PMTCT) programmes and since 2004 for all people with advanced HIV through ART programmes. Prior to the introduction of ART, the proportion of children younger than nine years declined in relation to all other age groups in a rural area of KwaZulu-Natal (Herbst et al. 2011). Since the introduction of PMTCT and ART services to the area in 2005, reduced under-five mortality rates have brought a reversal of this trend, with these infants now accounting for the single largest age group in the area (Herbst et al. 2011).

The legacy of apartheid

South Africa has one of the largest economies in Africa but shows characteristics of both a developed and developing country, with the greatest inequalities across both racial and geographical divisions (Swartz 2009). Deep inequity was inherited from the apartheid era policies of racial segregation throughout aspects of education, health care, employment and population resettlement. The Population Registration Act of 1950 divided the country into four major ethnic groups; African, Asian, White and Coloureds and non-Whites were geographically discriminated by the Group Areas Act, which allocated 'nation states' or 'homelands' by racial grouping (South African Department of Health 2003).

Exclusion from White-only welfare, education and job reservation policies placed households into financial obscurity, forcing many African men to relocate to urbanized areas for long periods in search of employment. When partners ceased to send income or were unable to earn enough to support the household, women were increasingly forced to enter employment to support their households, leaving less time for childcare (Swartz 2009).

Discriminatory provision of contraceptive methods under the 1974 National Family Planning Programme typically restricted African women to long-term hormonal injections. Justifiably, the programme was faced with resistance but it is important to note that many African women chose to adopt the available contraceptive methods in order to take responsibility for their own childbearing in a difficult economic climate. Governmental family planning programmes provided women the means to limit the size of their household relative to income, and contraceptive injections offered women the freedom to do so without permission from their partners. The result was increased contraceptive use but a prevailing disparity in childbearing found along closely aligned racial, geographical and socio-economic margins (South African Department of Health 2003; Cooper et al. 2004).

Fertility has reached below-replacement levels amongst the White and Indian populations, with a TFR of around 1.9 since 1989 (Chimere-Dan 1994) and 1.88 in 2005, respectively (Mokomane and Khan 2009). The Coloured population refers to a grouping typically of mixed African and other European or Asian heritage that have experienced a comparatively slower decline in fertility, with a TFR of 2.27 in 2006. Fertility remains highest amongst Africans of the four ethnic groups with a TFR of 2.92 in 2006, following a steady decline from 6.6 since 1960 (Statistics South Africa, Department of Population and social development 1998).

Prevalence of the HIV epidemic is also highly disparate across racial groupings with the heaviest burden amongst Africans (Shisana et al. 2010). Furthermore, this population accounts for 79.4 per cent of the total population but a disproportionate 95 per cent of the poverty gap, placing the greatest demand for health care amongst the most impoverished (Statistics South Africa 2010).

An era of ART and reproductive health policy

Since the first democratic election on 27 April 1994, healthcare delivery has transitioned towards the provision of holistic primary health care services. South Africa now has one of the most progressive reproductive healthcare legislation in the world, integrating reproductive health as part of a universal and free point of care service under the new National Department of Health (Mokomane and Khan 2009).

The South African Population Policy introduced in 1998 aimed to address previously neglected issues of maternal mortality, gender violence, unwanted and teenage pregnancies and the growing incidence of Sexually Transmitted Infections (STI) and HIV transmission. Yet progress was confounded by an era of AIDS-denialism between 1999 until 2008, with the health minister casting doubt over the association between HIV and AIDS and the efficacy of ART.

The reality was a delayed distribution of antiretroviral drugs and the provision of HIV education and prevention services under a series of

Table 10.2 Population HIV prevalence and amongst antenatal care attendees per province

Province	HIV prevalence (%) (2008)	HIV prevalence (%) amongst ANC attendees (2010)
KwaZulu-Natal	15.8	39.5
Mpumalanga	15.4	35.1
Free State	12.6	30.6
Gauteng	11.3	30.4
North West	10.3	29.6
Eastern Cape	9.0	29.9
Limpopo	8.8	21.9
Northern Cape	5.9	18.4
Western Cape	3.8	18.5
Total	10.9	30.2

Source: Adapted from Avert (NB Small sample sizes may limit precision in HIV prevalence data).

vertical programmes, resulting in many HIV-infected people being left untreated (Schneider and Fassin 2002). Accordingly, prevalence of HIV amongst women attending Antenatal Care (ANC) clinics has risen from just 1 per cent in 1990 to 30.2 per cent in 2010 with further regional differences in prevalence, approaching 40 per cent in KwaZulu-Natal (Table 10.2).

Determinants of fertility and HIV

The relationship between HIV and fertility is complex. Sexual exposure, contraceptive practice, reproductive tract infection and breastfeeding may simultaneously determine risk of HIV transmission and pregnancy. Socio-economic and cultural factors may then have opposing effects on these determinants of TFRs and incidence of HIV. While factors that influence sexual activity and contraceptive use will affect fertility and HIV incidence in the same way, the importance of the epidemic in shaping or modifying these mechanisms is highly speculated.

Historically, contraceptive use is by far one of the most important determinants of fertility in South Africa. In this section, we will explore the relative influence of the epidemic upon marriage and contraceptive use as examples of the classical determinants of fertility (Bongaarts 1978) applied to the South African context.

Avoidance of marriage and pre-marital childbearing

Traditionally, early age of marriage has been associated with childbearing almost universally across sub-Saharan Africa (Bongaarts 1978). However, falling rates mean that that marriage has lost much of its value as a determinant of fertility in South Africa. In 2006, a mere 4 per cent of women aged 15–19 years reported ever being married in comparison to an average 23 per cent across the continent (Bureau 2006). Retrospective studies indicate this fall in marital rates started as early as the 1980s as a consequence of repressive apartheid policies of labour migration, tribal homelands and living restrictions placed on most African couples (Harwood-Lejeune 2001; Hosegood et al. 2009). Ambiguity in the definition and changes in the legal recognition of customary marriages have created inconsistency in administrative and survey data, making exact estimates difficult to compare over time (Budlender et al. 2004). In consideration of these limitations, census data from 1996 to 2001 reported lower rates of marriage amongst Africans and Coloured compared to Whites and Asians, indicating a preference for delayed marriage or living with a partner or neither amongst the African population (Gustafsson and Worku 2006).

Avoidance of marriage has been attributed to differing gendered perspectives of marital roles, with a culture of female empowerment placing higher levels of education and employment at odds with marital rates (Gustafsson and Worku 2006). It has been suggested as a survival strategy for impoverished women (Muthwa 1995), while others suggest that a desire for marriage may remain for some but is prevented under difficult circumstances (Preston-Whyte 1993). Further, the expense of *lobola* or bride price may deter young men from marriage. The role of HIV in shaping a preference for delayed marriage has been speculated but lacks much empirical evidence. Fears of acquiring HIV could influence an avoidance of sexual unions, with a more careful partner selection resulting in delayed age of marriage as reported in Uganda (Asiimwe-Okiror et al. 1997), Zimbabwe (Gregson et al. 1997) and across sub-Saharan Africa (United Nations 2002). Alternatively, HIV could encourage childbearing if women enter an earlier sexual debut in order to quickly establish a long-term relationship or for financial support (Gregson 1994).

In South Africa, the high value placed on childbearing appears to take precedence, independent of marriage (Preston-Whyte and Zondi 1992). Relative cultural acceptance of childbirth outside of marriage has facilitated a rise in extramarital fertility rates, which differed only marginally to those of married women in 1996 (Chimere-Dan 1999) and 2001 (Moultrie and Timaeus 2001). The extent of extramarital fertility is primarily attributed to the high number of adolescent pregnancies (South African Department of Health 2003). World Bank data points to a decline in adolescent fertility rates estimated at 56.3 births per 1000 women in 2009 with many young men and women entering their sexual debut aged around 18 and 19 in rural KwaZulu-Natal (McGrath et al. 2009); yet the mean age of first birth has not increased despite the steady decline in fertility (Garenne et al. 2001).

The concept of pre-marital fertility has been extended to encompass women aged 15–26 years of age in an analysis of census data from a rural province of South Africa that revealed a bimodal pattern of fertility. Two distinct 'pre-martial' and 'marital' peaks of fertility at age 18 and 30 years (Garenne et al. 2001) point to higher rates of childbearing amongst adolescents followed by a period of postponement once a woman has been exposed to family planning services during antenatal care. In response to the HIV epidemic, improved uptake of reproductive health services particularly amongst youths could minimize levels of unplanned pregnancies and contribute to a decline in extramarital fertility.

Contraceptive use

The 2003 South African Demographic Health Survey found awareness of modern methods of contraception to be almost universal. Contraceptive prevalence using these methods since the 1980s has remained amongst the highest in sub-Saharan Africa with around 60 per cent of women aged 15–19 (Population Reference Bureau 2010) (Table 10.3).

Preference for modern contraceptive methods is exceptionally high in comparison with other sub-Saharan countries, and use of these methods has steadily increased across all racial groupings, with the exception of the White population group. African women reported increased use of modern contraceptives in 2003, reaching 63 per cent in comparison to a contraceptive prevalence of around 50 per cent in 1990. However, even in light of this increase, Africans, nulliparous women and people living in rural areas were less likely to report using contraception (Burgard 2004).

Sustained use of hormonal contraceptives for the postponement of childbearing is a key factor in driving the South African fertility transition, yet the high number of women relying solely on oral, injectable or sterilization methods places them at prolonged risk of acquiring an SIT (Timæus and Moultrie 2008). The contraceptive injection

Table 10.3 Contraceptive availability, use and awareness in South Africa (%)

Contraceptive	Availability	Current Use	Knowledge
Traditional methods		0.0	38.3
Lactational amenorrhoea	N/A	0.0	11.7
Periodic abstinence	N/A	0.0	19.1
Withdrawal	N/A	0.0	27.9
Other traditional	N/A	0.0	0.3
Modern methods		65.2	96.5
Oral contraception for women	Combined Oral Contraceptive (COC) pills and Progestogen-only Contraceptive (POP) offered free of charge at clinics and hospitals. Can also be purchased from pharmacies without prescription.	12.5	81.6
Contraceptive injection for women	*Nur-Isterate* is given every two months or DMPA (*Depo Provera/Petogen*) every three months.	33.2	88.3
Intrauterine device (IUD)	A small device that is inserted into a women's uterus and can prevent pregnancy for at least five years.	0.8	48.1
Condoms	Male condoms are free of charge at clinics and some public venues. Can also be purchased cheaply at most pharmacies and shops. Female condoms are available free of charge at a few designated clinics and for sale in some pharmacies.	Male 7.9 Female 0.3	Male 82.8 Female 57.0
Sterilization	Any person 18 years or above who is capable of consenting may be sterilised. The operation is free of charge at some community health centres and hospitals at every level.	Male 0.7 Female 14.4	Male 32.8 Female 49.8
Other services			
Emergency contraception	Pills are free of charge at clinics and hospitals and can also be bought without prescription at pharmacies.	–	–
Termination of Pregnancy	Termination of Pregnancy (TOP) legal in South Africa and available as a last resort.	–	–

Note: Missing values not measured by survey.
Source: Adapted from (Western Cape Government Family Planning) Data from 2003 DHS (South African Department of Health 2003).

offers women effective and longer term protection from unwanted pregnancies and has been increasingly utilized by younger women wishing to space births in respect to the age of current children, with 33.2 per cent of sexually active women opting for this method (Du Plessis 1996; South African Department of Health 2003).

Application of contraceptives for the purpose of birth spacing reflects a conscious decision in response to economic circumstances, improved education and female employment. As a result, the average birth interval has almost doubled to a period of 60 months creating a pattern of birth spacing unlike that of other sub-Saharan countries (Camlin et al. 2004). It has recently been suggested that this behaviour is actually one of postponement, as women defer childbearing for alternative reasons until an unspecified time point that eventually becomes permanent (Timæus and Moultrie 2008).

Literature documenting a change in contraceptive behaviour in response to HIV is inconclusive but suggests a minimal impact in South Africa. A 2005 study of South African women found that HIV-positive women were more likely to be dual contraceptive users, although 40 per cent of women with HIV did not use any form of contraception (Shisana and Simbayi 2008). When used appropriately, condoms are the only effective barrier to both pregnancy and transmission of HIV and other STIs, yet only 7.9 per cent of sexually active adults report current use. In line with the continental trends, the 2003 South African Demographic Health Survey (SADHS) survey revealed an encouraging growth in male condom use, indicating a shift in preference from other non-barrier methods in response to the risk of HIV and other STIs.

HIV and population fertility

The relationship between HIV and fertility is intricate; infection with HIV can bring about changes in a woman's desire and capacity to bear children, while a greater desire for children can increase the risk of HIV transmission when accompanied by a change in reproductive behaviour. Both physiological changes in the capacity to bear children and a behavioural response to a change in the desire for children amongst infected women will determine the aggregate impact upon fertility (Gray et al. 1998; Gregson et al. 2009). The overall effect of HIV on national fertility decline will be determined by the strength of its influence at each level of the population.

HIV-infected women

Clinical and population-based surveys describe an overall negative influence of the epidemic, with a 25–40 per cent reduced fertility amongst HIV-infected women versus uninfected women from Uganda, Zimbabwe, Tanzania, Rwanda and Democratic Republic of Congo (Allen et al. 1993; Ryder et al. 1991; Zaba and Gregson 1998; Zaba et al. 2003). This trend was reported for women of all age groups except 15–19-year olds and could be stronger amongst older women experiencing reduced fertility at later clinical stages (Ryder et al. 1991). Meanwhile, data from multiple sub-Saharan countries point to lower odds of pregnancy amongst HIV-infected women in the range of 0.74–0.84 (Carpenter et al. 1997; Glynn et al. 2001; Hunter et al. 2003) and even as low as 0.45 (Gray et al. 1998) before ART was made widely available, with less than half of this change attributable to physiological factors in one analysis (Young 2005). In light of improved access to treatment services, it is uncertain whether we will see fertility rates approach those of uninfected women.

Physiological changes

HIV-positive women may reduce their coital frequency or experience a diminished capability to carry a child to full term as the disease progresses (Gray et al. 1998). Advanced progression of the disease has been linked to increase risk of adverse birth outcomes such as miscarriage, spontaneous abortion, stillbirths and amenorrhoea (the absence of a menstrual period) (Gray et al. 1998), while production of sperm was also found to be lower in studies of HIV-positive men at both advanced HIV stages (Gray et al. 1998) and prior to AIDS progression (Martin et al. 1992).

A significant mechanism of sub-fertility amongst HIV-infected women is an increased risk of co-infection with STIs such as syphilis, Chlamydia or gonorrhoea (Bracher and Santow 2001). Co-infection can dramatically increase risk of pelvic inflammatory disease (Cates et al. 1988) leaving women unable to bear children after two episodes in 20 per cent of cases (Bracher and Santow 2001). However, one of the studies from Uganda found that current STI infection was not associated with pregnancy, while the effects of prior infection were not analysed (Gray et al. 1998). In the context of a HIV epidemic, STI prevalence could lead to reduced fecundity, while improvements in STI services may reduce this impact (Gregson et al. 2009).

Considering the absolute number of women at later stages of infection, physiological effects are unlikely to be a major determinant of fertility decline at the population level. It is more likely that changes in childbearing desire and reproductive behaviour in response to the HIV epidemic at the population level will influence aggregate fertility (Gregson et al. 2009; Young 2005).

HIV and the desire for children

For people living with HIV, concerns over future health, risk of transmission to future children and the welfare of existing children can deter a woman from fulfilling her reproductive potential (Rutenberg et al. 2000). This may be compounded by stigmatized views held by the community, discouraging fertility amongst HIV-infected women (Gregson et al. 2004; Rutenberg et al. 2000), and in South Africa, perceived negative attitudes of health workers have also been cited as deterring women from future childbearing (Cooper et al. 2007). Yet for many women, strong desires for parenthood override these concerns. Community, family and partner expectations place a high cultural value on a woman's fertility, and childbearing is also attributed to male status.

The desire for more children was reportedly low amongst HIV-positive women living in South Africa, although awareness of PMTCT was found to influence childbearing desires prior to ART availability (Peltzer et al. 2009) as reported in other sub-Saharan countries (Yeatman 2009; Young 2007). It is assumed that treatment knowledge could alleviate concerns of personal health and mother-to-child transmission, allowing women and men to reconsider their reproductive desires. Since PMTCT and ART programmes became nationally available in 2001 and 2004, a range of qualitative studies have explored the effect of ART on childbearing desire with mixed results.

ART use was strongly positively associated with women's fertility intentions in a survey of 459 HIV-infected men and women living in Cape Town, including those on ART and those not yet eligible for treatment (Cooper et al. 2009) and amongst women living in other developing countries (Kaida et al. 2006). Favourable attitudes to childbearing have been attributed to a longer duration of treatment (Cooper et al. 2007; Myer et al. 2007), although this had no impact on childbearing decision-making amongst women living in Soweto (Kaida et al. 2011). Furthermore, knowledge of treatment availability may influence reproductive decision-making differently by gender. Men have reported greater desires then women when accessing treatment (Myer et al. 2007), while women were more likely to express a wish for more children only when both ART and PMTCT were available (Cooper et al. 2007).

To see an effect on actual fertility trends, a shift in reproductive desires amongst people living with HIV must precede a change in reproductive behaviour. Before the introduction of ART, it was common to find that contraceptive use and fertility remain unchanged, irrespective of reported desire (Bova and Durante 2003; Gray et al. 1998; Rutenberg et al. 2000). However, the effect of ART on rates of pregnancy was quantified in a multi-country study of 4531 pregnant or recently postpartum HIV-infected women receiving PMTCT services across seven countries between 2003 and 2007. Those receiving ART were more likely to experience a pregnancy (9 per 100 person years) compared to women solely accessing PMTCT services (6.5 per 100 person years) with one of the biggest differences reported from South Africa (Myer et al. 2010). Another single study from Uganda found no such association (Maier et al. 2009).

The long-term impact of ART provision on national fertility rates in South Africa remains unclear, but it is likely that socio-economic factors may be of greater influence in a woman's decision to have more children even in areas of high HIV prevalence under a prevailing social importance of parenthood (Cooper et al. 2007, 2009; Nattabi et al. 2009). Furthermore, a survey of women in Zimbabwe found that despite an association between HIV status, fertility desire and incidence of pregnancy, 69 per cent of recorded pregnancies were unplanned (Feldman and Maposhere 2003). In the context of relatively low planning, a behaviour change amongst infected women alone would not be enough to drive a demographic transition to the extent seen in South Africa.

HIV uninfected women

The impact of the HIV epidemic on reproductive behaviour amongst uninfected women is more difficult to assess. A majority of the general population are uninfected and a range of factors act as proximate determinants of fertility at this level, while any change in patterns of childbearing attributed to the disease would be behavioural. In areas of high HIV prevalence, the epidemic could encourage earlier childbearing amongst uninfected women or those unaware of their status in order to 'insure' against the risk of infant mortality. Alternatively, many women may avoid marriage and sexual unions for fear of acquiring the disease. However, one analysis of Demographic Health Survey data from 13 countries revealed that childbearing amongst uninfected women was not altered in relation to community level HIV prevalence, suggesting very little behavioural response in the context of HIV (Juhn et al. 2008).

Population level

Multi-country Demographic Health Survey data presents a small or no impact of HIV prevalence on population fertility, even pointing to a positive association in high prevalence countries such as Kenya and Lesotho (Fortson 2009; Juhn et al. 2008). This effect was not tested for South Africa, but a high prevalence of HIV in the province of KwaZulu-Natal was found not to be a significant determinant of fertility decline in this area, coinciding with a reported stall in fertility decline up to 2005 (Moultrie et al. 2008).

An apparently minimal association between the epidemic and population level fertility is most likely explained by a heterogeneous behavioural response to HIV in the general population (Durevall and Lindskog 2011). It is important to distinguish the relative importance of physiological or behavioural changes amongst both people living with HIV and uninfected individuals living in areas of high HIV prevalence if we are to determine the childbearing effects for the South African population. As yet, there is no agreement on the direction of this response (Juhn et al. 2008).

Conclusion

The South African transition is one of the most established in sub-Saharan Africa. This chapter aimed to explore this transition in the context of a unique political history and strong socio-economic development and to consider the impact of one of the heaviest global burdens of HIV at each level of the population. Pregnancy and transmission of HIV share many of the same proximate determinants, while socio-economic and cultural mechanisms can act upon these determinants in opposing directions. To further complicate an association between fertility and HIV, physiological changes may limit the fertility of people living with HIV while changes in contraceptive use, sexual activity and desires for more children can occur amongst all levels of the population in response to the epidemic.

Continued fertility decline will be largely attributed to falling rates amongst African and Coloured women with contraceptives being applied for the purpose of birth spacing or even postponement under difficult economic circumstances. High extra-marital fertility elucidates a strong cultural importance for childbearing regardless of marital status. Yet for those wishing to limit their births a preference for hormonal contraceptives remains, despite the high risk of HIV acquisition or re-infection. Meanwhile, increasing trends in condom use indicates a shift in contraceptive preference rather than prevalence and with little overall impact on fertility.

The influence of this relatively recent HIV epidemic on fertility trends seems to be limited in South Africa, although the apparent stability could be masking a range of heterogeneous behavioural responses amongst the population, which may well be removed as we enter an era of ART. More research will be needed to fully understand the long-term implications of the epidemic.

References

Allen, S., Serufilira, A., Gruber, V., Kegeles, S., Van De Perre, P., Carael, M. and Coates, T. J. (1993) Pregnancy and contraception use among urban Rwandan women after HIV testing and counseling, *American Journal of Public Health,* 83: 705.

Asiimwe-Okiror, G., Opio, A. A., Musinguzi, J., Madraa, E., Tembo, G. and Caraël, M. (1997) Change in sexual behaviour and decline in HIV infection among young pregnant women in urban Uganda, *Aids,* 11: 1757.

Avert (2011) http://www.avert.org/safricastats.htm, date accessed 17 March 2011.

Bongaarts, J. (1978) A framework for analyzing the proximate determinants of fertility, *Population and Development Review,* 4: 105–32.

Bova, C. and Durante, A. (2003) Sexual functioning among HIV-infected women, *Aids Patient Care and Stds,* 17: 75–83.

Bracher, M. and Santow, G. (2001) Modelling some fertility effects of STDs and HIV/AIDS. Paper presented at the annual meeting of the Population Association of America, Washington, DC, 29–31 March 2001.

Budlender, D., Chobokoane, N. and Simelane, S. (2004) Marriage patterns in South Africa: methodological and substantive issues, *Southern African Journal of Demography,* 9: 1–26.

Bureau, P. R. (2006) The World's Youth 2006 Data Sheet, Washington, DC.

Burgard, S. (2004) Factors associated with contraceptive use in late and post apartheid South Africa, *Studies in Family Planning,* 35: 91–104.

Caldwell, J. C. (2000) Rethinking the African AIDS epidemic, *Population and Development Review,* 26: 117–35.

Caldwell, J. C., Caldwell, P. and Quiggin, P. (1989) The social context of AIDS in sub-Saharan Africa, *Population and Development Review,* 15: 185–234.

Camlin, C. S., Garenne, M. and Moultrie, T. A. (2004) Fertility trend and pattern in a rural area of South Africa in the context of HIV/AIDS, *African Journal of Reproductive Health/La Revue Africaine de la Santé Reproductive,* 8: 38–54.

Carpenter, L. M., Nakiyingi, J. S., Ruberantwari, A., Malamba, S. S., Kamali, A. and Whitworth, J. A. G. (1997) Estimates of the impact of HIV infection on fertility in a rural Ugandan population cohort, *Health Transition Review,* 7: 113–26.

Cates, W., Rolfs, R. and Aral, S. (1993) The pathophysiology and epidemiology of sexually transmitted diseases in relation to pelvic inflammatory disease and infertility. In: Gray R. H., Ledridon H. and Spira A. (eds). *Biomedical and Demographic Determinants of Reproduction* (Oxford: Oxford University Press).

Chimere-Dan, O. (1994) Determinants of racial fertility differentials in some urban areas of South Africa, *Journal of Biosocial Science,* 26: 55–63.

Chimere-Dan, O. (1999) Marriage and the fertility transition in South Africa. Paper presented at the African Population Conference, Durban, South Africa, 6–10 December.

Cohen, B. (1998) The emerging fertility transition in sub-Saharan Africa, *World Development,* 26: 1431–61.

Cooper, D., Harries, J., Myer, L., Orner, P. and Bracken, H. (2007) 'Life is still going on': reproductive intentions among HIV-positive women and men in South Africa, *Social Science and Medicine,* 65: 274–83.

Cooper, D., Moodley, J., Zweigenthal, V., Bekker, L. G., Shah, I. and Myer, L. (2009) Fertility intentions and reproductive health care needs of people living with HIV in Cape Town, South Africa: implications for integrating reproductive health and HIV Care services, *Aids and Behavior,* 13(Suppl. 1): S38–46.

Cooper, D., Morroni, C., Orner, P., Moodley, J., Harries, J., Cullingworth, L. and Hoffman, M. (2004) Ten years of democracy in South Africa: documenting transformation in reproductive health policy and status, *Reproductive Health Matters,* 12: 70–85.

Department of Population and Social Development (1998) *White Paper on Population Policy,* Government Gazette (ed.). Pretoria: Government Printer.

Du Plessis, G. (1996) Reproductive choice and motivation in South Africa, *South African Journal of Demography,* 6: 33–48.

Durevall, D. and Lindskog, A. (2011) Uncovering the impact of the HIV epidemic on fertility in sub-Saharan Africa: the case of Malawi, *Journal of Population Economics,* 24, 629–55.

Feldman, R. and Maposhere, C. (2003) Safer sex and reproductive choice: findings from, *Reproductive Health Matters,* 11: 162–73.

Fortson, J. G. (2009) HIV/AIDS and Fertility, *American Economic Journal-Applied Economics,* 1: 170–94.

Garenne, M., Tollman, S., Kahn, K., Collins, T. and Ngwenya, S. (2001) Understanding marital and premarital fertility in rural South Africa, *Journal of Southern African Studies,* 27: 277–90.

Glynn, J. R., Buvé, A., Caraël, M., Musonda, R. M., Kahindo, M., Macauley, I., Tembo, F. and Zekeng, L. (2001) Factors influencing the difference in HIV prevalence between antenatal clinic and general population in sub-Saharan Africa, *Aids,* 15: 1717.

Gray, R. H., Wawer, M. J., Serwadda, D., Sewankambo, N., Li, C., Wabwire-Mangen, F., Paxton, L., Kiwanuka, N., Kigozi, G. and Konde-Lule, J. (1998) Population-based study of fertility in women with HIV-1 infection in Uganda, *The Lancet,* 351: 98–103.

Gregson, S. (1994) Will HIV become a major determinant of fertility in sub-Saharan Africa, *Journal of Development Studies,* 30: 650–79.

Gregson, S., Zaba, B. and Hunter, S. C. (2009) The impact of HIV-1 on fertility in sub-Saharan Africa: causes and consequences, *asdf,* 113–117.

Gregson, S., Zhuwau, T., Anderson, R. M. and Chandiwana, S. K. (1997) HIV and fertility change in rural Zimbabwe, *Health Transition Review,* 7: 89–112.

Gregson, S., Zhuwau, T., Anderson, R. M. and Chandiwana, S. K. (2004) HIV and fertility change in rural Zimbabwe, *Health Transition Review,* 7(Suppl. 2): 89–112.

Gustafsson, S. S. and Worku, S. Y. (2006) *Marriage Markets and Single Motherhood in South Africa* (Tinbergen Institute Discussion Paper), University of Amsterdam.

Harwood-Lejeune, A. (2001) Rising age at marriage and fertility in Southern and Eastern Africa, *European Journal of Population/Revue européenne de Démographie,* 17: 261–80.

Herbst, A. J., Cooke, G. S., Bärnighausen, T., Kanykany, A., Tanser, F. and Newell, M. L. (2009) Adult mortality and antiretroviral treatment roll-out in rural KwaZulu-Natal, South Africa, *Bulletin of the World Health Organization,* 87: 754–62.

Herbst, K., Ndirangu, J. and Newell, M. (2011) Longer-term consequences on the population structure after changes in child mortality due to impact of ART and PMTCT programmes in a rural population in KwaZulu-Natal, SA. *18th Conference on Retroviruses and Opportunistic Infections* (Boston: Africa Centre for Health and Population Studies, UKZN).

Hosegood, V., Mcgrath, N. and Moultrie, T. A. (2009) Dispensing with marriage: marital trends in rural KwaZulu-Natal, South Africa 2000–2006, *Demographic Research,* 20: 279–312.

Hunter, S. C., Isingo, R., Boerma, J., Urassa, M., Mwaluko, G. M. P. and Zaba, B. (2003) The association between HIV and fertility in a cohort study in rural Tanzania, *Journal of Biosocial Science,* 35: 189–99.

Juhn, C., Kalemli-Ozcan, S. and Turan, B. (2008) HIV and fertility in Africa: first evidence from population based surveys, National Bureau of Economic Research Cambridge, Mass., USA.

Kaida, A., Andia, I., Maier, M., Strathdee, S. A., Bangsberg, D. R., Spiegel, J., Bastos, F. I., Gray, G. and Hogg, R. (2006) The potential impact of antiretroviral therapy on fertility in sub-Saharan Africa, *Current HIV/AIDS Reports,* 3: 187–94.

Kaida, A., Laher, F., Strathdee, S. A., Janssen, P. A., Money, D., Hogg, R. S. and Gray, G. (2011) Childbearing intentions of HIV-positive women of reproductive age in Soweto, South Africa: the influence of expanding access to HAART in an HIV hyperendemic setting, *American Journal of Public Health,* 101: 350.

Kalipeni, E. (1995) The fertility transition in Africa, *Geographical Review,* 85: 286–300.

Maier, M., Andia, I., Emenyonu, N., Guzman, D., Kaida, A., Pepper, L., Hogg, R. and Bangsberg, D. R. (2009) Antiretroviral therapy is associated with increased fertility desire, but not pregnancy or live birth, among HIV+ women in an early HIV treatment program in rural Uganda, *Aids and Behavior,* 13(Suppl. 1): S28–37.

Martin, P., Gresenguet, G., Herve, V., Renom, G., Steenman, G. and Georges, A. (1992) Decreased number of spermatozoa in HIV-1-infected individuals, *Aids,* 6: 130.

Mcgrath, N., Nyirenda, M., Hosegood, V. and Newell, M. (2009) Age at first sex in rural South Africa, *Sexually Transmitted Infections,* 85: i49–55.

Mokomane, Z. and Khan, N. (2009) Towards a 10-year review of the population policy implementation in South Africa (1998–2008) sexual and reproductive health and rights. In Department of Social Development, Pretoria, http://www.population.gov.za/pop_dev/index.php/Policy-+10/, date accessed: 5 April 2011.

Moultrie, T. A., Hosegood, V., Mcgrath, N., Hill, C., Herbst, K. and Newell, M. L. (2008) Refining the Criteria for Stalled Fertility Declines: An Application to

Rural KwaZulu Natal, South Africa, 1990–2005, *Studies in Family Planning,* 39: 39–48.

Moultrie, T. A. and Timaeus, I. M. (2001) Fertility and living arrangements in South Africa, *Journal of Southern African Studies,* 27: 207–23.

Moultrie, T. A. and Timaeus, I. M. (2002) Trends in South African fertility between 1970 and 1998, *Cape Town: Medical Research Council of South Africa, Burden of Disease Unit.*

Muthwa, S. W. (1995) Economic survival strategies of female-headed households, the case of Soweto, South Africa. *Journal of Gender Studies,* 3(2): 165–75.

Myer, L., Carter, R. J., Katyal, M., Toro, P., El-Sadr, W. M. and Abrams, E. J. (2010) Impact of antiretroviral therapy on incidence of pregnancy among HIV-infected women in sub-Saharan Africa: a cohort study, *PLoS Med,* 7: e1000229.

Myer, L., Morroni, C. and Rebe, K. (2007) Prevalence and determinants of fertility intentions of HIV-infected women and men receiving antiretroviral therapy in South Africa, *Aids Patient Care and Stds,* 21: 278–85.

Nattabi, B., Li, J., Thompson, S. C., Orach, C. G. and Earnest, J. (2009) A systematic review of factors influencing fertility desires and intentions among people living with HIV/AIDS: implications for policy and service delivery, *Aids and Behavior,* 13: 949–68.

Ndirangu, J., Newell, M. L., Tanser, F., Herbst, A. J. and Bland, R. (2010) Decline in early life mortality in a high HIV prevalence rural area of South Africa: evidence of HIV prevention or treatment impact?, *Aids,* 24: 593.

Peltzer, K., Chao, L. W. and Dana, P. (2009) Family planning among HIV positive and negative prevention of mother to child transmission (PMTCT) clients in a resource poor setting in South Africa. *Aids and Behavior,* 13: 973–9.

Population Reference Bureau (2010) World Population Data Sheet.

Preston-Whyte, E. (1993) Women who are not married: fertility, 'illegitimacy', and the nature of households and domestic groups among single African women in Durban, *South African Journal of Sociology,* 24: 63–71.

Preston-Whyte, E. and Zondi, M. (1992) Questionable issue: illegitimacy in South Africa. In: Burman, S. and Preston-Whyte, E. (eds). *Assessing Illegitimacy in South Africa* (Cape Town: Oxford University Press).

Rutenberg, N., Biddlecom, A. E. and Kaona, F. A. D. (2000) Reproductive decision-making in the context of HIV and AIDS: a qualitative study in Ndola, Zambia, *International Family Planning Perspectives*, 26(3): 124–30.

Ryder, R. W., Batter, V. L., Nsuami, M., Badi, N., Mundele, L., Matela, B., Utshudi, M. and Heyward, W. L. (1991) Fertility rates in 238 HIV-1-seropositive women in Zaire followed for 3 years post-partum, *Aids,* 5: 1521.

Schneider, H. and Fassin, D. (2002) Denial and defiance: a socio-political analysis of AIDS in South Africa, *Aids,* 16, S45.

Shisana, O., Council, H. S. R., Council, S. A. M. R., Centre for Aids Development, R., Evaluation and Diseases, N. I. F. C. (2010) *South African National HIV Prevalence, Incidence, Behaviour and Communication Survey, 2008: The Health of Our Children* (Cape Town: HSRC Press).

Shisana, O. and Simbayi, L. (2008) *South African National HIV Prevalence, HIV Incidence, Behaviour and Communication Survey, 2005*, Human Sciences Research Council.

South African Department of Health (2003) South Africa Demographic and Health Survey. Pretoria.

Statistics South Africa (2010) *Mid-year Population Estimates* http://www.statssa.gov.za/publications/P0302/P03022010.pdf, date accessed, 8 March 2011.

Swartz, L. (2009) Fertility transition in South Africa and its implications on the four major population groups, *asdf*, 487.

Terceira, N., Gregson, S., Zaba, B. and Mason, P. R. (2003) The contribution of HIV to fertility decline in rural Zimbabwe, 1985–2000, *Population Studies*, 57(2): 149–64.

Timæus, I. M. and Moultrie, T. A. (2008) On postponement and birth intervals, *Population and Development Review*, 34: 483–510.

Townsend, C. L., Cortina-Borja, M., Peckham, C. S., De Ruiter, A., Lyall, H. and Tookey, P. A. (2008) Low rates of mother-to-child transmission of HIV following effective pregnancy interventions in the United Kingdom and Ireland, 2000–2006, *Aids*, 22: 973.

United Nations (2002) HIV/AIDS and fertility in sub-Saharan Africa: a review of the research literature in Department of Economic and Social Affairs, P. D. (ed.).

Western Cape Government Family Planning (2011) http://www.westerncape.gov.za/eng/directories/services/11517/6473#02, date accessed 12 April 2011.

WHO (2010) UNAIDS. Towards universal access: scaling up priority HIV/AIDS interventions in the health sector. Progress report 2010. Geneva: World Health Organization.

The World Bank (2008) *Health Nutrition and Population Statistics (HNP)*, http://databank.worldbank.org/ddp/home.do?Step=*x*12&id=4&CNO=311, date accessed, 31 May 2011.

Yeatman, S. E. (2009) The impact of HIV status and perceived status on fertility desires in rural Malawi, *Aids and Behavior*, 13: 12–19.

Young, A. (2005) The gift of the dying: the tragedy of AIDS and the welfare of future African generations, *Quarterly Journal of Economics*, 120: 423–66.

Young, A. (2007) In sorrow to bring forth children: fertility amidst the plague of HIV, *Journal of Economic Growth*, 12: 283–327.

Zaba, B. and Gregson, S. (1998) Measuring the impact of HIV on fertility in Africa, *Aids*, 12: S41–50.

Zaba, B., Terceira, N., Mason, P. and Gregson, S. (2003) The contribution of HIV to fertility decline in rural Zimbabwe, 1985–2000, *Popul Stud (Camb)*, 57: 149–64.

11
Declining Fertility, Television and the (Mis)representation of Motherhood

Stuart Basten

Introduction

Television and celebrity are ubiquitous in the industrial world and, increasingly, in the developing world. Making the connection between television and childbearing preferences may seem a leap of faith, but recent studies are increasingly finding links (Basten 2010). This chapter briefly outlines the relationship between television and fertility in the developing world, then presents some recent research and thoughts on television in lower fertility settings to suggest how television could influence childbearing decisions. The over-arching message is that this relationship is woefully under-researched, especially given the ubiquitous nature of television and celebrity in the modern world.

Television and fertility in the developing world

Mass media interventions have been successful in changing and nurturing both public health activities and social and cultural norms. Family planning and reproductive health are two areas that have been widely used in mass media messaging for some time, particularly in high fertility settings in the developing world. In Nigeria, for example, a campaign using music videos with popular national artists promoting family planning began in 1989–90 and was found to have improved contraceptive use and intention as well as lowering desired family size (Bankole et al. 1996).

One particular genre has been exploited as a very successful means of 'edutainment', namely soap operas (Fung 2007). Some soap operas are designed explicitly to promote a family planning message, with perhaps the most famous examples of such soaps being found in Mexico. The first *telenovela* to promote family planning was a nine-month series entitled *Acompañame*, which was shown primetime, weekdays during 1977–78. As a result of its success, Mexican TV network *Televisa* commissioned four more family planning soaps that ran throughout the 1970s and 1980s – *Vamos Juntos* (We Go Together), *Caminemos* (Let's Walk), *Nosotros las Mujeres* (We the Women) and *Por Amor* (For Love) – during which period Mexico's population growth rate declined by 34 per cent. All of these shows were produced by Miguel Sabido, after whom the 'Sabido Methodology' of pro-social serial programming has been coined (PMC 2009). Indeed, Thomas Donnelly, then of USAID, stated in the 1980s that

> Throughout Mexico, wherever one travels, when people are asked where they heard about family planning, or what made them decide to practice family planning, the response is universally attributed to one of the soap operas that *Televisa* has done. The *Televisa* family planning soap operas have made the single most powerful contribution to the Mexican population success story.
>
> (PMC 2009)

Along with Mexico, *telenovelas* in Brazil have been studied intensively in terms of their relationship to family planning and fertility rates. Within three decades, television coverage rose from zero to become almost universal in urban areas and to almost 50% in rural households. Coterminous with this rise in *telenovelas* is a dramatic drop in Brazilian fertility rates from over 6.0 in 1960 to below 2.0 today (Dunn 2001).

As well as a generally better quality of script and production, the fundamental difference between the Brazilian *telenovelas* and those which follow the Sabido methodology is that the former did not explicitly promote family planning and population control (La Ferrara et al. 2008). Indeed, the advertising of contraceptive methods was illegal in Brazil until the late 1970s. Instead, the TV shows were vehicles for writers to express modern and liberal ideas. As such, recurring themes included

> freedom, criticism of religious and traditional values, consumption of luxurious goods, the portrayal of wealthy families, the display of new lifestyle, the circulation of modern ideas such as female emancipation in the work sphere, the female pursuit of pleasure and love even if through adultery, displays of homosexuality, criticism of machismo and emphasis on individualism.
>
> (La Ferrara et al. 2008)

Often this material related to family size preferences. Indeed, a content analysis of 115 *telenovelas* between 1965 and 1999 reveals that 72 per cent of the main female characters (aged <50) had no children at all, while one in five had only one – all, of course, in marked contrast to prevalent fertility rates in Brazil during much of this period (La Ferrara et al. 2008).

In Dunn's study of north-eastern Brazil, none of the women in the study said that media had changed their own childbearing behaviours or attitudes. However, evidence does seem to suggest that *the* telenovelas may have played a role. La Ferrara et al. sought to test more robustly the hypothesis that the smaller families presented on television influenced views on family size. They exploited the differences in the timing of entry into different markets by *Rede Globo*, the television network which, until the early 1990s, had an effective monopoly on *telenovela* production in Brazil. The study found that *Globo* presence was significantly associated with lower fertility after controlling for time and regional characteristics. This effect appears to be heightened among women of a lower socio-economic status, and among women who are in the middle or late phases of their childbearing careers, suggesting that television contributed more to *stopping* rather than *postponing* behaviour – a feature consistent with available demographic data for Brazil (La Ferrara et al. 2008). Interestingly, a similar effect was found among divorce rates, which also rose when the *Globo* signal was received in a given area (Chong and La Ferrara 2009).

Social soap operas have also been used in Asia. In India, *Hum Log* (tr. 'People Like Us'), which began broadcasting in 1984, averaged an audience of 50 million people. Set amongst a lower middle-class joint family, the serial promoted equality for women, family harmony and smaller family sizes. Epilogues related the content of each programme to viewer's daily lives. These epilogues were delivered by the famous Hindi actor Ashok Kumar and ended with an address to which letters regarding the programme could be directed (CIN 2009). As a result as Chatterji (2008) observes, 'viewers sent more than 400,000 letters, many of them addressed to the characters rather than to the actors and actresses.... Many of these viewers identified with one or more of the characters, and many commented on the social issues raised by the show'. A survey of 500 such letters written found that the great majority (92 per cent) were influenced in the intended direction and 7 per cent reported changes in behaviour as a result of the show. Furthermore,

> 53 per cent of respondents believed in copying positive role models identified in *Hum Log*, 23 per cent believed in copying negative

> role models. 70 per cent believed that women should have equal opportunities, 71 per cent said that family size should be limited, 64 per cent thought women's welfare programs should be encouraged. 33 per cent of the sample of 500 letters had their social attitudes influenced by the show.
>
> (CIN 2009)

A recent study has revisited the Indian context to examine in greater detail the impact of cable television on local communities (Jensen and Oster 2009). Indian television output has strongly featured soap operas, such as *Kyunki Saas Bhi Kabhi Bahu Thi* (tr. 'Because a mother-in-law was once a daughter-in-law too'), which, like the Brazilian *telenovelas*, are overwhelmingly set in urban locations. As such, rural viewers see a different society inhabited by (generally) more emancipated women. This research found that the introduction of cable television was related to significant decreases in domestic violence towards women and the preference for a son as well as increases in women's autonomy and decreases in fertility. This quantitative evidence confirms anthropological reports describing the perceived effect of introducing television on gender empowerment in India (Johnson 2001; Scrase 2002).

In sum, as television becomes more ubiquitous in the developing world, there is clearly an opportunity to use mass media as part of public health, family planning and general development policies. These messages can – and have – been blended to include both a presentation of a potential 'better life' through aspiration to education and gender empowerment and a sense of heightening the urgency of particular public health initiatives. In other words, such messages are able to balance the top-down imperatives of safe sex and HIV-AIDS prevention with the post-Cairo population consensus of reproductive rights.

A major caveat to this, however, is that the rapid growth of the Internet has the potential to supersede television as a primary point of contact for entertainment and information. However, given the extremely low levels of Internet access penetration in settings such as sub-Saharan Africa, this is unlikely in the short term (Internet World Stats 2012).

Media and the family in low fertility, industrialized countries

The evidence from developing countries strongly suggests that television can play an important, if often indirect role, in how families and individuals relate to family planning, public health and fertility (Basten 2010). But can this be translated to low fertility settings?

One argument for a role for television in demographic thought can be found in the so-called 'Low Fertility Trap Hypothesis', which posits that in a setting of falling fertility rates, a process of normalization and socialization occurs with smaller families not only being commonplace among friends, siblings and colleagues, but also in media representation. Once fertility falls below a certain level, and in the context of this cultural normalization, 'ideal family size would become lower, which in due course may result in further declining actual family size and still lower ideals in the subsequent generation' (Lutz et al. 2006, p. 18). Indeed, there are also occasions where society can change to leave television behind. Consider the British soap operas *EastEnders* and *Coronation Street*, which follows the families of two areas of London and Manchester. In both of these serial dramas, there is a deep interaction between neighbours on social, economic and romantic levels. However, this degree of neighbourliness in fact bears relatively little relation to contemporary urban Britain.

In this vein, it is important to understand how mass media in the developed world reflects and presents the family. Some work has approached this in terms of the presentation of childlessness and 'ideal families' on television, but the research in this area is very much underdeveloped (for an exception, see Sass 2004).

Possibly the most cited example of the discussion of family typology on television comes from the early 1990s and a speech by US Vice President Dan Quayle who, when discussing the reasons for the riots in Los Angeles in 1992, saw fit to mention the TV show *Murphy Brown*. According to Quayle,

> ...if a single mother raising her children in the ghetto, has to worry about drive-by shootings, drug-deals, or whether her children will join gangs and die violently, her already difficult task becomes impossible. It doesn't help matters when primetime TV has *Murphy Brown* – a character who supposedly epitomizes today's intelligent, highly paid, professional woman – mocking the importance of fathers – by bearing a child alone, and calling it just another 'Lifestyle Choice'.
>
> (Time 1992)

Goldstein et al. (2003, p. 491) observe that 'large families are not a feature of German or Austrian television (except through American imports)', implying that the USA's higher fertility rates are reflected in its media output. However, it is not as clear cut as this might suggest. For example, the genres in which families are presented in various forms are immense. These include animated presentations of dysfunctional families – *The Simpsons, American Dad, Family Guy, South Park*; reality shows featuring celebrity families – *The Osbournes, Hammertime, Keeping Up with the Kardasians*; the presentation of perpetually single adults in *Friends* and *Sex in the City* and, of course, the sitcoms based around strained but ultimately cozy family relationships, as in *My Family, Outnumbered, Married with Children*. As yet, a full content analysis of the changing presentation of family size, family typologies and attitudes towards children on television has not yet been performed. This is surely an important research priority.

We can also move our analysis beyond the representation of particular family types and consider more broadly the representation of celebrity parenthood – usually taken to be celebrity motherhood. This is a growing theme in both recent media studies and feminist works alike. In particular, a number of studies have focussed on the creation of an unrealistic representation of motherhood. In the next section, I explore some of these elements, and ask whether or not the misrepresentation of motherhood could shape individual decision making regarding childbearing and, in turn, play a role in shaping regimes of lower fertility in industrialized countries.

The 'attack of the celebrity moms'

The 'attack of celebrity moms' was the title of a chapter in Douglas and Michaels (2004) best-selling book *The Mommy Myth*, which took as its overall theme the 'idealization of motherhood and how it has undermined women'. This chapter is a withering attack on the culture of celebrity motherhood which, the authors claim, has 'bulldozed through American popular culture' since 2000 in the same way that 'motherhood and maternal practices became a national obsession in the 1980s and 1990s' (Douglas and Michaels 2004, p. 116).

For Douglas and Michaels, the cult of the celebrity mom is a direct rejection of the black humour favoured by feminists and women humourists of the 1970s and 1980s. They could, like Erma Bombeck, say that 'having children made your stomach and ass fall down to your knees, and that sometime all you wanted to do was murder the kids and bury them near the septic tank' (Douglas and Michaels 2004, p. 116). New celebrity moms have banished all such (exaggerated) negativity:

> Celebrity moms loved their kids unconditionally all the time; they loved being mothers all the time; they yearned for babies if they

> didn't have them and yearned for more if they did. They had everything under control and their children were perfect because celebrity moms always did everything right.
>
> (Douglas and Michaels 2004, p. 116)

Since the publication of *The Mommy Myth* in 2004, the proliferation of outlets for photographs, videos and stories with celebrity mothers has grown exponentially, not least through celebrity magazines – both on- and off-line. Indeed, the growth of Internet celebrity gossip sites has served to make the whole celebrity mom phenomenon far more interactive. *People* magazine, for example, has an entire section of its website solely dedicated to the newborn children of celebrities (http://celebritybabies.people.com/) with subsections including 'News, Photos, Celeb Style' (dedicated to both mother and child clothing) and a handy calendar of the due dates of celebrities and the birthdays of their offspring. Apart from being an unabashed opportunity for targeted advertising, the overall theme of the articles in such websites is in line with Douglas and Michael's observations in 2004, that everything is *perfect* in the lives of celebrity mums.

Many websites encourage users to rate celebrity moms according to their style and general attitude. One such site (www.babble.com) invites users to either 'Like' or 'Loathe' said celebrity moms in different categories – overall, 'busiest', 'most controversial', 'most stylish' and 'best playmate'. As the site states:

> Celebrity moms are the media's newest big thing – some are idolized and emulated, others criticized and ridiculed – but as a culture, we're clearly obsessed. We track every stage of their baby bumps, scoff at their post-baby bodies, drool over their kids' outfits and desperately search for any traces of normalcy that show us, Hey, they're just like me! Love them or loathe them, here are 50 we couldn't ignore. Now, it's your turn. Who'd we miss? Nominate your favorite – and least favorite – celebrity moms.
>
> (www.babble.com)

The most loathed appear to be women who, in some sense, have failed to conform the mothering ideal for one reason or another. The speed at which celebrities lose weight can be an especially onerous burden on the prospective mother. Halle Berry, Jennifer Lopez, Victoria Beckham and other high profile celebrity mothers quickly 'regained their figure' after childbearing, often citing the most casual methods for doing so. Heidi

Klum, for example, was famously back on the catwalk six weeks after her first birth, and modelling underwear eight weeks after her second.

While some celebrities are exceptionally fortunate in being able to 'regain their figure' without any effort – Myleene Klass, for example, resumed modelling three months after her first birth through 'breast-feeding and clever dressing' – the physiological similarities between even the most exalted celebrity women and everybody else suggests that many do, indeed, try rather harder. Enhanced financial resources allow celebrity mothers to invest in personal trainers, expensive and elaborate dieticians, the best clothes, flattering photographers and plastic surgery.

However, it has been suggested that there may be a number of potential ill-effects of this unrealistic presentation of post-pregnancy weight loss. The UK's National Institute for Health and Clinical Excellence recently published draft guidance on post-weight which explicitly cited celebrities:

> Women receive a wealth of sometimes conflicting advice on what constitutes a healthy diet and how much physical activity they should do during pregnancy and after childbirth. This comes not just from health professionals and official sources but from family, friends, the media and news media (such as social networking sites). For example, the press regularly publishes celebrity claims of unrealistic and rapid weight loss after pregnancy. This may create additional pressure on women to lose weight inappropriately at an already stressful time.
>
> (NICE 2010)

Furthermore, celebrity mothers frequently have another precious commodity, which so many mothers do not: time. Because of the effectively limitless supply of childcare available to celebrities, they are able to invest large amounts of time in achieving the image which they desire – both as celebrities and, of course, as mothers. This time can also be devoted to resuming their career very quickly.

Some recent surveys seem to give some evidence of the negative influence of celebrities. A 2010 Netmums/Royal College of Midwives survey of 6252 women found that 67 per cent of women were anxious about their weight after birth, and that 59 per cent blamed celebrities who lost their baby-weight quickly for making them feel more under pressure (Netmums 2010). Meanwhile almost 70 per cent of 9000 mothers surveyed by Netmums (2008) said they felt that the presentation of celebrity mums placed too much pressure on them to always look their best while trying to combine a family life with work demands. Furthermore, this concern had spread into the consumption with many women reporting impulse buys of celebrity-endorsed objects:

> I splashed out on a Storksak nappy bag – I mean, who really cares what a 'poo' bag looks like?!!
>
> I bought lots of seeds to grow my own veg. As if 2 jobs, 3 kids, a partner and house to look after aren't enough! Gwyneth Paltrow does it, why can't I????
>
> Burberry check baby outfits – I now cringe!!
>
> I tracked down a stupid hippy baby carrier I saw actress Rachel Weiss using which I still can't work out how to use!
>
> (Netmums 2008)

Unrealistic presentations of motherhood can not only leave women feeling disillusioned with their own lives, but can also lead partners, friends and families to have unrealistic expectations. As Douglas and Michaels suggest, the intention of such representation of celebrity motherhood is far less important than its effect:

> How is the reader [of celebrity magazines] supposed to feel, really, when the mother she is reading about has perfectly coiffed hair, is beaming ecstatically, has a hunky, rich husband allegedly fully involved in childrearing, an infant who sleeps through the night and never cried, and who actually weighs less than she did before getting pregnant, all because she ate bean sprouts, exercised, and prayed? You, meanwhile, are a 'sputum covered, exhausted slob in your bath robe' whose child 'screams from 4:00PM until 9:12PM, and then is up every hour-and-a-half during the night with diarrhea, night terrors and a missing blanket'.
>
> (Douglas and Michaels 2004, p. 119)

The implication here, then, is that if mothers 'fail to get with the program' then 'your kids will not make the grade, your husband won't look at you the way he used to, and, worst of all, other mothers will see you for what you are: an unworthy loser, a bad mother' (Douglas and Michaels 2004, p. 139).

Douglas and Michaels' rejection of celebrity motherhood is fundamentally grounded in a feminist, anti-consumptionist framework, which is clear from the title of their book. Their impressionistic analysis may also overestimate the influence of media on ordinary people's values and behaviour. However, in the high-pressure, consumption-based society of the twenty-first century where the cult of the celebrity is so strong – particularly in English-speaking countries – the misrepresentation of motherhood may feed into anguish about childbearing. The high expectations which these celebrities feed into can serve to heighten the pressures surrounding making one of the biggest decisions a person can take (see Chapter 15 in this book).

What we do not know, however, is whether any of this makes any real difference in terms of decision-making. Furthermore, it could be argued that the more interactive nature of Web 2.0 means that while images and stories of unrealistic celebrity moms are becoming more and more ubiquitous, so too are the opportunities for 'iconoclastic' behavior through forums, comments, blogs and personal websites. More careful research needs to be performed on both content analysis and surveying the extent to which the representation of motherhood by the media could play a role in shaping childbearing intentions.

The next section moves from the general presentation of families and mothers on television to the possible impact of a particular television genre, childbirth reality television.

The maternity ward-ization of birth

Giving birth in the developed world is safer today than at any point in human history. However, reported fear of the birthing process is higher than ever. There are, of course, many reasons for this, not least associated with the relative lack of occasions in the modern, industrial world where our health is genuinely at risk.

Birth fear is related to several factors such as lack of a social network, having an unskilled job or a vocational education, being a current smoker, young age, unemployment and past feelings of anxiety and depression (Laursen et al. 2008).

Additionally, some midwives and birth educators have suggested that the presentation of childbirth on television may have a role to play both in the reporting of enhanced fear of childbirth and in what one might call the 'super-medicalization of childbirth'. *Maternity Ward* on the US network TLC, one of the channel's most popular programmes, follows doctors and obstetricians at high-risk units across the United States. On *Maternity Ward*, as Ann Grauer remarks,

> No laboring women are depicted out of bed. Whether they are in early labor or pushing, they are flat on their backs. Machinery is

> everywhere. Blood pressure cuffs are on; electronic fetal monitors are strapped onto bellies. Legs are draped, and support people are off to the side. Heart-racing music plays whenever something 'dramatic' happens. The mothers look terrified...
>
> Within five minutes of watching the show, I am terrified for them. As the doctors move from room to room, viewers meet mothers and hear a little of their medical stories (almost all are considered 'high risk' by their health care providers). In the first room, for example, viewers meet a woman who has developed gestational diabetes. She's near her due date, so her doctor opts to induce labor, even though the mother's cervix is not ready. Will she make it through the labor? Will her baby be okay? Viewers will find out... after a commercial break. Almost four ads later, viewers witness the result: a 72-hour labor and a doctor who worries aloud whether or not the baby will be too tuckered and a Cesarean section will be necessary. But, viewers won't know for now. It's time for another commercial break.
>
> (Lothian and Grauer 2003)

Similar 'childbirth reality' shows have increased in number in recent years. A British example is *One Born Every Minute*, which featured on Channel Four (C4) for two seasons. The C4 website describes the show as follows:

> Every minute of every day, a baby is born in Britain. One Born Every Minute celebrates what it really feels like to become a parent, by filling a bustling maternity hospital with 40 cameras. Filming from the reception desk to the neo-natal ward; from the operating theatre to the birthing pool, this ground-breaking and tender new series observes the dramatic, emotional and often funny moments that go hand in hand with bringing a new life into the world, from the perspective of the soon-to-be parents and family, as well as the hospital staff.
>
> (Channel 4 2011)

Set in St Mary's Hospital, Southampton, the programme recently won a BAFTA award for best factual series and regularly draws more than three million viewers. While many harrowing scenes and relatively rare situations are shown, overall the show is generally balanced and, indeed, has received praise from various quarters. Sue Macdonald, education manager of the Royal College of Midwives stated that 'There have been some nice experiences and others where there has been more intervention. For the majority of women, birth is very normal and the programme makers need to continue to make sure they show that' (Saner 2011). Furthermore, the general response to C4's *One Born Every Minute* on Internet forums and comments on reviews of the programme seem to be generally positive (e.g. Mumsnet 2010). On the other hand, certain writers – especially doulas – have criticized the programme for its emphasis on pain. One doula, Sarah Johnson, wrote:

> Birth is persistently portrayed as scary, incredibly and pointlessly painful, dangerous, an emergency, a high-adrenalin medical situation from which a woman has to be rescued. If it isn't portrayed as a terrifying drama it is made comedic and ridiculous. The sense of slowly passing time which is inevitable with a first labour is never portrayed. The need for a quiet, protected, private environment (this is a physiological need, not simply an emotional one) is never referred to and the emphasis is entirely on 'things going wrong'.
>
> (Johnson 2010)

In 2010, the US version of *One Born Every Minute* set in Riverside Methodist Hospital in Columbus, Ohio, premiered on the *Lifetime* network. The show quickly became the channel's most-watched unscripted series premiere among women aged between 18 and 49, with a season average of 831,000 total viewers. It has recently been commissioned for a second series. However, after watching both British and American series, one is left in no doubt as to the very different approaches of the programme makers. The American version is far more dramatic, with a much more developed sense of drama portrayed through both content and presentation. The 'everyday goings on' at Riverside Methodist Hospital are presented in Table 11.1 and demonstrate the frequently dramatic nature of childbirth at Riverside. Even the respective websites show a completely different approach to childbirth, with the UK version showing a picture of a newborn baby in the masthead with the US version alternating between four terrified looking mothers and fathers shouting 'PUUUSH!', 'Never again!', 'Breathe hon!' and 'It huuuuurrrts!' (lifebegins.channel4.com/; www.mylifetime.com/shows/one-born-every-minute).

Online criticism of the US version does seem to be somewhat more heightened. In particular, there is much criticism from doulas who feel that the show demeans those women (and their partners) who opt

Table 11.1 Episode synopsis, season one, *One Born Every Minute, Lifetime* network, USA

Episode	Synopsis
1	Moms cope with labour pains in different ways in the premiere of this documentary series following the goings-on at a maternity ward in a Columbus, Ohio, hospital
2	A woman faces a serious complication during labor; a patient carries twins fathered by two different men.
3	A first time mom tries to joke her way through labor, but her delivery has the last laugh; two teenagers cram for the test of parenthood as they say goodbye to their childhood; a loving couple conquers the dreaded needle only to face a gut wrenching C-Section
4	An Iraq War veteran witnesses the birth of his second child; a woman's hopes for a girl come second to the child's safe delivery; and newlyweds endure a long labor.
5	A woman has to rely on her instincts when she leaves her birth plan at home; a mother of four has a complicated delivery; and a surrogate mother gives birth
6	A single mom's lip ring interferes with the birth of her second child; a woman leaves a bar to help her friend who's in labor.
7	Two sportscasters prepare to be parents for the first time; a woman who experienced a difficult prior delivery readies for the birth of twins; and a new mother deals with overwhelming fears.
8	A husband's parents try to be supportive; a large fibroid in a woman's birth canal causes trouble; and a couple hope to adopt twins.

Source: www.mylifetime.com/shows/one-born-every-minute

for natural birth procedures (Feministbreeder.com 2011). One midwife observed that

> Midwives, doulas and women seeking natural childbirth are frequently portrayed by these shows as weird or crazy hippies. One even showed nurses mocking a woman who wanted to labor in the shower and demeaning a couple that was trying to advocate for the type of birth they wanted.
>
> (Carlisle 2011)

Much of the evidence presented above derives from critics who have a defined self-interest in the promotion of natural child births. By contrast, some women feel that having all of the resources of the medical establishment at their side in the event of an emergency is extremely comforting. Indeed, a comment on the US version's website reads:

> I am a big fan of the UK version of this show and wish the US version lived up to its predecessor. The UK version manages to be an unintrusive and unbiased look into the goings on of the labor and delivery ward. With its judgmental editing and voice over, the US version offers quite a skewed view of birth. The show's production is obviously pro-epidural and tends to glorify medicated births while making the few mothers they show who want a natural birth look like lepers. It truly is a shame. I will continue to watch the UK version and avoid this one.
>
> (www.mylifetime.com/shows/one-born-every-minute)

However, in this context is the general distortion of deliveries in these shows. The vast majority of births pass off without particular event, with few difficulties or problems. The vast majority of women also do remember their birth plans and do not get the 'grapefruit sized fibroids' which affected a patient at Riverside. Labour generally lasts for a long time and, when things do go wrong, hospitals generally do not pipe dramatic music in a minor key into the surgery room. But for reality television at least, the average event is not enough. Therefore, while cameras record every minute of the birth experience, the final edited version which viewers are presented with is, perhaps inevitably, a roller-coaster ride of emotions covering joy and tragedy at breakneck speed.

We need far more research into understanding how young women are engaging with these representations of childbirth, and whether the new phenomenon of childbirth reality shows is educating, or misinforming their audiences. In turn, we can then see whether or not this plays any role in both childbearing decision-making and the fear of childbirth.

Theorizing television and demographic behaviour

To conclude, we can now combine existing research and the preliminary thoughts conveyed in this chapter in a hypothetical model of the interaction between television and fertility behaviour (Figure 11.1). This model suggests three stages of intent ranging from the explicit public health and family planning messages of government- or NGO-led initiatives, through indirect fertility messages of the *telenovelas* and

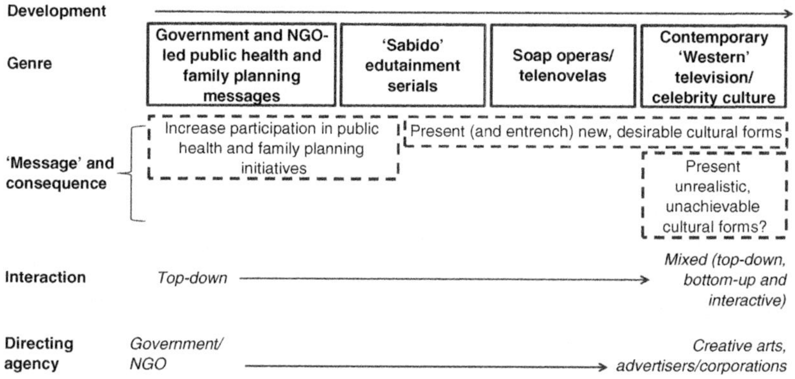

Figure 11.1 A hypothetical model of the interaction between mass media (television) and fertility behavior

soap operas of Brazil and India. It might be more useful to think of these genres in terms of how the creators intend an interaction with the audience. These range from a top-down message to an implicit recommendation. However, both of these approaches leave us somewhat puzzled when we reach low fertility countries. Partly, they also spread desirable images of parenthood. In addition, they can represent extreme and sensational events, as in reality shows, which may serve to educate, scare, or stimulate reflection and discussion. In some ways, this reaches into the very heart of just what the media does in terms of reflecting real or skewed (sometimes to an extreme degree) characteristics of its audience, and the possible feedback effect that that might have.

Conclusion

The evidence presented in this chapter emanates primarily from higher fertility countries and suggests that television could play a role, albeit indirectly, in attitudes towards family size. However, we know very little about the role of television – and by extension advertising and celebrity culture – in individual formation of ideas concerning childbearing.

It is vital, therefore, to foster a greater relationship between demography and the television and media industries, in conjunction with areas such as advertising, psychology and media, cultural and communication studies in order to gain a greater understanding of the possible interactions between the various presentations of family life on television, and the views held by, particularly, young people. Indeed, as other studies begin to probe the impact of both explicit and implicit mass media messaging on other walks of life such as voting behaviour (e.g. Ladd and Lenz 2009), consumption (Chavis and Leslie 2009), eating disorders (Becker 2004) and women's rights and sex stereotypes (Holbert et al. 2003), an analysis of this kind in relation to fertility behavior would be timely. Only by pursuing this research agenda will we be able to fully understand the role, and significance, of the media as a component of the 'Low Fertility Trap Hypothesis' and other theories of low fertility societies.

References

Bankole, A., Rodriguez, G. and Westoff, C. F. (1996) Mass media messages and reproductive behaviour in Nigeria, *Journal of Biosocial Science,* 28(2): 227–39.

Basten, S. A. (2010) Television and fertility, *Finnish Yearbook of Population Research,* XLV: 67–82.

Becker, A. E. (2004) Television, disordered eating, and young women in Fiji: negotiating body image and identity during rapid social change, *Culture, Medicine and Psychiatry,* 28(4): 533–59.

Carlisle, R. (2011) *Childbirth Reality TV Shows Overdramatize Labor and Delivery,* http://www.clinicaladvisor.com/childbirth-reality-tv-shows-overdramatize-labor-and-delivery/article/199417/, date accessed 1 April 2011.

Channel 4 (2011) *One Born Every Minute,* http://www.channel4.com/programmes/one-born-every-minute/episode-guide/series-1 (homepage), date accessed 27 March 2011.

Chatterji, S. (2008) *India Together: Looking Back at Hum Log,* http://www.indiatogether.org/2008/jul/wom-humlog.htm, date accessed 2 April 2011.

Chavis, L. and Leslie, P. (2009) Consumer boycotts: the impact of the Iraq war on French wine sales in the U.S., *Quantitative Marketing and Economics,* 7(1): 37–67.

Chong, A. and La Ferrara, E. (2009) Television and divorce: evidence from Brazilian novelas, *Journal of the European Economic Association,* 7(2–3): 458–68.

CIN (2009) 29th April 2009, *Hum log.* http://www.comminit.com/en/node/2220/print, date accessed 2 April 2011.

Douglas, S. J. and Michaels, M. W. (2004) *The Mommy Myth: The Idealization of Motherhood and How It Has Undermined All Women* (New York: Free Press).

Dunn, J. S. (2001) *Mass Media and Individual Reproductive Behavior in Northeastern Brazil.* Paper presented at the XXIV General Population Conference of the International Union for the Scientific Study of Population, Salvador, Brazil.

Feministbreeder.com (2011) *Lifetime TV Shows Us There's One (Unnecessary Intervention) Born Every Minute,* http://thefeministbreeder.com/lifetime-tv-shows-theres-one-unnecessary-intervention-born-every-minute/, date accessed 2 April 2011.

Fung, A. (2007) Intra-Asian cultural flow: cultural homologies in Hong Kong and Japanese television soap operas, *Journal of Broadcasting and Electronic Media,* 51(2): 265–86.

Goldstein, J., Lutz, W. and Testa, M. R. (2003) The emergence of sub-replacement family size ideals in Europe, *Population Research and Policy Review,* 22(5): 479–96.

Holbert, R. L., Kwak, N. and Shah, D. V. (2003) Political implications of prime-time drama and sitcom use: genres of representation and opinions concerning women's rights, *Journal of Communication,* 53(1): 45–60.

Internet World Stats. (2012) *Internet Usage Statistics for Africa,* http://www.internetworldstats.com/stats1.htm, date accessed 4 November 2012.

Jensen, R. and Oster, E. (2009) The power of TV: cable television and women's status in India, *Quarterly Journal of Economics,* 124(3): 1057–94.

Johnson, K. (2001) Media and social change: the modernizing influences of television in rural India, *Media, Culture and Society,* 23(2): 147–69.

Johnson, S. (2010) *Tokophobia and Toxic TV,* http://www.birthhypnosis.net/news-and-info-for-pregnant-and-new-mums/63-tokophobia- and-toxic-tv, date accessed 28 May 2010.

La Ferrara, E., Chong, A. and Duryea, S. (2008) *Soap Operas and Fertility: Evidence from Brazil,* Working Paper 172. Bureau for Research and Analysis of Development (BREAD), Duke University.

Ladd, J. M. and Lenz, G. S. (2009) Exploiting a rare communication shift to document the persuasive power of the news media, *American Journal of Political Science,* 53(2): 394–410.

Laursen, M., Hedegaard, M. and Johansen, C. (2008) Fear of childbirth: predictors and temporal changes among nulliparous women in the Danish National Birth Cohort, *British Journal of Obstetrics and Gynaecology,* 115: 354–60.

Lothian, J. A. and Grauer, A. (2003) 'Reality' birth: marketing fear to childbearing women, *Journal of Perinatal Education,* Spring, 12(2): vi–viii.

Lutz, W., Skirbekk, V. and Testa, M. R. (2006) The low-fertility trap hypothesis: forces that may lead to further postponement and fewer births in Europe, *Vienna Yearbook of Population Research,* 2006: 167–92.

Mumsnet (2010) *One Born Every Minute* – 16.3.10 at 9 pm/AllOnOnePage (355 Posts), http://www.mumsnet.com/Talk/telly_addicts/930397-, date accessed 24 March 2011.

Netmums (2010) *A Growing Problem? Weight in Pregnancy,* http://www.netmums.com/campaigns/A_Growing_Problem_Weight_in_Pregnancy.5616/, date accessed 24 March 2011.

Netmums (2008) *What about Me? Survey Results,* http://www.netmums.com/homelife/What_about_me_Survey_results.967/, date accessed 24 March 2011.

NICE (2010) *Dietary Interventions and Physical Activity Interventions for Weight Management before, during and after Pregnancy,* http://www.nice.org.uk/nicemedia/live/13056/49926/49926.pdf, date accessed 27 March 2011.

PMC (2009) *Sabido Methodolog,* http://www.populationmedia.org/what/sabido-method/, date accessed 24 April 2012.

Saner, E. (2011) How C4's One Born Every Minute made childbirth a reality TV hit, *The Guardian Online* (22 March 2011) http://www.guardian.co.uk/lifeandstyle/2011/mar/22/one-born-every-minute-tv-c4- childbirth, date accessed 27 March 2011.

Sass, E. (2004) *The Image of the Voluntarily Childfree: An Ethnographic Exploration of Media Representation and the Childless by Choice,* MA thesis, School of Mass Communications, University of South Florida.

Scrase, T. J. (2002) Television, the middle classes and the transformation of cultural identities in West Bengal, India, *Gazette,* 64(4): 323–42.

Time Magazine (1992) *Dan Quayle vs. Murphy Brown* (Monday, 1 June 1992) http://www.time.com/time/magazine/article/0,9171,975627,00.html, date accessed 1 April 2011.

Part III

What Will Be the Impact of Women Having Fewer Babies?

12
What Will Be the Impact on the Well-being of Children?

Ann Buchanan

> 'People are the real wealth of a nation.' With these words the 1990 Human Development Report (HDR) began a forceful case for a new approach to thinking about 'development'.
>
> (UNDP Report 2010, summary p. 1)

As someone who has spent much of her life working with, and researching into children and their well-being, I think now is the time to look to the future. What impact will declining fertility rates have on the world's children? In a world where there are more lone children or children with only one brother or sister how will this impact on their development? What do we know about the psychological and educational outcomes of lone children? What role do siblings play in family life and what will be missing if they do not have them? What stresses will they bear as they carry the aspirations of their parents and grandparents? How will this impact on their well-being? How will gender preference influence the future number of boys and girls? What consequences will there be on society in a world populated by children who may be more 'indulged'?

Overall the story is one of good news for children. Partly because of the decline in fertility, children of the world are less likely to die young, less likely to experience extreme poverty. Overall children are living longer, healthier and better educated. But hidden behind the good news are some darker stories. The international and national averages of child well-being hide gross inequalities, selective abortion as a result of gender preference and higher mortality for girls. For the individual lone child, psychological research suggests that the outlook is mostly positive. Lone children, disproving the stereotype of 'little emperors' and 'little princesses', are mainly sociable and high achievers. But here too there is also a darker side. In societies where a high value is placed on educational achievement, those who do not make the grade may be at risk of child abuse, high levels of stress and, in extreme cases, suicide.

This chapter will first take a macro-view of the impact of low fertility on children in the international context. It will explore the dramatic improvements, but it will also consider the evidence of less welcome, often unintended consequences. The second half of the chapter will explore the psychological impact on the child, both the good news and less good. The final section will consider how smaller families and greater prosperity is associated with more liberal values and the possible consequences of these changing values.

Taking a macro-view

In anticipating how children will fare in a world of low fertility, we need to be aware of the larger picture: in particular, the fast-moving global economic and social changes. As we saw in the Mumsnet responses, in Chapter 6, parents today are living and adapting to change. These associated trends are interacting with the decline in fertility and are strongly influencing child outcomes. As a recent document from the Economic and Social Council of the United Nations noted:

> The medium-term effects of fertility reductions on economic growth in both developed and developing countries are estimated to account for about 20 per cent of per capita output growth between 1960 and 1995. Declining fertility has also contributed to poverty reduction. Between 1960 and 2000, demographic change alone accounted for a 14 per cent drop in poverty levels in developing countries and could produce an additional 14 per cent reduction during 2000 to 2015.
>
> (United Nations 2011, p. 1)

The UN Development Report (UNDP 2010) notes rapid progress around the world as measured by the Human Development Index (HDI). This index measures development by combining life expectancy, educational attainment and income into a composite indicator. Are children living longer? Are they better educated? Are they less poor?

The world's average HDI has increased by 18 per cent since 1990 and 41 per cent since 1970 (UNDP 2010, p. 3). But not all countries have seen such rapid progress. Amongst those experiencing slower progress are countries with high birth rates and other areas struck by the HIV epidemic. Overall mortality rates have fallen faster in infants and children than in adults. If mortality rates of the 1970s were applied today, nearly

7 million more children would have died. The decline in infant mortality is faster in developed countries. In developing countries, where fertility and poverty is likely to be higher, there are eight times more infant deaths. So the good news is that children globally are generally healthier, better educated and less poor.

The darker side of the story is that the HDI does not measure the gross inequalities *within* countries. If we are concerned about the well-being of *all children*, we need to look beyond the national figures. The overall level of inequality in a country, region or population group – and more generally the distribution of consumption, income or other attributes which is an important dimension of welfare – can be indicated by the Gini Index. The index used by the United Nations Development Report (UNDP 2009), broadly speaking, measures difference in consumption between the richest 10 per cent in a country and the poorest 10 per cent. The lower the score, the smaller the difference between the richest and the poorest. While Norway topped the list under the HDI, their Gini index at 25.8 (UNDP 2009), assessed during 1992–2007, shows that there was a level of inequality which was marginally higher than Sweden at 25. Levels of inequality are considerably higher in the USA at 40.8, which is very similar to China at 41.5 (UNDP 2009).

What does this mean for children? For some in the developing world, this may mean lacking the basic essentials: food and health care. In the developed world, the basic essentials may be there but the impact of 'relative poverty' is more subtle. Psychologically, children are divided into the 'haves', 'have less' and 'have nots'.

Poverty as a predictor of child outcomes

Poverty is strongly associated with poor child outcomes. Inadequate nutrition impacts on both children's physical development, their ability to learn, and in adulthood their ability to work and be productive. Traditionally, large families have long been linked to child poverty and a range of negative outcomes for children. Hatton and Martin (2010), for example, concluded in a major study that the improvement in the health of UK children in the first half of the twentieth century was strongly based on the reduction of poverty associated with a reduction in family size. Bradshaw et al. (2006) found that UK children in large families had a poverty risk more than twice as high as children in small families. Further afield Bradshaw et al. (2010) confirms similar findings in a study in Georgia. While 23 per cent of children without siblings and 26 per cent of children with only one sibling are poor, the poverty rate jumps to 34 per cent for children with two siblings and to 44 per cent for those with three or more siblings. These findings are reflected in studies that have informed UNICEF (Gordon et al. 2005).

Smaller families, where this means less child poverty, have generally improved outcomes for children, but as we have seen, even in countries with low fertility, there are considerable inequalities. The important fact is that many small families are also poor. Brooks-Gunn et al. (1997) showed that in any given year, 1987–96, about one in five of all American children lived below the poverty threshold. In 1993, this figure was a little under $12,000 for a family of three people. What does 'poverty' mean? UNICEF quotes the European Union (1984) definition of poverty: 'the poor are those whose resources (material, cultural, and social) are so limited as to exclude them from the minimum acceptable way of life in the Member States in which they live' (UNICEF 2007, p. 6). For practical and statistical purposes, this has usually meant drawing national poverty lines at a certain percentage of national median income. There are many other definitions, but practically Brooks-Gunn et al. (1997, p. 2) found that families who were poor 'could not buy toys, books... parents who were poor might have poor emotional health, be more depressed more irritable leading to less consistent parenting, more punitive behaviour'. The hard fact of 'not having what other children have' interacts with poor parenting.

Family income and educational attainment is also strongly associated with educational outcomes for children (e.g. Blanden and Gregg 2004). In the United Kingdom, a simple measure of poverty is whether a child receives Free School Meals (FSMs) at school. Any child whose family is on one sort of welfare benefit or another is eligible to receive a free meal in the middle of the day at school. Children who receive FSMs do less well than those who pay for their own meals. In London, for example, the proportion of 11-year-olds reaching Level 4 – the expected level of attainment in English, Maths and Science – is between 30 per cent and 40 per cent lower among pupils eligible for FSMs than among other pupils (Department of Children Schools and Families 2010). These children may go on to fail in secondary school and later have difficulty in finding work.

Although some of the children on FSMs may come from large families, in the United Kingdom many of these families will be headed by a single (never married) or lone (separated, divorced or widowed) parent with between one or two children. In 2002 there were an estimated 1.75 million lone parents (single and separated, divorced or widowed) in the United Kingdom with about 2.9 million dependent children. The United

Kingdom has the highest rate of teenage parents (age 15–19) in Europe. The socio-economic and health impacts of lone parenthood in the case of teenage mothers are likely to be particularly negative. Evidence shows that former teenage mothers show higher levels of physical and mental ill health by the age of 30. Across countries the lone parent is particularly disadvantaged (de Paz Nieves et al. 2009).

The gender debate – the preference for boys

Another dark fact of fertility decline is the impact of gender preference. In strongly patriarchal societies, where the cultural and economic value of sons is at a premium, the preference for a son manifests itself in many ways, ranging from differential allocation of household resources, medical care and neglect of girl children to female infanticide. In addition, with the increasing availability of ultrasound in the mid-1980s, sex determination followed by sex-selective abortion began to become widespread (Miller 2001).

Men normally have higher mortality rates than women throughout life, and age-specific sex ratio declines gradually as age increases. Therefore, in most countries in the world there are more women than men, and normal sex ratio in the general population is around or below 100. In 2005, in North and South America, Africa, Europe and Oceania, sex ratio in the general population was around 100 or lower (UNFPA CHINA 2007).

'Normal' sex ratio *at birth* is in general between 103 and 107 male live births per 100 female live births. Countries that are known to have a high male-female sex ratio include South Korea (peak of 115.2 in 1943), India (112 in 2004) and China (120.5 in 2005) (UNFPA CHINA 2007).

In China according to the five censuses and three 1 per cent population sample surveys, sex ratio in the general population has been high throughout the last 50 years (UNFPA CHINA 2007).

Sex ratio at birth in China has increased over the past two decades, from 107.6 in 1982 to 120.5 in 2005. There is a major difference between urban and rural populations with more boys being born in rural areas. In 2005, sex ratio at birth of rural areas reached 122.9. Sex ratio at birth of urban areas, however, has also increased dramatically, from 109.9 in 1990 to 117.1 in 2005 (UNFPA CHINA 2007).

Generally, the sex ratio of second and later children is around the normal sex ratio at birth. However, in countries with an imbalance in sex ratio at birth, the imbalance increases remarkably with the rise in birth order. In South Korea in 1994, sex ratio at birth for the first birth was normal at 106.1, but increased to 114.3 for the second and 205.6 for the third birth. In 1992, sex ratio for the fourth birth in South Korea was an astonishing 229 (Hesketh and Xing 2006).

Since the early 1980s, the use of sex-selective abortion has increased in many Asian contexts. Estimates indicate that several million female foetuses were aborted in the last two decades of the twentieth century (Miller 2001). Since the 1980s, the ultra-sound B machine has gradually become accessible and affordable, making it possible to identify the sex of the foetus. While sex selection for non-medical reasons was made illegal in most countries since the 1990s, it still continues to be used.

Korea, however, has managed to reduce the trend. In a study by the World Bank (Chung and Das Gupt 2007), the most important factor in the changing attitudes towards girls appeared to be the radical shift in the country's economy, which opened the doors to women in the workforce and dismantled long-held traditions. The Korean government played a small role starting in the 1970s. After growing alarm by the rise in sex-preference abortions, leaders mounted campaigns to change people's attitudes, including one that featured the popular slogan 'One daughter raised well is worth 10 sons!' In 1987, the Korean government banned doctors from revealing the sex of a foetus before birth. But experts say enforcement was lax because officials feared too many doctors would be caught. Demographers say the rapid change in South Koreans' feelings about female babies gives them hope that sex imbalances will begin to shrink in other rapidly developing Asian countries. Similar programmes to promote the value of the girl child are being tested elsewhere and in various areas in China (Buchanan 2009).

Meanwhile, discriminatory treatment against girls, especially access to medical care, has also contributed to excess female child mortality. In the world as a whole, the death rate for boys of all age groups is higher than those of girls because of biological factors. Normally, the male to female ratio of mortality rate for children under five years is greater than one. Some countries with a high sex ratio in the general population are however witnessing lower than expected mortality in boys under five. In India in 1998, the sex ratio of mortality rate for age one to four was 0.687, that is less boys but more girls were dying than expected. In Pakistan, the ratio for age one to four was 0.70 during 1982 and 1986, and 0.63 during 1997 and 2008. What this means is that better care for boys around infancy and in early childhood means more boys are surviving in adulthood than girls. A study in India has shown that girls with older sisters are subject to the highest risk of mortality (Arnold et al. 1998).

These issues raise further concerns. In countries with a shortage of girls this may impact further on the security and safety of women, and the girl child's right to life, participation and development may be denied. An imbalanced sex ratio may stimulate sexual violence, abduction and rise in the trafficking of women and girls. It is also predicted that many men may fail to get married due to a shortage of women. In China they talk of 'Bare Branches', the young men who are unlikely to find a wife (Jin 2010). As my guide in a rural area of China said to me: 'who will marry me? I am small, not good-looking and I do not have a grand apartment or car. Girls all want these things today.' In China there is concern that dissatisfaction amongst these young men will not be conducive to a harmonious society (Hesketh and Xing 2006).

How will lone children fare? The micro-picture

Moving from the macro-picture of the impact of low fertility, we may wonder how individual lone children fare. What impact does having no brothers or sisters have on the modern child? Historically, only children have been portrayed as having undesirable personalities and social behaviours. History is replete with harsh stereotypes of the self-centred, selfish only child. Stanley Hall, one of the early developmental psychologists in the USA, reportedly said that to be an only child 'was a disease in itself' (Fenton 1928).

Concern grew in China following the one child policy that there would be a nation of 'little emperors' and 'little princesses'; children so overindulged by their parents that they would be unable to function in a group setting. As Jones notes in Chapter 4, the one child family is very common in other East Asian countries where there have been no such policies.

Despite historical views, psychological research demonstrates that the earlier negative opinion of the lone child is not supported. Toni Falbo from the USA, in a series of high quality studies, has spent much of her academic career disproving the stereotype of the self-centred, selfish only child. In a meta-analysis (Falbo and Polit 1986) of 115 studies measuring achievement, adjustment, character, intelligence, parent-child relationships and sociability, only children surpassed all others except first-borns on achievement and intelligence, and across all developmental outcomes only children were found to be indistinguishable from first-borns and people from small families. However, she found, as with all families, that parent–child relationships were critical.

In 2009, Falbo, Kim and Chen explored the sibling status effects on health in later life in a study of 3968 graduates of 1957, who had taken part in the Wisconsin Longitudinal Study. She found that although there were differences in health status in later life (oldest and only children were generally healthier), these were probably best understood as reflective of educational attainments, higher economic status or origin.

More recently she has been exploring the academic performance and personality traits of only children in China. In the Chinese study, only children from the town of Beijing had higher scores in achievement and height when compared to their peers with siblings. Children from the rural area of Jinil Province, however, did not show the only-child advantages in achievement. None of her analyses indicated only children had undesirable personalities as judged by teachers and mothers. The difference seen between urban and rural children may be more to do with income and educational opportunities than family size (Falbo and Poston 1993).

Doh and Falbo (1999) undertook a further study in Korea. This compared the social competence of sixth graders who had no siblings with those who did. The three factors of social competence considered in this study were: popularity, sociability, and brattiness. 'Brattiness', an interesting new measure, was identified by four questions 'Often becomes angry when playing with his/her friends'; 'has everything his/her own way when playing with his/her friends'; 'sometimes reacts with temper tantrums'; 'tends to be selfish'. Only children were found to score similarly to others on popularity and sociability, but scored worse than others on the 'Brattiness' scale. Although Fablo felt there may be a cultural explanation for this finding, it may be worth further exploration.

What difference do siblings make?

Traditionally, the wider family has always been at the front line of family support. In a study using data from the National Child Development Study (Buchanan and Ten Brinke 1997), the wider family was the first port of call for a range of problems. The question here is what difference do siblings make? A key issue is whether they give support to each other as they progress through life. Basically, the findings are mixed but in adversity and in later life sibling support appears to be important.

Dunn et al. (1994) using the Cambridge Sibling Study tracked sibling relationships from pre-school through childhood and early adolescence and found that some children were affectionate and supportive to their siblings, whereas others were extremely hostile and aggressive. They found considerable continuity of sibling positive and negative behaviours seen from early childhood into adolescence. Where there were family adversities, maternal illness, marital disharmony and divorce and/or difficult stepchildren relationships, relationships between siblings became closer. In Boer and Dunn (1992), it was shown that across the life span, the majority of individuals reported feeling close to their siblings, yet only a small number depended on their siblings for intimate companionship or for financial, emotional or physical assistance when they were adults. However, certain life experiences (e.g. never marrying, having no children, becoming widowed or experiencing divorce) could produce closer contact and greater feelings of closeness among siblings. For the majority of siblings, their interaction with adult brothers and sisters was positive and appeared to lead to the development of an affectionate life-long bond.

Earlier work by Cicirelli (1982) noted that most siblings feel close to others, with the least closeness between brothers and sisters and the most between sisters. He hypothesized that siblings were socialized within the family in early life to behave in a certain way, and these behaviours continue through the life span. Van Gaalen, Dykstra and Flap (2008) in a study using the Netherlands Kinship Panel Study note that 'the sibling tie is the family relationship with the longest duration'. Although parental relationships are essentially dyadically based, they are subject to the influence of the network in which they are embedded. Siblings may be an important part of that network. Wellmann and Wortley (1989) in a study of Toronto social networks found kin were providing five types of sibling support: emotional aid; services; financial aid; companionship, housing or job information; and complementary parenting to children. Nearly a quarter of emotionally supportive relations were provided by siblings.

As with all family relationships, Fingerman, Hay and Birditt (2004) note that close family relationships can be both the best of ties and the worst. Family members who become overly involved with an individual stressful life event may exacerbate the stressor effect.

Stress

Falbo's (e.g. Falbo and Polit 1986) research demonstrates that only children are generally social and well adjusted, when compared with children with siblings. Much of her earlier research took place in the

USA with local samples. Although education is highly valued in the USA, culturally the value attached to attainment is particularly high in some Asian societies. For only children, in the highly competitive environment of Beijing and other East Asian countries, this may have come at a heavy price.

The Confucian tradition, so central in many Asian societies, emphasizes education and study (e.g. Legge 1893). Confucius disparaged those who had faith in intuition and argued that the only real understanding of a subject comes from long and careful study.

It is one of the enduring global dilemmas, that as standards of health, education and wealth rise (Layard 2006), levels of happiness fall and the numbers of those with mental health problems increase. Children in the fast developing tiger countries brought up under the Confucian tradition may experience additional stressors to achieve, and only children, who must satisfy the aspirations of all their grandparents, may be under particular pressure. Hesketh, Zhen, Lu Dong, Jun and Xing (2009) undertook a study of 2191 9–12-year olds in primary school in urban and rural areas of the Zheijiang Province in Eastern China. The vast majority of these children were 'onlys'. Eighty-one per cent worried 'a lot' about exams; 63 per cent were afraid of punishment by their teachers; and 73 per cent were physically punished by their parents. They noted particular concerns about the 8 per cent of children who scored near maximum points on the stress scale. The authors concluded that the competitive and punitive educational environment led to high levels of stress and psychosomatic symptoms.

In an earlier paper Hesketh et al. (2002) noted that the suicide rate in China is estimated to be around three times the global average, with women in the 15- to 24-year-old age group particularly vulnerable. In her study of 1576 adolescents, one-third of the students had suffered symptoms of severe depression, with 16 per cent admitting to suicide ideation and 9 per cent to actually having attempted this. There was very little professional help available. Most young people sought help from family and friends.

World values survey: changing family values

Another feature of rising Gross Domestic Productivity (GDPs) is a globalization of family values. The dilemma here is that although we may welcome some of these changes, they pose particular problems in societies who have depended on intergenerational cohesiveness to support their elderly.

One important source of this information is based on global surveys of mass values and attitudes. From 1981 to 2007, the World Values Survey and the European Values Study carried out five waves of representative national surveys covering almost 90 per cent of the world population. The values survey demonstrates that the views of people living in rich countries differ markedly from those of low-income societies across a wide range of norms (Inglehart and Welzel 2009). The differences run along two dimensions. The poorer countries generally support traditional values (emphasizing religion, traditional values about family and parenthood, respect for obedience to authority values; they tend to reject abortion and have high levels of national pride), while the richer generally support more secular values. The other dimension is 'survival versus self expression'. In poor countries, survival gives top priority to economic and physical security and conformist social norms. In richer countries, self-expression values give high priority to freedom of expression, gender equality and tolerances of homosexuals and minorities. The findings show that to a remarkable degree, the values and beliefs of a given society reflect its level of economic development. When the positions of given countries in successive waves of the values survey from 1981 to 2007 are compared, one finds that almost all of the countries that experienced rising per capita GDP also experienced predictable changes in their values.

The challenge to Asian Confucian values

Recently studies, for example, from Korea (Sung 1990), Taiwan (Wang 2011), Japan (Yamato 2006) and China (Ting 2009) are showing that Asian attitudes to elder care are changing. These changes may be related to greater longevity in the elderly, higher numbers of women working, better education and greater social and geographic mobility. But one of the reasons attributed to changing values is that the declining fertility rate has placed heavy responsibilities on lone children (Ting 2009).

As we see in Chapter 13 (Harper), the increasing numbers of elders and the 'democratic deficit' is a worldwide concern. The stereotypical view is that modern Western cultures valued individualism and independence, whereas Asian cultures value familism, filial piety and interdependence within the family. It is felt that the development of the welfare state in modern westernized societies emerged from the Western cultural emphasis on individualism and independence (Yamato 2006), whereas in East Asian societies the family is the fundamental unit for people's welfare (Liu and Keding 2000).

In post-war Japan, however, social changes have transformed people's attitudes and more people are seeing elderly dependence on children as less desirable (Yamato 2006). In Taiwan (Wang 2011), as the country's fertility rate has dropped dramatically since 2005 (Net Fertility Rate is now near one), the idea of sending elderly parents to an institution has become more acceptable. Whereas in 1985, 91.6 per cent felt this was very wrong, only 46.5 per cent considered it so in 2005. In Japan (Yamato 2006), there is evidence that the elderly are now more reluctant to accept financial support from their children. In Hong Kong, in a major review of the literature on filial piety, the author notes that socio-demographic changes make it increasingly difficult for families to take care of elderly members, and these changes have fundamentally altered the relationships between adult children and their parents (Ting 2009).

Globalization has accelerated the erosion of filial piety, but whether this is the result of young people adopting Western secular values or whether it is the result of children from smaller families being able to be more self-centred and individualistic, is debatable.

Conclusion

As noted at the beginning of the chapter, the macro-picture shows that the impact of declining fertility is generally good news for children. With smaller families, more will survive infancy and childhood; fewer families will be economically challenged, and more children will be healthier and better educated. There remains a big divide between those who have, those who have less, and those who have little. Poverty impacts in many ways but in both the developed and developing world, those who have less have poorer health, poorer education and can remain socially excluded from the wider society. Policies that move to bring about greater well-being for all children, especially those in disadvantaged areas, will bring further advantages both to the families and, as will be discussed later, a society's economic development. Some of these poor families are also small families.

The darker side of the decline in fertility is that gender preference may, in some societies, lead to selective abortion of female foetuses and discrimination and poor health care for girl children. Interventions, however, are showing that it is possible to reverse attitudes and to increase the value attributed to the female child. Selective abortion may also lead to a surplus of men who will be unable to find wives and with this comes the possibility of increased levels of violence and instability.

Psychological research also reports good outcomes for lone children and children of smaller families. Lone children, contrary to the stereotypes, are generally shown to be high achieving, sociable and competent but with a possible tendency to 'brattiness'. The paradox is that worldwide, despite improving levels of health, wealth and education, populations are less 'happy', and growing numbers are succumbing to mental illness. For many lone children, educational aspirations of parents and grandparents has led to high levels of stress, and for a few this has resulted in higher than expected levels of mental illness and suicide. Global studies (Patel et al. 2007) show that mental disorders account for a large proportion of the disease burden in young people in all societies. Addressing young people's mental-health needs is crucial if they are to fulfil their potential and contribute fully to the development of their communities.

The increased economic well-being that is associated with smaller families is also associated with a dramatic change in values. Across the world, as fertility declines and families are generally better off, there has been a global shift from more traditional values (emphasizing religion, family and parenthood and respect for obedience to authority tending to reject abortion, and having high levels of national pride) to more secular values. There has also been a dramatic shift from values emphasizing survival (where top priority is given to economic and physical security and conformist social norms) to self-expression values where priority is given to freedom of expression, gender equality and greater tolerance of homosexuals and minorities. Although cultural values influence these considerations, the World Values Survey has shown that as prosperity increases, values become more liberal. In Asian societies where filial piety has, in the past, ensured good care of the elderly, erosion of Confucian values and a growing reluctance to care for parents may cause considerable problems. As already shown, research studies are showing that the state is less able to rely on 'filial piety' to support their elderly.

Apart from the care of the elderly, it is debatable whether these changing values are good news or bad. It is certain that all authorities to date feel they are unlikely to be reversed. The brave new world may be more a self-centred global community. There will be more divorces and more children born outside marriage. The State in all societies may have to step in to help care for those unable to look after themselves. But against that there will be greater gender equality, more liberal attitudes to homosexuals, and more acceptance of immigrants. Overall, bankers permitting, the world will be more prosperous, children better educated and healthier and fewer babies will die.

Maybe this will give us the opportunity to focus on the children who in the past have not done so well. This may not happen for traditional humanitarian reasons, but it will happen because every child will be needed. The economic reality of a shrinking workforce will force us to do what we have to do to maximize the potential of every child and make time for children. But that is the subject of the last chapter (Chapter 18).

References

Arnold, F., Choe, M. K. and Roy, T. K. (1998). Son preference, the family-building process and child mortality in India. *Population Studies*, 52: 301–15.

Blanden, J. and Gregg, P. (2004). Family income and educational attainment: a review of approaches and evidence for Britain. CEEDP, 41. Centre for the Economics of Education, London School of Economics and Political Science, London, UK.

Boer, F. and Dunn, J. (eds) (1992). *Children's Relationships with Siblings: Developmental and Clinical Issues*. Hillsdale, NJ: Erlbaum.

Bradshaw, J., Chzhen, Y., Gugushyili, D. and Hoelscher, P. (2010). Child Poverty in Georgia. Working Paper No. EC 2412, University of York, http://www.york.ac.uk/inst/spru/research/extreme/CP5.pdf

Bradshaw, J., Finch, N., Mayhew, E., Ritakallio, V. and Skinner, C. (2006). *Child Poverty in Large Families*. Bristol: Policy Press.

Brooks-Gunn, J., Duncan, G. J. and Maritato, N. (1997). Poor families, poor outcomes: the well-being of children and youth. In J. Brooks-Gunn and G. Duncan (eds) *Consequences of Growing Up Poor* (pp. 1–17). New York, NY: Russell Sage.

Buchanan, A. (2009). Student's MSc thesis, Department of Social Policy and Intervention, University of Oxford.

Buchanan, A. and Ten Brinke, J. (1997). *What Happened When They Were Grown Up?* York: Joseph Rowntree Foundation/York Publishing.

Cicirelli, V. G. (1982). Sibling influence throughout lifespan. In M. E. Lamb and Sutton-Smith (eds) *Sibling Relationships: Their Nature and Significance across the Lifespan* (pp. 267–84). Hillsdale, NJ: Lawrence Erlbaum.

Chung, W. and Das Gupt, M. (2007). Why is son preference declining in South Korea? The role of development and public policy, and the implications for China and India. Policy Research Working Paper 4373. The World Bank, Washington DC, USA.

de Paz Nieves, C, Otano, C., Coutts, A. and Suhrcke, M. (2009). Lone parents in the UK: the impact of the New Deal for Lone Parents (NDLP) on socioeconomic and health inequalities (Background Report to the Marmot Review). Research Report.

Department for Children Schools and Families 2008–09 (2010). National Pupil database. www.londonspovertyprofile.org.uk/indicators/topics/low-educational-outcomes/statistical-releases-from-dcsf-dcsf-performance-tables/, accessed 12 March 2012.

Doh, H. S. and Falbo, T. (1999) Social competence, maternal attentiveness and overprotectedness: only children in Korea. *International Journal of Behavioral Development,* 23(1): 149–62.

Dunn, J., Slomkowski, C. and Beardsall, L. (1994). Sibling relationships from the preschool period through middle childhood and early adolescence. *Developmental Psychology*, 30: 315–24.

Falbo, T. and Polit, D. (1986). Quantitative review of the only child literature: research evidence and theory development. *Psychological Bulletin*, 100: 176–89.

Falbo, T. and Poston, D. L. (1993). The academic, personality, and physical outcomes of only children in China. *Child Development*, 64: 18–35.

Falbo, T., Kim, S. H. and Chen, K. (2009). Alternate models of sibling status. Effects on health in later life. *Developmental Psychology*, 45(3): 677–87.

Fenton, N. (1928) The only child. *Journal of Genetic Psychology*, 35: 546–56.

Fingerman, K. L., Hay, E. L. and Birditt, K. S. (2004). The best of ties, the worst of ties: close, problematic, and ambivalent social relationships. *Journal of Marriage and the Family*, 66: 792–808.

Gordon, D., Irving, M., Nandy, S. and Townsend, P. (2005). Multidimensional measures of child poverty. International Conference on The Many Dimensions of Poverty, 29–31 August 2005, Brasilia, Brazil.

Hatton, T. and Martin, R. (2010). The Effects on stature of parents, family size and birth order: British children in the 1930s. *Oxford Economic Papers*, 62(1): 157–84.

Hesketh, T., Ding, Q. J. and Jenkins, R. (2002). Suicide ideation in Chinese adolescents. *Social Psychiatry and Psychiatric Epidemiology*, 37(5): 230–5.

Hesketh, T. and Xing, Z. W. (2006). Abnormal sex ratios in human populations: causes and consequences. *Proceedings of the National Academy of Sciences of the United States of America*, 103(36): 13271–5.

Hesketh, T., Zhen, Y., Lu, L., Dong, Z. X., Jun, Y. X. and Xing, Z. W. (2009). Stress and psychosomatic symptoms in Chinese school children: cross sectional survey. *Archives of Disease in Childhood*, 95(2): 136–40.

Layard, P. R. G. (2006). *Happiness: Lessons from a New Science*. New Jersey: Penguin Group USA.

Inglehart, R. and Welzel, C. (2009). Development and democracy: what we know about modernization today. *Foreign Affairs*, 8: 33–41.

Jin, Xiaoyi (2010). Aggregation of bare branches and public security in rural communities: findings from survey in hundreds of villages. Paper for the conference on Family Change in the Wake of Demographic Transition. Institute of Population and Labor Economics, CASS September 17–18, Beijing.

Legge, J. (1893). *Lun Yu (The Analects)*. Oxford: Clarendon Press.

Liu, W. T. and Keding, H. (2000). Critical issues of caregiving: east-west dialogues. In William T. Liu and Hal Keding (eds) *Who Shall Care for the Elderly? An East-West Value Divide* (pp. 1–23). Singapore: Singapore University Press.

Miller, B. D. (2001). Female-selective abortion in Asia: patterns, policies, and debates. *American Anthropologist*, 103(4): 1083–95.

Patel, V., Flisher, A. J., Hetrick, S. and McGorry, P. (2007). Mental health of young people: a global public-health challenge. *Lancet*, 369: 1302–13.

Sung, K.-T. (1990). Measures and dimensions of Filial Piety in Korea. *The Gerontologist*, 35(2): 240–7.

Ting, K.-F. (2009). A Review on the literature on Filial Piety, Central Policy Unity, Government of Hong Kong. http://www.cpu.gov.hk/chs/documents/new/press/Filial%20Piety%20Literature.pdf, accessed 12 March 2012.

UNFPA CHINA (2007). *Sex Ratio – Facts and Figures*, UN China: UNFPA.

UNICEF (2007). Child poverty in perspective: an overview of child well-being in rich countries, Innocenti Report Card 7, 2007. UNICEF Innocenti Research Centre, Florence, CEF.

United National Development Programme (2009). UNDP Report 2009 Gini Index http://hdrstats.undp.org/en/indicators/161.html, accessed 12 March 2012.

United National Development Programme (2010). UNDP Report 2010. http://hdr.undp.org/en/reports/global/hdr2010/chapters/en/, accessed 12 March 2012.

United Nations (2011). Commission on population and development to discuss impact of growing disparities. UN Economic and Social Council POP/990. http://www.un.org/News/Press/docs/2011/pop990.doc.htm, accessed 12 March 2012.

Van Gaalen, R. I., Dykstra, P. A and Flap, H. (2008). Intergenerational contact beyond the dyad: the role of the sibling network. *European Journal of Ageing*, 5: 19–29.

Wang, K. Y.-T. (2011). Child care and elder arrangements in Taiwan. *Journal of Comparative Social Welfare*, 27(2): 165–74.

Wellmann, B. and Wortley, S. (1989). Brothers' keepers: situating kinship relations in broader networks of social support. *Sociological Perspectives*, 32: 273–306.

Yamato, R. (2006). Changing attitudes towards elderly dependence in postwar Japan. *Current Sociology*, March 2006, 54(2): 273–91.

13
Falling Fertility, Ageing and Europe's Demographic Deficit

Sarah Harper

Introduction

By the middle of the twenty-first century, the proportion of young people globally will have fallen to less than 20 per cent. Correspondingly, the proportion aged over 60 will have increased to more than one-fifth, standing at some 2 billion older adults. This increase is through a combination of two demographic trends: falling fertility, which reduces the percentage of younger people in the population, and falling mortality, which has increased average life expectancy, and thus the number of people surviving to older and older ages. A trend which started in Europe over 200 years ago has now spread across the globe to all regions bar sub-Saharan Africa, fuelled by a fall in Total Fertility Rates (TFR), that is, the number of children per reproductive women, requiring 2.1 for replacement. In 1950, Europe's TFR was 2.5 children per reproductive woman. This has fallen to 1.5 (2010). Future fertility is difficult to estimate: projected TFRs are between 1.34 and 2.34 children per woman by 2045 (Lutz et al. 2001). Alongside the well-recognized low fertility of Western Europe, with all countries below replacement level, and southern Mediterranean countries in particular at 1.2 and 1.3, we see a similar pattern emerging in Asia. Singapore and Korea have now fallen to below 1.2, while Hong Kong, at below 1, now has the lowest TFR in the world. Even the Islamic countries of Pakistan and Afghanistan with current TFRs of 4.0 and 6.6, respectively, are predicted to halve to just above replacement by 2050. Thus the number of children being born per women has fallen significantly – with most countries in Europe, and many in Asia and the Americas now having below replacement level fertility, with less than two children per woman of reproductive age. TFR in Vietnam and Thailand, for example, has now dropped to below that of many EU countries. Some demographers have expressed the hypothesis that a very low fertility rate could become irreversible (Lutz et al. 2005).

The economic impact of these figures will be felt at the national, regional and global levels. Particularly concerning is the effect in low and middle income countries, which are now showing signs of population ageing driven by falling fertility and are likely to have European-style old age structures by the middle decades of the century. Interest focuses around the demographic deficit caused by this ageing. It is argued that population ageing leads to both a decline in economic activity, due to the proportionate fall of young workers in the population, and growth in economic burden, due to increased requirement for pensions and health care. This is based on the perception that human capital and productivity increasingly decline at older ages, particularly beyond age 70, and that disability and ill health increases at older ages.

The global proportion aged under 15 fell from 34 per cent in 1950 to 27 per cent in 2010 and is predicted to stand at 20 per cent by 2050. This has been accompanied by an increase in older people. In 1950, the global percentage of people aged over 60, 65 and 80 was 8 per cent, 5 per cent and 0.6 per cent, respectively. In 2010 this had reached 11 per cent, 8 per cent and 1.5 per cent, and is predicted at 22 per cent, 16 per cent and 4.3 per cent by 2050. The historically unprecedented relationship of a world with older people (aged 60 or over) than children (aged under 15) will be reached by the mid-century. This has already been reached in the developed regions, where in 2010 21 per cent were aged 60 or over, and 17 per cent aged under 15, and this is projected to stand at 33 per cent and 15 per cent by 2050, when there will be twice as many older people as young. Here the proportion of 'working age' (15–59) will decline from 62 per cent to 52 per cent. The proviso here is that by 2050 age 60 may no longer be a meaningful definition for 'old age', and the 'working age' population may be significantly extended beyond these boundaries. Corresponding figures for the less developed regions were 6 per cent in 1950, 8 per cent in 2010, 20 per cent by 2050 for those aged 60 or over, and 37 per cent in 1950, 30 per cent in 2010, 20 per cent by 2050 for those aged under 15. By the middle of the century, there will thus be equal young and old dependents in these regions both standing at one-fifth.

Across all regions, declining fertility will eventually lead to a shift in the support ratio between the workers and the elderly dependents, and it is argued that this will result in slower economic growth, inadequate investment in human capital, inefficiency in labour markets, reduced consumption and unsustainable public transfer systems providing pensions and long-term care. This is because an individual's needs and contributions vary over their lives. People tend to consume more when they are young (goods and education) and old (health) and produce more in their middle years (economic productivity). Thus, as a country moves from large proportions of working adults to large proportions of older people, it will experience slower economic growth. This chapter will consider in some detail the arguments around the so-called 'demographic deficit', taking the case of Europe.

Europe's falling fertility

There should be no surprise that fertility has fallen so significantly in Europe, as the current age structures, which we now face, are those associated with the late stage of the *demographic transition* (Bloom et al. 2003; Pool 2005). There is significant debate both around the drivers of this transition and the identification of a *second demographic transition* (Bongaarts and Feeney 1998; Bucht 1996; Cliquet 1991; Lutz and Goldstein 2004; Van de Kaa 1987; Vaupel and Lundström 1996). Typically associated with economic development is the decrease in both mortality and fertility rates. Mortality rates fall first, including infant mortality, enabling the survival of large birth cohorts into adulthood. Then due to a variety of interrelated factors fertility rates fall. There seems to be a strong relationship between falling infant mortality and women's choice to bear few babies. This arises when mothers realize that if they bear eight babies and all survive then they will have to raise eight children. Their preference is to raise a smaller number of healthy children in whom they can invest. Education of girls enables them to gain skills and to enter the economic labour market; they are introduced to different ways of living, which do not include endless childbearing. It also reduces the age of first marriage. In particular, it changes people's mindsets so they are more open to ideas around family planning and delaying and spacing children. This was termed 'Ideational Change' by Caldwell, who identified this as the foremost factor in reducing TFRs. As fertility falls, population growth levels of; the profile of the population ages, as late-life mortality rates fall and individuals survive to increasingly older ages.

If we take an age structural change perspective, we can view population change in terms of a shift between providers and dependents – the dependency ratio – and how this will typically move from a large percentage of young to a large percentage of old dependents during the demographic transition. Some have raised concern that this will lead to a so-called 'demographic deficit', whereby societies will not have sufficient younger workers to drive their economies and to support their increasingly older populations.

Dependency ratios

Dependency ratios are a useful measure of those in and out of economic productivity.

Elderly Dependency Ratios (EDR) measure the number of persons of working age (aged 15–64) per person aged 65 or over. For many countries, the rise in the EDRs will be significant. It is forecasted to almost double in Africa, Europe, Northern America and Oceania and to almost triple in Asia, while it will be more than triple in Latin America and the Caribbean. By 2050, the ratio of persons aged 65 or over to those of working age is projected to grow from currently 6:100 to 11:100 in Africa, from 10:100 to 27:100 in Asia, from 10:100 to 31:100 in Latin America and the Caribbean, from 16:100 to 30:100 in Oceania, from 19:100 to 36:100 in Northern America and from 24:100 to 47:100 in Europe. The next decade will thus see a rapid shift towards increased EDRs in most industrialized countries. The EU-25 EDR is set to double and reach 51 per cent by 2050, as the working-age population (15–64 years), decreases by 48 million between now and 2050, and the EU-25 will change from having four to only two persons of working age for each citizen aged 65 and above (European Commission 2006). Many see the *demographic deficit* as having negative implications for Europe (Lee and Mason 2010). The concerns fall into two broad themes. Some argue that a decline in population numbers due to falling fertility, particularly in the percentage of young people and thus young workers, will lead to a decline in economic activity. The second group argue that this fertility decline is leading to population ageing, with a growing economic burden arising from the increased need for pensions and health care.

Falling fertility leads to decline in economic activity

There is an assumption that declining populations can have dramatic negative effects, via declining demand on economic growth and employment (Chesnais 1998; Fina-Sanglas 2000). This they argue can have negative psychological effects on investors, which may affect some strategic activities such as the building industry, and slow down the growth of many other markets to the detriment of the productive economy (Fina-Sanglas 2000). This is, however, contested by those who argue that in a modern, industrial economy aggregate demand depends on aggregate incomes rather than on the number of people. It is also argued that in a modern, open economy the extent of the markets does not depend on the number of domestic consumers (Holzmann 2002).

On the more positive side, authors such as Fougere and Merette (1999) suggest that with declining birth rates some of the costs of caring and educating these are reduced, and these savings may be shifted to other parts of the economy. For example, as the overall cost of schooling falls when there are fewer young people, it is possible to shift these savings into the more intensive training of the young. This they argue may lead to subsequent productivity growth. Others argue that the demand for employment will shift from one sector to another as the population shifts from young to old. In particular, given that falling fertility is occurring alongside increased longevity, there will be an increased demand for elder care services, and this will increase overall productivity and drive the economy.

In terms of productivity, there is also considerable evidence that older workers will stay in the labour market and be productive for far longer than in recent decades. As Harper (2010) and Bloom et al. (2010) have pointed out, with higher levels of education, skills and training, future cohorts of older men and women will be able to maintain high levels of productivity, given supportive and conducive working environments. Perhaps the most significant implication for older workers and their employers is the change in work capacity with age. Whilst this is by no means universal, physical, mental and social capabilities may undergo some degree of change, and the extent to which this impacts on health and safety will depend very much on the nature of the work. For example, those involved in sedentary clerical work may be less affected than those who are involved in work of a very physical nature, for example, lifting or handling equipment and/or patients. Notwithstanding that general health promotion is important (Naumanen 2006) in light of evidence that lifestyle is a major contributor to all risk mortality (see previous sections), chronological age is no longer a reason to exclude older workers from the workforce. Impairments can be mitigated by good ergonomic designs (Benjamin and Wilson 2005). For example, a study by Reynolds et al. (1998) points out significant cohort and time effects. According to the study, adults born in the late 1940s and 1950s will probably be in better cardiovascular condition but worse musculoskeletal health in comparison to current cohorts of older people.

Similarly, much research has been undertaken by the Finnish Institute of Occupational Health, which argues that productivity can be maintained if work demands change as workers change with age – known as productive ageing (Ilmarinen 2001). The work ability index reveals how well a worker can perform his or her tasks and that productivity may be increased through modifications to the work environment (employer) and lifestyle (employee). In other words, the demands of the job need to be adapted to meet the functional capacity of the worker (Griffiths 2000). There are three main risk factor groups: 'physical demands that were too high', 'stressful and dangerous work conditions' and 'poorly organised work' (Ilmarinen 1995). Work ability is not just about functional ability but includes workload effects (subjective and objective) and the nature of tasks, that is, demands and amount of control or autonomy. All these many be addressed in a modern working environment and thus counter the demographic deficit of declining younger workers.

Falling fertility leads to population ageing with the economic burden of pensions and health care

The second side of the demographic deficit argument is that falling fertility leading to the ageing of the population as a whole will impact upon the capacity of societies to finance pensions and long-term health and social care. This will depend both on the growth of labour productivity and on the employment rate. Average annual growth in the EU between 2004 and 2010 was 2.4 per cent, which was projected to fall to 1.2 per cent by 2030 due to the reduction in the working age population. It is argued that the EU will have to increase its productivity to compensate for this (European Commission 2006).

However, the future direction of EU productivity and employment rates is unclear, and future structural changes in the labour market are contested. Some argue that technological advances will reduce future employment opportunities, while others contest that growth in the service sector will absorb job losses arising in post-industrial European economies. These will be influenced by such variables as female participation rates, entry and exit rates and structural changes in the labour market.

It is projected that the working-age population in the countries of the Organisation for Economic Cooperation and Development (OECD) will rise by 1.9 per cent between 2010 and 2020, compared to the 8.6 per cent growth seen between 2000 and 2010 (IOM 2010). The IOM reports further predict that while the incoming (20–24) working-age cohorts in OECD countries were about 32 per cent larger on average than the outgoing retiring (60–64) ones in 2005, the situation in 2015 will be substantially different, with the incoming labour force cohorts being scarcely 2 per cent larger. By 2020 they will be some 9 per cent smaller. For almost half of the OECD countries, the outgoing cohorts will be larger than the incoming ones in 2015.

However, recent projections from Eurostat show that although the working-age population will begin to fall from 2010 onwards, the total number of persons in work in the EU-25 will continue to increase until around 2017. More than two-thirds of this increase will be the result of cohort change as a higher number of future high educated women enter the labour force. The remainder is predicted to arise from the increase in older workers, particularly the 55–65 age group, which has over the past three decades withdrawn prematurely from the EU labour market through early retirement. Delaying future retirement is clearly an option, particularly for Europe where early retirement rates are high. An increase in the effective retirement age will be supported by higher levels of educational and health status of successive future cohorts. This argument clearly links into the early discussion around increasing productivity of older workers and their retention in the labour market.

As we noted earlier, there is considerable informal productivity that is not recorded in the formal economic literature. Harper and Leeson (2010) show for Europe, and Bloom and Canning (2004) for the United States, the extensive downward transfers made by older people to their adult children and grandchildren within families. It has also been estimated by the same group that within the United Kingdom alone some 4 billion is contributed to the UK economy by voluntary work done by older adults alone, and a further 11–57 billion in unpaid caring for older people and grandchildren.

Conclusion

As was stated earlier, there should be no surprise that fertility has fallen so significantly in Europe, as the current age structures which we now face are those associated with the late stage of the demographic transition. This has led to some concern, especially by economists that some regions, and Europe in particular, will be negatively impacted by its 'demographic deficit'. As this chapter has discussed, however, many of these fears are unfounded and do not adequately take into account the role that older people play both in the formal and informal labour market. Declining fertility is good for the planet in the long run as it reduces the maximum population that the earth will have to support. As we transition to a low fertility world, we shall meet challenges, such as the demographic deficit, but these may be overcome by policies which facilitate and encourage the potential of all adults to contribute to society, whether through the labour market or informally through communities and families.

References

Benjamin, K. and Wilson, S. (2005) *Facts and Misconceptions about Age, Health Status andEmployability*, HSL/2005/20 (Buxton: Health and Safety Laboratory).

Bloom, D. E. and Canning, D. (2004) Global demographic change: dimensions and economic significance, in *Global Demographic Change: Economic Impacts and Policy Challenges*. Proceedings of a symposium, sponsored by the Federal Reserve Bank of Kansas City Jackson Hole, Wyoming.

Bloom, D. E., Canning, D. and Fink, G. (2010) Population aging and economic growth, in M. Spence and D. Leipziger (eds) *Globalization and Growth: Implications for a Post-Crisis World* (Washington, DC: World Bank), pp. 297–328.

Bloom, D. E., Canning, D. and Sevilla, J. (2003) The demographic dividend: a new perspective on the economic consequences of population change, *RAND Population Matters Monograph Series* (Santa Monica, CA: RAND Corporation).

Bongaarts, J. and Feeney, G. (1998) On the quantum and tempo of fertility, *Population and Development Review*, 24: 271–91.

Bucht, B. (1996) Mortality trends in developing countries: a survey, in W. Lutz (ed.) *The Future Population of the World. What Can We Assume Today?* Revised Edition (London: Earthscan), pp. 133–48.

Chesnais, J. C. (1998) Below-replacement fertility in the European Union (EU-15): facts and policies, 1960–1997, *Review of Population and Social Policy*, 7: 83–101.

Cliquet, R. L. (1991) *The Second Demographic Transition. Fact or Fiction?* (Strasbourg: Council of Europe).

European Commission (2006) *The Demographic Future of Europe – From Challenge to Opportunity* (Luxembourg: Office for Official Publications of the European Communities).

Fina-Sanglas, L. (2000) Europe's population and labour market beyond 2000: main issues and policy implications, in A. Punch and D. L. Pearce (eds) *Europe's Population and Labour Market beyond 2000, Population studies, 33* (Strasbourg: Council of Europe Publishing), pp. 43–111.

Fougere, M. and Merette, M. (1999) Population ageing and economic growth in seven OECD countries, *Economic Modelling*, 16: 411–27.

Griffiths, A. (2000) Designing and managing healthy work for older workers, *Occupational Medicine*, 50: 473–7.

Harper, S. (2010) Demographic challenges and social security – societal challenges and the capacity to adapt: social security in an ageing world, *International Social Security Association*, 63: 1–11.

Harper, S. and Leeson, G. (2010) Global ageing survey, volunteering, OIA Working Paper.

Holzmann, R. (2002) Can investments in emerging markets help to solve the aging problem?, *Journal of Emerging Market Finance*, 1: 215–41.

Ilmarinen, J. (1995) Aging and work: the role of ergonomics for maintaining work ability during aging, *Advances in Industrial Ergonomics and Safety*, VII: 3–17.

Ilmarinen, J. E. (2001) Aging workers, *Occupational and Environmental Medicine*, 58: 546.

IOM (2010) World Migration Report 2010.

Lee, R. and Mason, A. (2010) Fertility, human capital, and economic growth over the demographic transition, *European Journal of Population/Revue Européenne de Démographie*, 26: 159–82.

Lutz, W. and Goldstein, J. (2004) How to deal with uncertainty in population forecasting?, *Special Issue of International Statistical Review*, 72: 1–4.

Lutz, W., Sanderson, W. and Scherbov, S. (2001) The end of world population growth, *Nature* 412: 543–5.

Lutz, W., Skirbekk, V. and Testa, M. R. (2005) The low-fertility trap hypothesis: forces that may lead to further postponement and fewer births in Europe, *Vienna Institute of Demography Research Paper* No. 4.

Naumanen, P. (2006) The health promotion model as assessed by ageing workers, *Journal of Clinical Nursing*, 15: 219–26.

Pool, I. (2005) Age-structural transitions in industrialized countries, in S. Tuljapurkar, N. Ogawa and A. Gauthier (eds) *Riding the Age Waves: Responses to Aging in Advanced Industrial States* (Berlin: Springer Verlag), pp. 3–21.

Reynolds, S. L., Crimmins, E. M. and Saito, Y. (1998) Cohort differences in disability and disease presence, *The Gerontologist*, 38: 578–90.

Van de Kaa, D. J. (1987) Europe's second demographic transition, *Population Bulletin*, 42: 1–59.

Vaupel, J. W. and Lundström, H. (1996) The future of mortality at older ages in developed countries, in W. Lutz (ed.) *The Future Population of the World: What Can We Assume Today?* Revised Edition (London: Earthscan), pp. 278–97.

14
The Impact on Mothers: Managing the Competing Needs

Ann Buchanan

Introduction

As David Reher notes in Chapter 2, 'throughout history the family has been a cornerstone of society'. It has been responsible for having and raising the next generation, educating the young and supporting its vulnerable members. For many women in the past, in both the developed and developing world, looking after children and caring for those who could not care for themselves was a lifelong task. With smaller families, and in particular the advent of 'the pill', women were better able to control their fertility and with this came a 'quiet revolution' (Goldin 2006). It was distinguished by women wanting to widen their horizons; to establish an identity independent from their husbands and to have greater involvement in decision making outside the home. In the developed world, the key factors were the growth of formal employment for women, education for all children and further education for women, and rising rates of divorce and family breakdown. These trends are vividly illustrated in Chapter 6 by young mothers in the United Kingdom. Today, we can see trends in the developing world following a similar pattern. However, with these changes comes a new dilemma. With women freer to pursue interests outside the home, who was to care for the children and who was to care for the increasing number of elders highlighted by Harper in the previous chapter. The paradox is that with smaller families there is a greater need for substitute carers.

The first part of this chapter explores changes in women's social and economic roles in both the developed and developing world. It considers how the advent of schooling, providing both reliable care and education for the young, presented a partial solution, but preschool, after-school and holiday care remained problematic. The second part of the chapter explores the development of substitute child care in both the developed and developing world. As always, family care is the first port of call. In particular, it examines the dilemmas of relying on sibling care, grandparent care and the care of those children 'left behind', while their parents work in other countries or areas. The third part of the chapter considers the impact of rising standards of parenting amongst the general population supported by the new theology of 'intensive parenting'; finally, this chapter considers how the 'sandwich generation' balance out their various responsibilities including caring for elders.

The quiet revolution: the growth in women's employment

Goldin (2006), tracing the development of women's employment in the United States, maintains that the modern economic role of women emerged in four phases. The first three were evolutionary; the last was revolutionary. In the evolutionary changes, women had limited horizons; they worked because they needed the money; or they worked to fill a passing phase before marriage. In the last phase, from the late 1970s, women's occupation and employment began to define their fundamental identity and worth. It involved a change from 'jobs' to 'careers'. In the 1970s, young women in their late teens upwardly revised their expectations of working when they were older. Eighty per cent predicted labour force participation when aged 30. Their revised expectations of future employment led to young women investing more in their education, and in the 1970s and 1980s girls narrowed the attainment gap between girls and boys in science and maths. They planned for college, and high status and/or high earning jobs after graduation. There was a notable increase in the fraction of females training for the professions, in particular business administration, dentistry, medicine and law (Goldin 2006). However, lack of adequate childcare was a major barrier to employment for a sizeable number of women both in the middle and upper income ranges and even more so for the low-income and single-parent families (Bloom and Steen 1990).

In the developing world, women have always worked and indeed in agrarian societies they trained their children to work alongside them (Whiting and Edwards 1992). These women contribute to the family smallholding and may not have received formal payment for their work (Donahue 1999). The recognition that much of women's work in the developing world is overlooked, undercounted and undervalued is not new. Statistics on women's work do not count unpaid domestic labour, subsistence farming and informal income-generating activities. In a survey in Egypt in 1993, Donahue (1999) found that only 16 per cent of currently married women were involved in nonfamilial employment, with a further 14 per cent involved in other income generation activities. However, some 78 per cent were involved in subsistence production and 99 per cent in housework. As in all societies the work available to these Egyptian women was partially determined by the needs of the household and their educational level. Those in paid employment generally had a higher average level of education.

In 1997, women made up 31 per cent of the official labour force in developing countries and 46.7 per cent worldwide (United Nations 1997). In 1950 only one-third of women in the United States of working age had a paid job. Today, two-thirds do, and women make up almost half of the United States' workforce. In the emerging East Asian economies, for every 100 men in the labour force there are now 83 women (The Economist 2006). However, the overall picture of the global capacity to tap the productive potential of its people is one in which nearly half (48.4 per cent) of the productive potential of the female population remains untapped (compared to 22.3 per cent for men) (International Labour Office 2010).

Women's involvement in domestic work

Those trying to measure women's work have attempted to estimate the extent of domestic work undertaken by women (Bittman et al. 2003). Wives do much more housework than husbands. For example, time-diary data on housework, excluding childcare, show that in 1992 Australian husbands averaged 11 hours per week, while their wives averaged 23 hours. Comparable data from the United States show husbands doing 13 hours per week while wives do 18 (Bittman et al. 2003). As Shelton and John (1996) note in a review of US literature:

> The most notable characteristic of the current division of household labor is that, whether employed or not, women continue to do the majority of housework.
>
> (Shelton and John 1996, p. 301)

Shelton and John (1996) note that a fairly consistent conceptualization in the literature of 'housework' refers to unpaid work to maintain family members and/or home. The assumption is that if the employed mother cannot care for the children, it is she who has to arrange alternative care and undertake the main share of household tasks.

In the West, we have heralded the arrival of the 'New Dad'. Certainly amongst college-educated parents, fathers are enjoying an increasing role in childcare (Welsh et al. 2004), but in middle England, fathers' roles have changed little. In a study of young people in England and Wales, it was found that a father's major role was confined to 'being there', and to bring out the 'big guns' to protect their children, for example, if they were being bullied at school (Welsh et al. 2004). Bittman et al.'s (2003) study shows that in Australia and the United States, as women start to earn more than men, there is a change in the amount of housework or childcare men undertake, but this is only marginal. In general, women spend at least twice as much time compared to men in care work.

Changing families

A less welcome side of the 'quiet revolution' is the increase in family breakdown. Lester (1996) in a study of 27 nations showed that divorce rates from 1950 to 1985 rose in 25 out of the 27 countries. Nations with higher divorce rates in 1950 had steeper rises in the divorce rates by 1985. More recent figures from the US Census Bureau of International Statistics (2011) in 12 advanced economies show a decline in both marriage and divorce rates between 1980 and 2008. In the United States, for example, the marriage rate in 1980 was 15.9 per 1000 population, while in 2008 it was 10.6. The divorce rate over the same period declined from 7.9 to 5.2. Only in Denmark and Sweden did the marriage rate increase. In Sweden, the divorce rate dropped marginally despite the increase in marriages, whereas in Denmark it stayed the same. The UN (2006) World Statistics suggest that, as societies evolve, there is an increase in the rate of divorce. The more evolved the country's society and economy, the higher the rate of divorce. The United States, despite the recent decline, still has the highest rate of divorce worldwide. In developing nations like India, Saudi Arabia and other third-world countries, divorce is still a social taboo. Greater awareness of equality between men and women has been associated with an increase in the divorce rates (UN 2006).

Gavin Jones, in Chapter 3, notes the substantial increase in divorce rates in East Asian countries. In Confucianist societies in the past, divorce carried a considerable stigma, and the pressure to remain in a disharmonious marriage for 'the sake of the children' and also for the sake of appearances and family honour was very strong. Jones suggests that factors such as the increasing economic independence of women, and the pressures (and widened range of contacts) in the big city environments in which an increasing proportion of East Asians live, are influencing divorce trends. More controversially, Jones suggests that there is evidence that East Asian societies are becoming more individualistic and less governed by Confucianist norms.

The rise in lone parenthood

With the changing trends in partnership formation and dissolution, the likelihood that children grow up in a household without both parents has increased (OECD 2011), although in most Organisation for Economic Cooperation and Development (OECD) countries, on average more than 80 per cent of children live with both their mother and their father. In Belgium, Estonia, Latvia and the United Kingdom, this figure drops to between 64 per cent and 68 per cent. On average around 14 per cent of children in OECD countries live with their mother alone. In the United Kingdom, this figure is 20 per cent. There has also been a sharp rise in the number of children born outside marriage. The OECD rate tripled from 11 per cent in 1980 to 33 per cent in 2007 (OECD 2011).

On average across OECD countries, more than six out of ten mothers with dependent children (0–16) are in paid employment. The rates vary, from below 50 per cent to around 75 per cent or more in the Nordic countries (OECD 2011). Virtually all mothers take a short break from paid work just before birth and during the first few months after a child's birth. After this, differences in parental leave and childcare arrangements contribute to different labour force behaviour. It is when the mother first returns to work that the need for alternative care of her new baby impinges. OECD (2011), in the foreword to its report *Doing Better for Families* asks some pertinent questions: Is family policy developing in a changing family context? Across nations, what are the best ways of helping adults to have the number of children they desire? What are the effects of parental leave schemes on female labour supply and on child well-being? What difference do different ways of supporting families influence women's employment and family and child outcomes? Are childcare arrangements a barrier to the employment of mothers and how can flexible workplace options help? Mumsnetters' views in Chapter 6 vividly highlight the policy challenges. More detailed discussion on these key issues will be seen in Chapter 18:

'Making time for children' and in Chapter 16 by Anne Gauthier on family policy and fertility.

Education for children – partial solution to the child care problem

The development of universal primary education offered the first opportunity for safe out-of-home care for children while mothers worked.

Kenny (2008) in a historical review of global education remarks on the spectacular expansion in basic school. Whereas in 1830 only a few children in the United States received primary education and the great majority of the world's children received no formal education at all, by 1870 somewhere between 12 and 23 per cent of the world's children were enrolled in school and by 1950 this figure had increased to 47 per cent. In 2002, global net primary enrolment was around 87 per cent (World Bank 2010). In England, there had been calls for universal education for both boys and girls up to the age of 18 from the seventeenth century (Hill 1991), but the expansion of primary education in Europe and United States had to wait until the mid to the end of the nineteenth century for education of children to become a legal requirement. Elsewhere in the world, progress was very slow prior to the First World War. By 1940, for example in Africa, Cameroon's enrolment stood at 4.1 per cent, and Kenya at 35 per cent. In 1930 Iran's enrolment was just 3.8 per cent, while China's was 10 per cent and Japan's 61 per cent (Kenny 2008). In 2004, except for sub-Saharan Africa, most countries have enrolment rates of above 80 per cent (UNESCO 2006).

As the numbers of children in school increased, women were freer to engage in outside employment. Of course, the fact that children received primary education did not mean that the hours children attended school compared with working hours.

Worldwide, 85 per cent of children in the last grade of primary school go on to attend secondary school. There are two regions that have rates below this global average: Eastern and Southern Africa (67.1 per cent) and West and Central Africa (52.4 per cent). Transition rates are highest in the industrialized countries (98.2 per cent) and in Eastern Europe and the countries of the Commonwealth of Independent States (CIS) (96.1 per cent) (International Education Stats 2005). There are major gender disparities in the number of children enrolled in secondary school. One of the reasons for this is that girls of secondary school age are often kept at home to care for young siblings.

Options for childcare

The advent of full-time universal school from ages 5–7, in most parts of the world did not, of course, solve the problem of who will care for the children before they are old enough for primary school, care for them after-school and care during the holidays.

The challenges and dilemmas of family care

Across the world, many children spend time with a childcare provider other than their parents and school. In the United States, for example, in 2010, 48 per cent of children aged 0–4 with employed mothers were primarily cared for by a relative – their father, grandparent, sibling, other relative – while the mother worked. Twenty-four per cent of these children spent most of their time in a centre-based arrangement (day care, nursery school, preschool or Head Start). Fourteen per cent were primarily cared for by a non-relative in a home-based environment, such as a family day care provider, nanny, babysitter or *au pair* (ChildStats 2011). Educated parents, who may both be working, who presumably had better jobs and could afford the costs, were more likely to use centre-based care or home-based care with nannies and/or *au pairs*.

Care by siblings

In the developing world, while parents are at work, the need for substitute caregivers for younger siblings places many children – usually girls – at risk of being kept out of, or needing to drop out of, school. If a family can afford school fees for only one child, it will likely be a boy who attends. If someone needs to fetch water or do housework instead of going to school, a girl will likely be chosen. If someone needs to stay home to care for younger siblings or sick or infirm household members, this will most likely be a girl: girls will also most likely be withdrawn from school early in adolescence as the age of marriage approaches (UNICEF 2000, Millennium report). A particular dilemma is that the young woman sacrifices her education and the possibility of employment and a better future for herself.

Grandparent care

Care by grandparents poses fewer concerns. Fergusson et al. (2008), in a study using longitudinal data, found that the popular belief that the extended family was no longer an important part of British life was not borne out. Indeed, they found grandparents played a significant role in the care of their young grandchildren (Fergusson et al. 2008). When it came to older adolescents (11–16 years), Buchanan and Griggs (2009) reported a similar finding. Indeed, these young people, whom many assumed would be spending their spare time with their peers, were dropping by Granny for tea, for help with their homework, or for general advice about life and their futures. These grandparents appeared to be taking over many of the parental tasks (Tan et al. 2010).

In most societies, care by grandparents is traditionally the first port of call for help (Buchanan and Ten Brinke 1997). In 2010 in the United States, some 20 per cent of childcare for the 0–4s was provided by grandparents. The Grandparent Association in the United Kingdom (2009) *estimate* that the 13.5 million grandparents in the United Kingdom provide some 60 per cent of all the childcare be it full-time or part time (The Grandparents' Association 2009), and one child in every hundred children lives with a grandparent.

Buchanan and Griggs (2009) found that grandparent involvement was associated with higher levels of well-being in their adolescent grandchildren. The results for the grandparents were, however, more mixed. Clarke and Roberts (2004) showed that, although most grandparents rated the relationship with their grandchild as 'one of the most important in my life', the harsher reality of grandparenting was that some felt that their help was taken for granted and that they were asked to do too much. Others found it hard to find the additional finance and energy needed to care for youngsters when living on a reduced pension and with poor health (Buchanan and Griggs 2009).

In the developing world, multigenerational households have been seen as the traditional way to serve the needs of care-giving for both the young and the old. Living in the same dwelling conveyed a much closer interaction and a sense of shared living (WHO 2002). Many grandparents still live with an adult child, especially in Asia. Historically, multigenerational households have been associated with family businesses, especially farming and shop keeping in western industrial societies.

In Africa, as we have seen in Chapter 11, the ratios of very young, adults and elderly have been affected by war, HIV/AIDS and other stressors, so that elderly people have become responsible for a large number of young children (Settles et al. 2009). The number of grandparents caring for AIDS orphans in developing countries has doubled over the last ten years, and up to half of the world's 15 million AIDS orphans are being cared for by a grandparent. The majority of older caregivers are women, who face serious financial, physical and emotional stress due to their belated care-giving responsibilities (WHO 2002).

Children left behind

Perhaps a more worrying solution to women's work and child care are the children 'left behind', while their parents work elsewhere or in another country (Cortes 2007). Estimates of the numbers of children affected are difficult to obtain. In Moldova, for example, in 2005, official information released by the Moldovan Ministry of Education showed 33,157 children of school age were 'left behind' by both parents. Bryant (2005) suggests that 3–6 million children have been left behind by Filipino parents, with either a mother or father working overseas; the equivalent figure for Indonesia is something like one million, and for Thailand half a million. These figures suggest that roughly 10–20 per cent of Filipino children have a parent working overseas. In China, with the challenges faced by migrant workers in the cities, many parents choose to leave their children in their hometowns. Until very recently, it was estimated by the Chinese government that there were around 20 million children 'left behind' in the countryside. Many of these children are cared for by a grandparent or other family member and might only see their parents once or twice a year (Yang 2006).

Traditionally, the remittances sent home facilitated extra benefits for children, such as schooling, but children left behind by migrating parents who are not able or willing to support them financially over a long period of time experience particularly poor outcomes (De la Garza 2010). Overall, family breakdown appears to be the most negative consequence of parental migration. Children whose parents are absent also have more responsibilities in their households, and this sometimes ends up in an overwhelming load of duties for the child. There is considerable evidence that children left behind are also more prone to psychological and emotional stress, feelings of abandonment and low self-esteem (De la Garza 2010). But it has to be remembered that in areas of extreme poverty, when the migrant parent(s) send remittances back to the carers, this may improve the standard of living for the child (Cortes 2007).

Preschool care and early years' education

As we have noted, the advent of primary schooling starting at ages 5–7, in most parts of the world, was important in facilitating a mother's ability to work. But the question remained: Who was to care for the children before they were old enough for school, after school and during the holidays?

As Esping-Andersen notes in Chapter 17, the extensive research in the United States and elsewhere on the benefits of early childhood education has been important in the development of preschool services in the developed world. Longitudinal studies, such as that from the HighScope Perry Pre-school study (Schweinhart et al. 2005), were able to demonstrate not only significant cognitive benefits for the children, but also, over 40 years, particularly for disadvantaged children, substantial economic returns. Further evidence from the growing research on the brain (Glaser 2000) demonstrated the importance of quality early years' care, and the potential harm of leaving young children in seriously neglecting environments.

In the United Kingdom until relatively recently, the provision of publicly funded education and care for children below compulsory school age at five was a local matter. Many local authorities provided nursery schools and nursery classes for children over the age of three, and/or admitted children to primary school at the age of four, but they were not obliged to do so and provision was patchy. Some children attended private fee-paying nursery schools and classes or voluntary sector playgroups, which kept fees affordable by relying on volunteer and community support. Full-time day-care, where available, was provided mainly by the private sector and had to be paid for by parents (Eurydice 2009).

An entitlement to part-time preschool education was introduced for all four-year-olds in 1999 and for all three-year-olds in 2004. Free provision has since been extended to some two-year-olds in deprived areas. From April 2008, local authorities had a new duty to secure sufficient childcare for working parents (Eurydice 2009).

In Europe more widely, a distinct feature of childcare services has been their diversity (Eurofound 2006). For example, a review of EU childcare statistics in 2002 found 136 formal types of childcare in the 15 European countries, ranging from the lowest number of types in Greece (four) to 14 in the United Kingdom. In the other member states, the number of types ranged from between 5 and 11 (Eurostat 2002). Since the enlargement of the EU in May 2004, which brought about a growth in informal childcare, this range has widened further. An underlying driver of this diversity has been the distinction made across Europe, with a few exceptions, between care and education. The cost of different childcare services, whether borne by individuals indirectly through taxation or directly through fees, remains a key determinant in the type of provision chosen by parents in the EU. Some studies concluded that the 'best' outcomes for early years' children are derived from formal childcare; others argue that 'close-parenting' leads to better outcomes, while some conclude that there is little difference between formal and informal childcare (Eurofound 2006). Whereas increasing the coverage and accessibility of childcare services was at the top of the political agenda in many member states during the 1990s, the focus of childcare policy in the immediate future is shifting towards improving the quality of services. Research shows that there is a significant relationship between quality of childcare and positive outcomes for children (Sylva et al. 2003). As working mothers become more informed, they are likely to insist on quality when they come to choose early year care for their offspring.

Despite the convincing argument for the importance of early childhood care, more than 200 million children under five years of age in developing countries do not reach their developmental potential (McGregor et al. 2007). One of the difficulties in investing in early childhood years is the fact that early childhood interventions are wide ranging in their domains. There are basic health and nutrition interventions, as well as education interventions. Researchers and practitioners in the health discipline may have few connections with those in the education discipline. While health practitioners tend to emphasize child survival, educationalists tend to emphasize child development. While the former tend to emphasize the youngest age, zero to three, the latter tend to emphasize the later age, three to five or until primary school entry age.

Nonoyama-Tarumi (2010), in a study using household survey data from the third round of Multiple Indicator Cluster Surveys of 31 developing countries, found overall, when combining three- and four-year olds, on average, one in five (19.7 per cent) children participated in some kind of organized form of early learning programmes. However, there was a wide range across countries, from 2.2 per cent of Burkina Faso in Africa to 88.1 per cent of Belarus. She concluded that many countries were lagging far behind in reaching international goals and commitments.

After school and holiday care

Childstats (2011) notes that in the United States as children get older, many parents allow them to spend time in unsupervised situations.

In the United States older children are often left to care for themselves: 2 per cent of children aged 5–8, 11 per cent of children aged 9–11 and 36 per cent of children aged 12–14 were regularly in self-care situations.

While there has been a considerable focus in the United Kingdom on the early years, adolescents' needs have received much less attention. This may change following the UK riots in 2011. Certainly, media reports suggest that the government is willing to draw in expertise from the United States and elsewhere. At the Family Research Centre, Harvard University, they are so concerned about the importance of out-of-school time, that there is a special department devoted to studying the issue. The following summarizes some of their findings:

> 'Does Participation in after School Programs make a Difference? Yes! A decade of research and evaluation studies, as well as large-scale, rigorously conducted syntheses of many research and evaluation studies, confirms that children and youth who participate in after school programs can reap a host of positive academic, social prevention and health benefits'. Harvard Family Research; (2008) After school programs in the 21st century.
>
> (Harvard Family Research 2008. Executive summary, p. 1)

Given the situation in the United Kingdom, it is not hard to imagine that there might be significant benefits from a longer school year. It would certainly make parents' concerns about what to do with their young people while they work easier to manage. In addition, young people may avoid the stigma of obtaining a criminal record before they leave school.

Children in especially difficult circumstances

In many parts of the world, some children are effectively parent-less. UNICEF in the mid-1980s and 1990s became increasingly concerned by a group of children categorized as 'Children in Especially Difficult Circumstances' (CEDC): the homeless, orphaned, living and working on the streets, affected by conflict and disabilities, those suffering from violence, abuse, exploitation and neglect. Increasingly, children affected by HIV or AIDS fell into this category. Some of these CEDC children were, in fact, not parent-less, but for one reason or another, they had parents who were not able to care or protect them effectively. It was recognized that these children increasingly faced considerable risks to their health and well-being (UNICEF 2009, *The State of the World's Children*), and international and state intervention was necessary in order to protect them.

It is not the purpose of this chapter to consider the various strategies set in place to care for these children. The central message here, however, is that in the final analysis, both international communities and nation states have the responsibility to care for or protect children living in situations of high risk.

The new theology of parenting research

The 2010 riots in London and other large cities in the United Kingdom have been blamed on poor parenting. Parents, and when we say parents we are, in most cases, talking about mothers, will always be blamed for their children's misdemeanours. This was a strong theme in the Mumsnet chapter. The puzzle in the United Kingdom is that despite the concern about parenting, overall standards of parenting have improved. Gardner et al. (2012) in a review of parenting trends over 20 years (1986–2006) found that although there was more divorce, more lone parents and increased maternal employment, young people in 2006 reported that their parents monitored them more closely than youth in 1986. For the vast majority, parental standards in care and supervision had improved. Women's work both in caring for the children and working outside the home has not been made easier by the new parenting science. Since the 1990s, there has been an accelerating trend towards increasingly 'intensive' mothering with a focus in child-rearing advice to maximize the children's brain development through ample and appropriate stimulation in the early years (Wall 2010). For time-poor parents, this had added to their pressures and perhaps increased their reluctance to have larger families.

The sandwich generation

Although this is not the focus of this book, a further challenge is elder care. Many parents in their 50s and 60s find themselves caught in the financial and emotional squeeze of the 'sandwich generation' (Grundy and Henretta 2006). The shift from the high mortality and high-fertility family to a low-mortality and low-fertility society has resulted in an increase in the number of generations and a decrease in the number of living relatives within these generations. In the West, at the beginning of the twentieth century between 4 per cent and 7 per cent of people in their 60s had at least one parent still living. Today, this figure is nearly 50 per cent. This has become known as the 'beanpole' family (Bengtson and Martin 2001). At the same time young people are choosing to delay transitions in adulthood, such as leaving the parental home, achieving full economic independence from parents, marriage and the birth of their first child. The number of individuals therefore who will live for part of their lives as members of three and four generation families is increasing, as is the proportion of grandparents among western populations. Grandparents Plus, report that 28 per cent of *grandparents* in the United Kingdom, caring for grandchildren under 16 are effectively in a *double* 'sandwich' – looking after older relatives as well as helping out with their own children and grandchildren. Overall one in five (19 per cent) grandmothers and 14 per cent of grandfathers provide more than ten hours childcare per week. One in five (21 per cent) children are cared for by grandparents each week (Grandparent Plus 2012).

But this is only part of the story. As recently as 1990, only 25 per cent of those between 18 and 24 lived with their parents. By 2000, the number had gone up to 52 per cent and with the ongoing recession this figure is likely to increase (O'Brien 2012). At the centre of this 'squeeze' will be the working and active middle generation and the grandparents. Just as women shoulder much of the childcare responsibilities within two-parent households even when both parents are working, the same is true for elder care (Ward and Spitze 1998). Evidence suggests that sandwiched workers were significantly more likely to be stressed than those who provided care for just one generation (Williams 2004). These workers felt that their situation could be helped by government policy and workplace support including flexible hours, ability to telework and information about community resources (Williams 2004).

With changing demographic trends, the number of women in this 'sandwich' or 'double sandwich' is likely to increase. As Sarah Harper notes in Chapter 13, the particular challenge is to encourage all elders to continue contributing to society, whether through the labour market or informally through communities and families and to facilitate their staying healthy for as long as possible.

Conclusion

In the developed and developing world, many will decry 'the quiet revolution', and deplore the changes in women's social and economic roles. 'Things were better in the old days'. The central issue is, for whom were they better? 'Children got better care when their mothers did not work'. We need to remember that many children live at home in less than ideal circumstances.

In the main, societies the world over have had a somewhat ambiguous stance towards women's employment. The male breadwinner model is deeply ingrained in many parts of the globe. But the quiet revolution has a momentum of its own and will keep on rolling. Indeed, as we will see in Chapter 18, as the number of children falls, and the growing number of elderly need to be cared for, there will be strong economic reasons for nation states to capitalize from women's employment.

How will families arrange for the care of their children? If we look into the crystal ball, it is likely that fathers will increasingly lend a hand. Indeed in some circumstances, it may be easier for women to obtain employment than men. Across the world, as in the past, family members, especially grandparents, will be the first port of call. Hopefully, societies will ensure that older sisters do not have to care for their siblings but are free to go to school. It is likely that increasing numbers of children, especially in economically disadvantaged areas will be 'left behind' with often over-stretched elderly carers as their parents migrate to obtain work. Whether this brings a better quality of life for the children may depend on the remittances sent home. Services will be needed to support these carers.

The development of preschool and early years' education is likely to develop apace. As we will see in Chapter 18, the joint pressure from the evidence of young children's brain vulnerability, combined with the known economic savings from state investment in early years care, is likely to be a strong argument for a further development of services. Economic arguments will also make a strong case for investment in primary and secondary education in those parts of the world where it is lacking. Perhaps, the forgotten quarter has been the supervision and care of adolescents, particularly where parents do not arrange this.

Today, the new parenting research hypothesizes that many of children's problems are related to poor parenting. 'Nature', however, interacts with 'nurture' and the environment. In the United Kingdom, and most likely elsewhere too, parenting standards are a continuum. At one end, there is 'intensive' parenting, which is largely practised by the better-off middle classes. At the other end, there are the poorer parents with poorer mental health. Gardner et al. (2012) found that poorer parenting was often associated with poorer parental mental health, and this in turn was linked with more behaviour problems in young people. In the extreme, such parenting is very harmful to children. The challenge for all societies is to bring the two ends of the spectrum together.

But caring is not confined to providing for and nurturing the next generation. Families have always been responsible for looking after their more elderly members, although in developed societies this responsibility is increasingly shared with the state. However, even in the West, parents and grandparents can find themselves caught in 'the sandwich generation' struggling to meet the demands of both their parents and their children and grandchildren.

The challenge for all societies is to help parents manage all their caring responsibilities, so that family life brings benefits; women can work; children can thrive in high-quality alternative provision and elders are provided for. Families and women, in particular, cannot do this on their own.

References

Bengtson, V. L. and Martin, P. (2001) Families and intergenerational relationships in aging societies: comparing the United States with German-speaking countries. *Z Gerontol Geriatr*, 34(3): 207–17.

Bittman, M., England, P., Sayer, L., Folbre, N. and Matheson, G. (2003) When does gender trump money? Bargaining and time in household work, *American Journal of Sociology*, 109(1): 186–214.

Bloom, D. and Steen, T. (1990) The labor force implications of expanding the child care industry, *Population Research and Policy Review*, 9(1): 25–44.

Bryant, J. (2005) *Children of International Migrants in Indonesia, Thailand and the Philippines, Review of Evidence and Policies*, Innocenti Working Paper, UNICEF, Innocenti Research Centre, Florence.

Buchanan, A. and Griggs, J. (2009) *My Second Mum and Dad*. Grandparents Plus, http://www.grandparentsplus.org.uk/wp-content/uploads/2011/03/%C3%A2%E2%82%AC%C5%93My-Second-Mum-and-Dad%C3%A2%E2%82%AC%C2%9D-research-report.pdf, date accessed 12 March 2012.

Buchanan, A. and Ten Brinke J-A. (1997) *What Happened When They Were Grown up? Outcomes from Parenting Experiences* (York: Joseph Rowntree Foundation).

ChildStats (2011) *America's Children: Key National Indicators of Well-Being, 2011*, http://www.childstats.gov/americaschildren/famsoc3.asp, date accessed 12 March 2012.

Clarke, L. and Roberts, C. (2004) The meaning of grandparenthood, and its contribution to the quality of life of older people, in A. Walker and C. Henessey (eds) *Growing Older: Quality of Life*, 188–208 (Buckingham: Open University Press).

Cortes, R. (2007) Children and women left behind in labor sending countries: an appraisal of social risks, *Global Report on Child Migration*. Child Migration Research Network, www.childmigration.net/files/Rosalia_Cortes_07.pdf, date accessed 6 November 2012.

De la Garza, R. (2010) *Children Left Behind: A Multidimensional Perspective*. Social and Economic Working Paper, UNICEF Policy, Advocacy and Knowledge Management, Division of Policy and Practice, http://www.unicef.org/socialpolicy/

files/Postscript_Formatted Migration_Development_and_Children_Left_Behind.pdf, UNICEF, date accessed 12 March 2012.

Donahue, D. (1999) Measuring women's work in developing countries, *Population and Development Review*, 25(3): 543–76.

The Economist (2006) Women in the workforce. The importance of sex. Forget China, India and the internet: economic growth is driven by women, http://www.economist.com/node/6800723, date accessed 12 March 2012.

Eurofound (2006) *Childcare Services in the EU – What Future?* European Monitoring Centre on Change, http://www.eurofound.europa.eu/emcc/content/source/eu06015a.htm?p1= ef_publication&p2= null, date accessed 12 March 2012.

Eurostat (2002) *Feasibility Study on the Availability of Comparable Childcare Statistics in the European Union*, Luxembourg, Office for Official Publications of the European Communities, http://www.uni-mannheim.de/edz/pdf/eurostat/02/KS-CC-02-001-EN-N-EN.pdf, date accessed 12 March 2012.

Eurydice (2009) *Early Childcare in Europe, Tackling Social and Cultural Inequalities*. Eurydice – Network on education systems and policies in Europe EACEA, European commission.

Fergusson, E., Maughan, B. and Golding, J. (2008) Which children receive grandparental care and what effect does it have?, *Journal of Child Psychology and Psychiatry*, 49(2): 161–9.

Gardner, F., Collishaw, S., Maughan, B., Scott, J., Schepman, K. and Hagell, A. (2012) Trends in parenting: can they help explain time trends in problem behaviour? in A. Hagell (ed.) *Changing Adolescence: Social Trends and Mental Health* (Bristol: Policy Press).

Glaser, D. (2000) Child abuse and neglect and the brain, *Journal of Child Psychology and Psychiatry*, 41(1): 97–116.

Grandparent Plus (2012) Report of seminar, http://www.grandparentsplus.org.uk/conferences-and-seminars, date accessed 1 May 2012.

Goldin, C. (2006) *The Quiet Revolution That Transformed Women's Employment, Education, and Family*, Ely Lecture, American Economic Association Meetings, Boston, MA (Jan. 2006), published in *American Economic Review, Papers and Proceedings*, 96: 1–21.

Grundy, E. and Henretta, J. (2006) Between elderly parents and adult children: a new look at the intergenerational care provided by the 'sandwich generation', *Ageing and Society*, 26: 707–22.

Harvard Family Research (2008) Year-Round Schooling. Executive summary, p. 1, http://www.edweek.org/ew/issues/year-round-schooling/, date accessed 12 March 2012.

Hill, C. (1991) *The World Turned Upside Down: Radical Ideas During the English Revolution* (London: Penguin).

International Education Stats (2005) *Transition from Primary to Secondary Education*, http://huebler.blogspot.com/2005/07/transition-from-primary-to-secondary.html, date accessed 12 March 2012.

International Labour Office (2010) *Women in Labour Markets: Measuring Progress and Identifying Challenges* (Geneva: International Labour Office).

Kenny, C. (2008) *The Global Expansion of Primary Education*. Center for Global Development. Center for Global Development [PDF] from psu.edu.

Lester, D. (1996) Trends in divorce and marriage around the world, *Journal of Divorce and Remarriage,* 25(1–2): 169–71.

McGregor, S., Cheung, Y., Cueto, S., Glewwe, P., Richter, L., Strupp, B. and the International Child Development Steering Group (2007) Developmental potential in the first 5 years for children in developing countries, *Lancet,* 369: 60–70.

Nonoyama-Tarumi, Y. (2010) *Early Childhood Development in Developing Countries: Paper Commissioned for the EFA Global Monitoring Report 2011, The Hidden Crisis: Armed Conflict and Education, UNESCO* 2011/ED/EFA/MRT/PI/06, http://unesdoc.unesco.org/images/0019/001912/191223e.pdf, date accessed 12 March 2012.

O'Brien, S. (2012) How to Avoid Sandwich Generation Problems. *Senior Living,* http://seniorliving.about.com/od/babyboomers/a/sandwich-generation.htm, date accessed 30 April 2012.

OECD (2011) *Doing Better for Families,* OECD Publishing, http://dx.doi.org/10.1787/9789264098732-en, date accessed 12 March 2012.

Schweinhart, L. J., Montie, J., Xiang, Z., Barnett, W. S., Belfield, C. R. and Nores, M. (2005) *Lifetime Effects: The HighScope Perry Preschool Study through Age 40,* Monographs of the High Scope Educational Research Foundation, 14 (Ypsilanti, MI: HighScope Press).

Settles, B. H., Zhao, J., Mancini, J., Doneker, K., Rich, A., Pierre, S. and Oduor, A. (2009) Grandparents caring for their grandchildren: emerging roles and exchanges in global perspectives, *Journal of Comparative Family Studies,* 40(5): 827–41.

Shelton, B. A. and John, D. (1996) The division of household labor, *Annual Review of Sociology,* 22: 299–322.

Sylva, K., Siraj-Blatchford, I. and Taggart, B. (2003 [2010]). *Assessing Quality in the Early Years* (Stoke on Trent: Trentham Books).

Tan, J-P., Buchanan, A., Flouri, E., Attar-Schwartz, S. and Griggs, J. (2010) Filling the parenting gap?, Grandparent involvement with UK adolescents, *Journal of Family Issues,* 31(7): 992–1015.

The Grandparents' Association (2009) The Grandparent Association, http://www.grandparents-association.org.uk, date accessed 12 March 2012.

UNESCO Institute for Statistics (2006) Global Education Database, October 2006, http://huebler.blogspot.co.uk/2006_09_01_archive.html, date accessed 12 March 2012.

United Nations (1997) Women at a Glance, http://www.un.org/ecosocdev/geninfo/women/women96.htm#labour, date accessed March 2012.

United Nations (2006) World Statistics (2006) Table 25. Divorces and crude divorce rates by urban/rural residence: 2002–2006, http://unstats.un.org/unsd/demographic/products/dyb/dyb2006/Table25.pdf, date accessed 12 March 2012.

UNICEF (2000) Millennium report. Goal: promote gender equality and empower women, http://www.unicef.org/mdg/index_genderequality.htm, date accessed 12 March 2012.

UNICEF (2009) *The State of the World's Children* (New York: UNICEF).

US Census Bureau of International Statistics (2011) http://www.census.gov/prod/2011pubs/12statab/intlstat.pdf, date accessed 12 March 2012.

Wall, G. (2010) Mothers' experiences with intensive parenting and brain development discourse, *Women's Studies International Forum*, 33(3): 253–63.

Ward, R. and Spitze, G. (1998) Sandwiched marriages: the implications of child and parent relations for marital quality in midlife, *Social Forces*, 17: 1889–208.

Welsh, E., Buchanan, A. Flouri, E. and Lewis, J. (2004) *'Involved' Fathering and Child Well-being: Fathers' Involvement with Secondary School Age Children,* National Children's Bureau for the Rowntree Foundation Parenting in Practice series.

Whiting, B. B and Edwards, C. P. (1992) *Children of Different Worlds: The Formation of Social Behaviour* (Cambridge, MA: Harvard University Press).

Williams, C. (2004) The Sandwich Generation, Perspectives 5-12, Statistics Canada, Catalogue 75-001-XIE http://ivt.crepuq.qc.ca/popactive/documentation2005_A/2004/2004-09-01.pdf, date accessed 30 April 2012.

World Bank Education Statistics Newsletter (2010) Indicator 2.1: Net enrolment rate in primary education. http://siteresources.worldbank.org/EXTEDSTATS/Resources/3232763-1197312825215/EdStatsNewsletter16.pdf, date accessed 12 March 2012.

World Health Organisation (2002) *The Impact of Aids on Older People in Africa,* WHO. http://whqlibdoc.who.int/hq/2002/WHO_NMH_NPH_ALC_02.12.pdf, date accessed 12 March 2012.

Yang, Q. (2006) 农村留守儿童教育问题探讨 Educational problems of left-behind children in rural areas, *China Labour Bulletin*, http://www.clb.org.hk/en/node/100459, date accessed 12 March 2012.

15
Baby Fever and Longing for Children

Anna Rotkirch

From the pill to 'baby fever'

In most societies, sexual maturation has been closely followed by marriage and childbearing. In the Hadza of Tanzania who are hunter-gatherers, women reach sexual maturation at 16.5 years, marry around 17, and have their first child at 19 (Marlowe 2011, p. 151). Similarly, in contemporary India many poor women experience sexual maturation, marriage and childbearing before they turn 16 (Raj, Saggurti, Balaiah and Silverman 2009).

The contraceptive pill, introduced in 1960 famously helped women and couples to enjoy sex without the constant fear of unwanted pregnancy. At first, modern and effective contraceptives were adopted side by side with the view that children belong to life and at least to marriage. One Danish woman who married in the 1960s remembers throwing the sheet with pills over board as the ship left for her honeymoon cruise. The gesture was spontaneous, as little planned as unproblematic, nothing she needed to discuss or even inform her husband about. Marriage implied children, just as children implied marriage or social stigma. Thus it had been for centuries, notwithstanding the widespread use of other means of contraception by couples who wished to space or stop childbearing.

European women of the Post-War era typically had their children in their 20s. Thus for much of the twentieth century and in many poorer parts of today's world, major regrets in women's lives related to marrying early and having too short a time with their spouse before the children arrived. Travels, educational paths and romantic years were irrevocably lost due to parenting.

Then, with the sexual revolution in Western countries the reproductive landscape changed. Less conventional lifestyles including single persons or homosexual families gained in social visibility and acceptance. For the first time in history, people could quite freely choose which parts they desired from the partner(s)-marriage-children package. The women's movement taught that womanhood is not tied to motherhood and that female creativity and self-realization may often be hampered by husbands and children. As we saw in Chapter 14, women also entered the labour markets with full force during the last decades of the twentieth century, with a simultaneous growth of the time spent by both men and women in education.

Substantial sexual and reproductive rights, including the right to divorce, remarry and to induce abortion, were perceived to be self-evident. As a result, having intercourse became easier and having children became in many ways more complex (Wager 2000). Parenthood started to be postponed to later ages and surrounded by increasing ambivalence. Both single and married people may wonder whether they should have children at all, when, and with whom. Ponder how a British woman describes her long way to motherhood. She first started thinking about babies as a young adult, and eventually gave birth to a child at the age of 37:

> There was no desperation for a baby, just a sensation, a constant presence that grew over the years. When I was younger, I didn't give children much thought. Neither did most of my friends, so a lot of us were amused when, around our early twenties, we suddenly started noticing babies, imagining motherhood, having dreams about being pregnant. We put it down to biology and then put it out of our minds, knowing our biological clocks had plenty of time to run. We assumed men, relationships, maybe marriage, would come along. If not, something else would. There are always ways of having children, we reasoned, and got on with all the other things in life.... For me, however, the men, the relationships, the marriage, didn't materialise.... But as the interest in relationships waned, so the desire to have children grew.
>
> (McCallin 2011)

This woman never found a suitable partner and eventually decided to use donated sperm in artificial insemination in order to have the child she craved. Her story illustrates how the focus of childbearing decisions has shifted from the issue of contraception to the issue of conception.

This shift includes a new emphasis on the emotional longing for a child. How to find not only the time for a child, but the right time and the right partner before it is biologically too late, is nowadays a constant theme in lay talk and the media (e.g. Clark-Flory 2012). As norms fade, the importance of feelings in guiding decision-making increases. New expressions, such as 'baby lust', 'baby fever' or 'baby angst' have entered the vocabulary of European languages. For instance, in early 2012 the number of blogs featuring the key word 'baby lust' was 7,700,000. The first results in my search were all personal, diary-like entries written by women, among these one mother longing for a third child she had decided not to have, and a childless woman who was ambivalent about motherhood, although her baby fever kept her awake at night. In comparison, 'contraception' yielded 10,100,000 blogs and 'contraceptive pill' 508,000 blogs, most by religious institutions or medical companies.

This chapter discusses the emotion of longing for a child or 'baby fever' and possible solutions available to those who face obstacles in having a child. With falling fertility rates, I will argue that, at both a societal and human level, we need to expand our approach to family planning to include advice not only about contraception, but also about having children. The emphasis put here on involuntary childlessness in the wealthy countries is not in any ways intended to disregard the acute need for contraception and reproductive rights that still exists in many countries.

How widespread is 'baby fever'?

While the value people and societies attach to children is broadly acknowledged in social research, the emotion of longing for a child has been little explored (but see Miller 1986; Thomson 1997; Thomson et al. 1990). To date, we have qualitative and survey data on strong longing for children only from Finland (Rotkirch et al. 2011) and smaller-scale psychological studies from the United Kingdom and United States (Brase and Brase 2011). These studies show that both men and women may feel a strong longing to have a child of their own and that this is related to their actual childbearing. Baby longing is not, however, experienced by everybody.

Lay talk also often equates longing for children with something instinctual and natural. Take, for instance, one online comment to *The Guardian* article quoted above. A woman who has suffered from infertility writes: 'We are designed, life is designed, sex is designed for women to give birth.' The commentator is certainly right that during human evolution, heterosexual intercourse has been designed to produce children, and parents have evolved to respond to their newborn babies. However, this does not mean that evolution has selected that baby longing should become a strong universal instinct – clearly it has not. Most parents in human history have had their children before they had the time or opportunity to long for them. Paradoxically, today some women hesitate to have children if they lack a strong urge to do so. Especially in the United States, there is a strong sense that the right feelings should guide your major decisions in life (see Pikul 2011 for a personal description of this situation) – if you do not long for a child, you may decide not to have one at all.

Survey data shows the expected association between having ever longed for a child and being a parent. Childless people have longed for a baby less often than parents have, while parents of several children have longed most frequently of all (Figure 15.1). Thus baby longing often triggers the decision to try and have a child, or appears while the couple is trying to achieve pregnancy or waiting for the child to be born. However, we should again note that not all people who become parents have had 'baby fever'. It is not a universal feeling and cannot be counted on as a sign about when you should become a parent.

Men, women and baby longing

Among childless women in Finland, most have longed for a child at least once. By contrast, the majority of childless men have never longed to have a child of their own. Ten per cent of childless men and 20 per cent of childless women said they had frequently longed for a child (Figure 15.1).

The gender difference is crucial when we want to understand the emotional challenges of unwanted childlessness. Although both sexes may long strongly for a child – contrary to some popular misconceptions that only women do – the emotion does appear to be both more common and more intense among women.

For instance, nearly half of both men and women reported having strongly longed for a baby once or several times in their life. But men had twice as often never felt any baby longing, and twice as seldom longed frequently (22 per cent of women but 42 per cent of men had never longed for a child, while 28 per cent of women and 13 per cent of men had longed several times) (Rotkirch et al. 2011, see Brase and Brase 2011 for similar results).

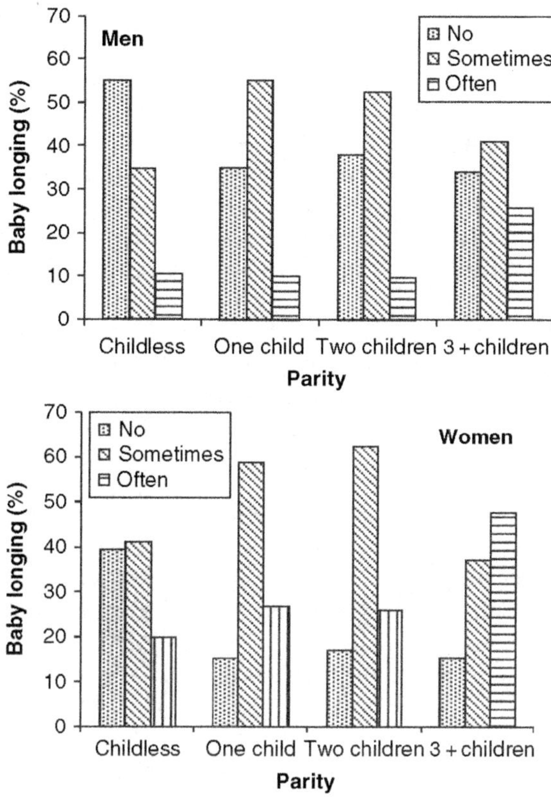

Figure 15.1 Strong longing to have a child of one's own ('baby fever') by sex and parity, 20–59-year-old men (n = 532) and women (n = 877), family barometer, 2007, of 20–59-year-old Finns
Rotkirch et al. (2011).

When asking Finnish men during in-depth interviews whether they had felt 'baby fever' and whether they thought that men in general could feel it, the answers were very varied. While no respondent questioned the view that women can get baby fever, they were more uncertain about men. Some respondents did not believe that men longed for babies, at least not in the sense of 'fever'. Other men, however, used the expression to describe the experiences of themselves or their friends (Rotkirch et al. 2011).

Interestingly, men and women have first felt baby longing in similar circumstances. The most usual situation was when the couple were trying to have their first child. However, men's longing was more often triggered by trying to make his partner pregnant or in no particular situation, while women had more often felt it since youth or due to specific triggers, such as when a friend or a sibling had a baby (Rotkirch et al. 2011.).

Qualitative evidence reported in Rotkirch (2007) also indicates that women's baby longing may often be deeper, more physical, and may, if prolonged, more easily turn into an obsession. Women describe baby fever as a *'painful longing of my whole being'*, an *'unbelievable aching'*, *'anxiety and sorrow'* or *'a pleasant longing and a burden'*. The desire is compared to natural disasters and biological drives. It was a 'tsunami', a 'wall', an equivalent to 'the male sexual urge to discharge, although in my case it aimed directly at the end result, the baby'. Baby fever may also be located in the body. The womb may 'burn', 'pinch' and 'convulse', the breasts 'feel heavy when I see a baby' or 'became sensitive and hard'.

An American woman compares it to falling madly in love:

> It was as instant as it was surprising. I remember it vividly. It was such a strong physical feeling. The thought of having a baby suddenly made my pulse race, my pupils dilate and my breathing go quick and funny. It was exactly like falling madly in love. It was completely irrational and powerful. It was absurd and awesome. Lust is the perfect way to describe the feeling.
>
> (Data collected via Pikul 2011)

Similar stories and descriptions are easily found from the wealth of baby fever blogs. For instance, one blog post describes recurring dreams at night:

> We're not planning to have a family anytime soon. Kids have never been high on my priority list. Yet, recently, I've been dreaming of babies.... There's always a crisis in these dreams. I either cannot clothe or feed the baby, or I've discovered that unbeknownst to me, I've had a child and have been keeping it in a suitcase for months.... The payoff for these horrors comes every night, when I hold my hungry, unfeedable child and feel his or her warm weight in my arms, or against my ribs, or on my hip. I inhale the sweet, and sometimes, sour odors of the child's body. I know it's mine. And then I wake up, and – as upset as I was when I realized that I was a mother – I am just as disappointed that the child is gone.
>
> It's a hell of a roller coaster to ride every night.
>
> (O'Connell 2012)

Why is baby longing more common today?

The concept of 'baby fever' appears to have spread in some societies in the 1990s. Earlier expressions, such as 'broodiness' in English, do exist. Nevertheless people from older generations may find the term 'baby fever' not just strange but incomprehensible and disturbing. For instance, a Finnish woman born in the 1940s commenting on baby lust wondered that what she saw as women's 'cruel destiny' has for many younger women become a privilege and right to be defended:

> Always when people talk about infertility treatments and women's right to them I get a difficult and unreal feeling. It is completely impossible for me to understand that some people really on purpose, without saving any effort and employing all means, strive for a situation that I very early on learnt to see as a cruel but unavoidable destiny.
>
> (Quoted in Rotkirch 2007)

Why do we nowadays pay more attention to baby longing? One main reason is that the period of young unattached adulthood has stretched in both directions. First, maturation is reached earlier. The age of reaching sexual maturity has, due to improved nutrition and higher childhood weight among other factors, declined in rich countries. Today, girls in the United Kingdom have their first menstruation on average when they are between 12 and 13 years old, while it was over one year later in early twentieth century (Morris et al. 2011). The sexual maturation of boys arrives somewhat later but has shifted to younger ages in a similar way (Goldstein 2011). Earlier sexual maturation leads to earlier sexual interest and earlier age at first sexual intercourse. Interestingly, it is also related to earlier attraction to babies, at least among girls (Maestripieri et al. 2004). This attraction to babies is, unsurprisingly, part of the emotion of having a baby fever (Brase and Brase 2011).

Second, people are becoming parents increasingly later, often in their late 20s (see Chapter 5 for further discussion of postponement of first births). Therefore, contemporary developed societies have more years of potential childbearing but no children. For the minority of people who have longed for children since youth, these may feel like very long years. Another consequence of postponement of parenthood is that a higher proportion of people will remain childless against their will, due to lack of a partner or to infertility (te Velde et al. 2012).

Longing for babies is often attributed to social norms and pressure from kin and peers. There is no evidence yet for this assertion. True, people who choose not to have children often feel misunderstood and excluded. However, people with baby longing, in Rotkirch's study (2007), did not feel they confirmed to social norms, often to the contrary. For instance, longing for a child when 'too young' may feel like breaking social expectations. Some younger women complain that their parents and boyfriends belittle or ignore their feelings, and say that only women in their 30s are 'allowed' to talk about 'biological clocks'. Another woman describes a desperation verging on depression as her boyfriend did not want to have children 'too early':

> I don't even know when I first felt symptoms of baby fever, it has always been so clear to me that I want children, in one way or another. In such an unfashionable way in today's society, I felt myself deficient and poor without children. In my circle of friends, which has until recently been quite child hostile, I was the somewhat strange exception.... At 24 I was already at a point where I felt my life did not advance, it was wasting itself, and something had to happen.
>
> (Quoted in Rotkirch 2007)

Another Finnish woman in her early 20s described seeing a baby on the cover of a magazine, while she was waiting to renew her contraceptive pills in the drug store, and starting to cry from baby longing. (This anecdotal evidence begs the question whether contraceptive pills, which suppress ovulation and hormonally mimic pregnancy, could possibly fuel the longing for a baby.)

A person's income or education does not appear to influence the experience of baby longing (Rotkirch et al. 2011), neither is baby fever related to stereotypical feminine traits (Brase and Brase 2011). Other primates such as female baboons also exhibit strong attraction to infants at certain life stages (Silk 2003). These results indicate that social pressure hardly explains the spread of baby longing.

In sum, while the time span available to long for a child and the social attention surrounding childbearing decisions are new, the emotion itself is probably no historical novelty. In comparing attitudes to childlessness and parenthood across the globe in the 1890s, Edward Westermarck (1891) noted that the former is universally stigmatized while the latter is associated with parental pride. The sorrow from childlessness is also frequently mentioned in fairytales and must have been familiar to people living centuries ago.

Baby longing as an argument with self, spouse or biology

The function of baby longing may be to signal the best time for a child. Such signals can be directed at the individual her- or himself, at spouses, or at the physiological obstacles created by infertility.

Many women feel baby lust as a real struggle between body and mind, between baby craving and rational life plans. We remember the quote above with the American woman who did not have children but dreamt of them every night. A Finnish woman of the same age repeats that description almost verbatim:

> As I became 28 years old I started having dreams about children almost every night. I had a restless feeling all the time, just as if my womb would have demanded something I did not agree with. I started thinking about having a child, although I knew that I did not want it under any circumstances.

We do not know how these struggles end, but it is clear that they at least make the woman reconsider her plans for childbearing. Next, if she decides she wants a child, comes the task of making her partner agree. Demographic studies show that couples often have similar fertility intentions (e.g. Thomson and Hoem 1998; Thomson et al. 1990). However, the spouses may have reached these intentions by preceding sex differences in the intensity of longing. The social media abounds with discussions of women needing to persuade more reluctant men. In my qualitative study of baby fever in Finland, some women explicitly mentioned the opposition of the father candidate, while a few women said their partners had tried to persuade them to have children. Women with reluctant partners told about increased sexual desire and using conscious seduction at the fertile moments in the menstrual cycle. Other means ranged from small hints in passing, discussions and planning, arranging birthday parties for other children (!), all the way to making the partner choose between a child and a divorce. A few women also wrote about sexual infidelities, falling in love with a new partner and actual divorce as a consequence of their baby longing. No woman mentioned deceiving the man with contraception, but a few men described such a situation (Rotkirch 2007).

However, when measuring childbearing intentions in Finnish couples, only 6 per cent reported that they and their spouse had very different opinions. It seems that spouses eventually agree on whether to have (more) children or not, or break up.

When asked what consequences baby fever had in the lives of the respondents, men's baby longing was reported to result in a child less often than women's longing. Both men and women said that women's longing had more influence on the couple's childbearing decisions (Rotkirch et al. 2011).

Finally, the wish for a child can stumble upon difficulties of achieving pregnancy. This chapter will conclude with looking at the solutions available for couples who long for a child and have decided to try and have one, but suffer from infertility.

Coping with unwanted childlessness

If a woman or a couple tries to achieve pregnancy without succeeding, the amiable talk of 'baby lust' or 'baby angst' acquires darker shades. Women describe feeling like *'a dried branch'*, *'a mere empty skin shell'* or *'as lacking viscera'*. They mentioned fear of death and loneliness, low self-esteem and envy – symptoms approaching those of clinical depression (Heckhausen and Wrosch 2002; Rotkirch 2007).

When first starting to long for children, people often become drawn to infants, children or baby things. Prolonged longing may lead to the opposite: a withdrawal from pregnant women and friends with children, to the point of ending the relationship as too painful. Female jealousy when the best friend has a child and the other cannot is not uncommon, can destroy lifelong friendships, and be no less intense than jealousy over a partner, maybe even stronger.

Most people who wish for children wait for the right partner to have children with, and renounce having children if she or he is not found. The trivial but nevertheless often overlooked truth is that for single men and homosexual male couples, either a consenting woman or adoption is required in order to become a father. But also among women, the lack of a suitable partner is the single most prevalent reason for remaining without a child. In various surveys, lack of partner is estimated to explain more than half of childlessness. As discussed in more detail in Chapter 5, this does not necessarily mean that no suitable partner was ever around, but when the partner was there, it did not feel it was the right time to have a child. When the time did feel right, the couple may have separated (Wager 2000).

As with any loss, involuntary childlessness leads to sorrow, which may turn into rage and depression, and may also be successfully coped with. One study found that after age 40, women who continued to wish for a child, although this life goal grew increasingly unrealistic scored lower in psychological well-being, while those who managed to disengage from their former life plans were much more satisfied (Heckhausen and Wrosch 2002).

When the adjustment to childbearing plans is being made by two spouses, the question is at what point each of them wants to stop and renounce further plans of childbearing, and how this impacts the psychological health of the other. Existing scattered evidence indicates that women are typically ready to go further and try more different solutions than men in order to have a child. Having a genetic descendant also appears to be more important for men than for women when they discuss infertility treatments (Waxman 2009). Thus women on average can be more prepared to try to overcome childlessness by adoption, or with the aid of infertility treatments, which include using sperm or egg cells from other than the prospective parents.

International adoption

Adoption is found in all known societies as well as in other species, such as lambs and the big apes. Indeed, one may speculate that if baby longing has evolved and served a function in our evolutionary past, it could have been to facilitate the motivation and bonding of the adoptive parent (Rotkirch 2008). As Harald Euler (2011, p. 191) stresses, we are used to thinking of adoptive parents as 'strangers from outside the family who were identified by a social agency'. However, in traditional societies and especially in Africa, close kin typically served as adoptive and foster parents. Among the Hadza hunter gatherers in Tanzania, the same word is used for 'mother', maternal aunt and paternal aunt, probably because the aunts so often ended up in maternal roles (Marlowe 2011). Usually, the maternal grandmother, or the maternal aunt, is most likely to act as foster parents in kinship foster. Kinship foster care placements are becoming increasingly favoured in Western countries as well (Hegar and Scannapieco 1999).

International adoption took off in the 1950s and has been increasing until the last decade. If the first emphasis was on saving poor unwanted children and providing them with a better life, as the demand grew, adoption shifted to become rather a way for parents to satisfy their own longing for a child. Nowadays adoptive parents are briefed that adopting a child is no less 'selfish' than having it the natural way. International adoption goes from poor countries to richer, which makes it a complex phenomenon: it can be approached as everything from a 'global gift' to a form of neo-colonialist exploitation (Selman 2002).

In the latter half of the twentieth century, international adoptions steadily increased. The number of children adopted reached 45,000 in 2004. In that year, the USA received a record high of 23,000 children through international adoption, accounting for over 1 per cent of all children that year. But adoption rates have dramatically declined since, in the United States by over 25 per cent (Selman 2009). While the demand is growing, the supply of children to be adopted (particularly the most desired children, that is, healthy babies) is diminishing. Since fertility is declining worldwide, there are fewer babies that do not have willing adult caretakers. For instance, Russia and China, who both exported many babies for adoption in the 1990s, have witnessed increasing living standards and have grown more concerned about their population prospects. Many poor countries provide foster homes within the countries. Some have also changed their policies for ideological reasons. More countries put strict demands on the age, gender, sexual orientation and marital status of the prospective adoptive parents, excluding many potential mothers and fathers. Thus, China requires since 2006 that adoptive parents are a married heterosexual couple, excluding adoptions by homosexuals and single women. Inter-country adoption also faces criticism from adult adoptees themselves, and of being related to the international trafficking of children, for example, from war zones, when it can be hard to establish who is really orphaned and who is not. It is of utmost importance that international adoptions follow the standards set by the Hague convention (1993) on the rights of children.

The decline in children offered for adoption means that it is no longer an easy way to have children: it has turned into a long, expensive and emotionally draining quest with uncertain outcomes (Högbacka 2008). By contrast, the improved success and broadened methods of infertility treatments provide a more sure way to have a child.

Infertility treatments

A couple who has tried to conceive for one year (or sometimes two years) is counted as having experienced infertility. The prevalence of infertility thus defined is estimated to affect over 70 million women in the world, of whom about 40 million have sought treatment. This equals a median of 9 per cent of infertility in countries from which evidence is available, with wide differences between them (Boivin et al. 2007). Secondary infertility, or fertility problems relating to second or higher order children, should be added to this number but is harder to measure.

The proportions of biologically sterile couples in Western countries have apparently not increased dramatically during the last decades, although the effects of, for example, environmental pollution and chemicals on sperm quality remain unclear. Instead, postponement of parenthood to later ages partly account for the increased number of involuntary childless couples. One study estimated that the proportion of infertility in couples had more than doubled in European countries as an effect of delaying parenthood, rising from 2–3 per cent in 1970–85 to 6–7 per cent in 2007. Its effect on overall fertility is nevertheless small; only around 0.04 of total fertility rates is estimated lost to infertility due to postponement (te Velde et al. 2012).

However, the same study also estimated that if all of these couples wanted and could access infertility treatments, the effect of postponement would be neutralized. In other words, what parents lose in fecundity with age may be helped with advances in reproductive medicine. Since the introduction of in-vitro fertilization in the mid-1980s, infertility treatments have progressed rapidly. The treatments have become less invasive and safer for both mother and children, and the probability of successful pregnancies is higher (Carson et al. 2011; Gnoth et al. 2011). The effect of infertility treatments on overall fertility vary from around 1 per cent in the United States to 2–3 per cent in Northern Europe (Carrell and Peterson 2010, p. 715).

A recent review found that assisted reproductive technologies could help half of the women who tried during three menstrual cycles to give birth to a child. If they continued with the treatments, as many as two of three women ended up having a healthy child. The authors conclude that 'most couples with infertility problems can be treated successfully if they continue treatment' (Gnoth et al. 2011). Since the topic has gained in public visibility, more couples know how to seek help in time.

However, around three of four couples facing infertility choose not to have treatments. The choice often relates to the nature of treatment offered. Most usual procedures are assisted reproduction or in-vitro fertilization, which may be more or less invasive for the patient and have various side effects. Many also do not start such treatments due to religious or ethical reasons, or because they lack the required economic resources.

Another problem is that infertility treatments may not be accessible to people who are not clinically infertile, such as single women and lesbian couples. Interestingly, even in a highly tolerant and liberal country such as Sweden, single women are not allowed to receive artificial insemination, and this decision is supported by a large part of the population. While public morality may easily condemn 'selfish' women, the women concerned blame men for failing to show up as reliable partners. One woman writing on the site of *The Guardian* in 2011 reflects:

> Sorry guys, you have let us down, yet I find it is you who are the harshest critics.... The IVF counselor said that in all the 15 years that she had practiced that there wasn't one woman who wanted to do this alone by choice, all had wanted a partner. Not one.

Yet more complex ethical and social issues arise when infertility treatments involve donated sperms or egg cells, or when the baby is born by a surrogate mother. At the extreme, a foetus is conceived by donated sperm and donated eggs and carried by a surrogate mother, after which the social parents adopt their child. Here the border between infertility treatment and inter-country adoption is irrevocably blurred.

To conclude: family planning as planning for children

This chapter has discussed how our prolonged life span and broader set of choices in life create a new space for baby longing. The importance that 'baby fever' has acquired in today's reproductive discussions reflects how challenging it may feel to find time, or make time, for parenthood.

There are theoretically more ways to become a parent today, through different family constellations, infertility treatments and adoption. However, there are currently higher demands than opportunities for adoption, and although the success rate of infertility treatments are constantly improving, more and more people suffer from childlessness at least at some point in their lives, due to physiological problems or the lack of a partner.

The issue of conception is so different from the issue of contraception, that the older generation and general public has been quite slow in grasping the extent of the despair related to unwanted childlessness. As one British woman commented on *The Guardian*'s website: 'There is little comment in society on the pain of being unable to have or lose children, for whatever reason.' Another woman agreed: 'Feminism did great things for us women, in terms of jobs and votes, but it has had a detrimental effect on maternity, it pushed our main aim in life to the side.'

While it is unfair to blame feminism for all the changes affecting women during the last three decades, the last quotation does raise an interesting point. In the 1970s, few predicted that individual self-realization would lead to growing agony and despair over decision making, and that unwanted childlessness would grow to such proportions.

Given a choice, most women and men would ideally want at least one long-term partner and 2–3 children (OECD Family database SF2.2). This basic trend is sometimes forgotten when rightfully praising the variety of families including childfree lifestyles that have become possible and more accepted during the so-called second demographic transition.

Indeed, with regards to parenthood the blessings of the second demographic transition have been mixed. During the 'first' demographic transition the lives of families undeniably improved: more infants survived, women gained greater control of their childbearing. The numbers of childless women also fell. But since the late 1960s and the shift to below replacement fertility, the development of parenthood seems harder to evaluate in positive terms only. True, there is less discrimination by gender, ethnicity and sexual orientation, but there are also more fragile unions, more men and women who are single against their will, and consequently more people who would have time for a family but feel the time passing them by.

Longing for a child but being unable to have one can turn into an obsession and negatively affect mental health and marital satisfaction. This appears to happen more easily among women.

Nevertheless, we have seen that men's and women's baby longing is not a question of binary categories but of degrees. For both sexes, baby fever typically appears when they have the first child. That a sizeable minority, including mothers and fathers with many children, had never strongly longed to have a child serves as a reminder that baby longing is not as universal as, for instance, the ability to fall in love.

Social and psychological services need to support individuals and couples in their childbearing decisions or in coping with involuntary childlessness. Obviously, the support should not aim at any specific solution but in helping people make the choices that suit them best. After the famous pioneering work by Bombardieri (1981), there are an increasing number of popular books on taking the 'the baby decision', but few if any of these insights are incorporated into professional training programmes. Many professionals are nervous about the risks of raising the question in the wrong and intrusive way. More studies are needed regarding which contexts are best for discussing family desires and plans in the broader sense – peer groups, social services or, for example, student medical services?

References

Boivin, J., Bunting, L., Collins, J. A. and Nygren, K. G. (2007) International estimates of infertility prevalence and treatment-seeking: potential need and demand for infertility medical care, *Human Reproduction,* 22(6): 1506–12. Doi: 10.1093/humrep/dem046.

Bombardieri, M. (1981) *The Baby Decision. How to Make the Most Important Choice of Your Life* (New York: Rawson Associates).

Brase, G. L. and Brase, S. L. (2011) Emotional regulation of fertility decision making: what is the nature and structure of 'baby fever'? *Emotion,* advance online publication, 15(8). Doi: 10.1037/a0024954

Carrell, D. T. and Peterson, C. M. (eds) (2010) *Reproductive Endocrinology and Infertility: Integrating Modern Clinical and Laboratory Practice* (New York: Springer).

Carson, C., Kelly, Y., Kurinczuk, J. J., Sacker, A., Redshaw, M. and Quigley, M. A. (2011) Effect of pregnancy planning and fertility treatment on cognitive outcomes in children at ages 3 and 5: longitudinal cohort study, *BMJ, 343.* Doi:10.1136/bmj.d4473.

Clark-Flory, T. (2012) I've got baby fever, *Salon,* 22(4), http://www.salon.com/2012/04/22/the_science_of_baby_fever/, date accessed 12 November 2012.

Euler, H. A. (2011) Grandparents and extended kin. In C. Salmon and T. K. Shackelford (eds) *The Oxford Handbook of Evolutionary Family Psychology* (Oxford: Oxford University Press), pp. 205–17.

Gnoth, C., Maxrath, B., Skonieczny, T., Friol, K., Godehardt, E. and Tigges, J. (2011) Final ART success rates: a 10 years survey, *Human Reproduction,* 26(8): 2239–46. Doi:10.1093/humrep/der178.

Goldstein, J. R. (2011) A secular trend toward earlier male sexual maturity: evidence from shifting ages f male young adult mortality, *PLoS ONE,* 6(8): e14826.

Hague adoption convention (1993) Convention on protection of children and co-operation in respect of intercountry adoption, http://www.hcch.net/index_en.php?act=conventions.textandcid=69, date accessed 3 March 2012.

Heckhausen, J. and Wrosch, C. (2002) Developmental regulation before and after a developmental deadline: the sample case of 'biological clock' for childbearing, *Psychology and Aging,* 16(3): 400–13.

Hegar, R. and Scannapieco, M. (1999) *Kinship Foster Care: Policy, Practice, and Research* (Oxford: Oxford University Press).

Högbacka, R. (2008) The quest for a child of one's own: parents, markets and transnational adoption, *Journal of Comparative Family Studies,* 39(3): 311–30.

Maestripieri, D., Roney, J. R., De Bias, N., Durante, K. M. and Spaepen, G. M. (2004) Father absence, menarche and interest in infants among adolescent girls, *Developmental Science*, 7: 560–6.

Marlowe, F. (2011) *The Hadza Hunter-gatherers of Tanzania* (Berkeley: University of California Press).

McCallin, J. (2011) The father's a viking, The Guardian, family, Saturday 5 February 2011, http://www.guardian.co.uk/lifeandstyle/2011/feb/05/sperm-donation-denmark-artificial-insemination#start-of-comments, date accessed 6 May 2011.

Miller, W. B. (1986) Proception: an important fertility behaviour, *Demography*, 23: 579–94.

Morris, D. H., Jones, M. E., Schoemaker, M. J., Ashworth, A. and Swerdlow, A. J. (2011) Secular trends in age at menarche in women in the UK born 1908–93: results from the Breakthrough Generations Study, *Paediatric and Perinatal Epidemiology*, 25: 394–400.

O'Connell, A. J. (2012) Baby fever: it's real, it's weird, and it's the reason I'm still awake. Blog posted 3 April 2012. http://ajoconnell.wordpress.com/tag/baby-lust/, date accessed 12 November 2012.

OECD Family database SF2.2: Ideal and actual number of children. http://www.oecd.org/els/social/family/database, date accessed 10 January 2012.

Pikul, C. (2011) The clockwatcher: how do you know when – or if – you should have a baby?, *American ELLE magazine*, February: 164–6.

Raj, A. Saggurti, N. Balaiah, D. and Silverman, J. G. (2009) Prevalence of child marriage and its effect on fertility and fertility-control outcomes of young women in India: a cross-sectional, observational study, *The Lancet*, 373(9678): 1883–9.

Rotkirch, A. (2007) All that she wants is another baby? Longing for children as a fertility incentive of growing importance, *Journal of Evolutionary Psychology*, 5(1–4): 89–104.

Rotkirch, A. (2008) What is 'baby fever'? Contrasting evolutionary explanations of proceptive behavior. In T. Meleghy, P. Meyer and H.-J. Niedenzu (eds) *The New Evolutionary social Science: Human Nature, Social Behaviour, and Social Change* (Boulder, CO: Paradigm Publishers), pp. 147–58.

Rotkirch, A., Basten, S., Väisänen, H. and Jokela, M. (2011) Baby longing and men's reproductive motivation. *Vienna Yearbook of Demographic Research 2011*, 9: 283–306.

Selman, P. (2002) Intercountry adoption in the new millennium; the 'quite migration' revisited, *Population Research and Policy Review*, 21: 205–25.

Selman, P. (2009) The rise and fall of intercountry adoption in the 21st century, *International Social Work*, 52(5): 575–94.

Silk, J. B. (2003) Natal attraction in adult female baboons (*Papio cynocephalus ursinus*) in the Moremi Reserve, Botswana, *Ethology*, 109(8): 627–44.

te Velde, E., Habbema, D., Leridon, H. and Eijkemans, M. (2012) The effect of postponement of first motherhood on permanent involuntary childlessness and total fertility rate in six European countries since the 1970s, *Human Reproduction, advance access*. Doi: 10.1093/humrep/

Thomson, E. (1997) Couple childbearing desires, intentions, and births, *Demography*, 34(3): 343–54.

Thomson, E. and Hoem, J. M. (1998) Couple childbearing plans and births in Sweden, *Demography,* 35(3): 315–22.

Thomson, E., McDonald, E. and Bumpass, L. L. (1990) Fertility desires and fertility: hers, his, theirs, *Demography,* 27(4): 579–88.

Wager, M. (2000) Childless by choice? Ambivalence and the female identity, *Feminism and Psychology,* 10: 389–95.

Waxman, A. Q. (2009) *Gender Differences and Their Influence on the Desire for Genetic Relatedness during Infertility Treatment* (San Francisco Bay: Alliant International University).

Westermarck, E. (1891) *The History of Human Marriage*. London: Macmillan.

Part IV

A Look into the Crystal Ball: Possible Responses

16
Family Policy and Fertility: Do Policies Make a Difference?

Anne H. Gauthier

In view of persistent very low levels of fertility (as discussed in Part I of this volume), many governments in Europe and other industrialized countries have been asking the questions of how best to support families and, in some cases, how to also encourage young people to have more children? Perhaps ironically, in the 1960s some of the same governments were instead concerned by their rapidly increasing population and high fertility (Gauthier 1996). Today, however, the situation is very different: not only has fertility remained below replacement level for more than three decades in numerous countries, but the spectre of a rapidly ageing population is also raising great worries among governments (Burnett 2007; Cowell 1993; Zeller 2010).[1] Whether or not governments should be concerned by this situation and whether or not they should actually intervene to raise fertility are however difficult questions which raise complex economic and ethical issues. In this chapter, we do not venture on that terrain but instead focus on the seemingly simple question: Can policies influence fertility?

We address this question by first reviewing the empirical evidence regarding the effects of policies on fertility. The overall conclusion of this review is that while policies appear to have a positive impact on fertility, the magnitude of this impact is very small. Moreover, the effect is often on the timing of births rather than on the total number of births. In view of this conclusion, we then devote the second section of this chapter to the possible explanations of this finding. In particular, we discuss the role of various elements that may influence the decision to have a child.

The empirical evidence

To start with, it is important to stress that very few countries have a comprehensive and well-coordinated family policy. In most cases, countries have instead patchwork of measures to support families, including direct and indirect cash transfers, leave entitlements and related cash benefits, as well as in-kind benefits and services. Moreover, it should be remembered that in most countries, family policies do not have an explicit pro-natalist objective and instead pursue a variety of goals including gender equality and poverty reduction. In other words, while some governments may implicitly aim at supporting individuals in their fertility decision, increasing fertility is rarely a stated objective. Whether or not policies can in fact increase fertility remains nonetheless a topical question.

So what do we know about it? The empirical literature on this topic is rapidly growing, and it is useful to distinguish three 'generations' of studies. The first generation was based mainly on indirect observations linking policies on the one hand and fertility on the other. For example, many argued that the fact that the level of fertility in France during the baby boom years and the following baby bust was higher than in most other European countries was the result of the strong French family policy introduced from the 1930s.[2] The policy, it was estimated, was responsible for a fertility rate that was about 10 per cent higher than in other countries (Dumont and Descroix 1988). Other studies pointed to the case of East Germany as evidence of the impact of policies on fertility. This argument was based on the observation that following the introduction of a series of family policies measures in East Germany in the 1970s, the fertility trends in East and West Germany started to strongly diverge. In this case, policies were estimated to have increased completed fertility by 0.1 to 0.3 children per woman (Chesnais 1987). While convincing, these studies were however relatively simple methodologically, and more importantly they failed to take into account other societal changes that may simultaneously have influenced fertility.

The second generation of studies came in the 1980s and 1990s when more complex data and more complex methodologies were used. For example, Blanchet and Ekert-Jaffé (1994), on the basis of data from 11 European countries for the period 1970–83, estimated that family benefits as equal to those provided in France resulted in higher fertility level of about 0.2 to 0.3 children per woman. Using a similar methodology and a larger number of countries, Gauthier and Hatzius (1997) concluded that a 25 per cent increase in cash benefits would result in a long-run increase in fertility of 0.07 children per woman. In general, studies published during this period concluded to a positive impact of policies on fertility but of a relatively small magnitude (see the review by Gauthier 2002 for more details). However, these studies were also limited, especially in view of their reliance on aggregate data (at the country level). In particular, these studies were unable to analyse whether different population subgroups responded differently to policies, and whether the impact of the policies was mostly on the timing of births or on the total number of births (the so-called tempo vs. quantum effect).

The third generation of studies published since the 1990s have attempted to address these methodological limitations by mainly using individual-level data.[3] By following individuals over time, these studies aimed at assessing whether changes in policies increased the likelihood of people having a child. In general, these studies also concluded to a positive impact of policies on fertility but provided more details regarding the impact of specific policies. With regard to cash benefits, studies overall suggest that continuous types of transfers (such as family or child allowances) as well as birth grants (also known as baby bonus) do result in an increase in fertility (Thévenon and Gauthier 2011). Some studies found however no such effect. For example, a recent study by Kalwij (2010) found no effect of financial transfers on completed family size on the basis of an analysis of 16 European countries. Studies on the impact of cash benefits further conclude that such benefits tend to affect mainly the timing of births rather than the completed fertility (Thévenon and Gauthier 2011). In other words, people tend to take advantage of the policy by having children sooner rather than later, but do not necessarily end up having more children.[4]

With regard to leave entitlements and related benefits (such as maternity, parental and childcare leave), recent studies suggest that more generous support is associated with higher fertility (Duvander et al. 2010). However, when the duration of the leave and the related cash benefits granted during the leave are examined separately, it appears that long leaves have a negative effect on fertility, while cash benefits have instead a positive or non-significant effect (Hilgeman and Butts 2009).[5] Finally, with regard to the provision of childcare facilities and related transfers, the evidence remains rather mixed with some studies concluding to a strong positive effect of childcare availability on fertility (Rindfuss et al. 2007), while others concluding to the absence of such an effect (Hank and Kreyenfeld 2003).

In view of this empirical evidence, it is perhaps surprising that policies do not appear to have a larger impact on fertility: surprising because by reducing the direct and indirect costs of children, and by helping parents to more easily combine work and family, one could expect policies to have a more systematic and larger influence on fertility. As discussed further, there are however numerous reasons that may explain this finding. The next question addressed in this chapter is therefore: why don't policies have a larger impact on fertility?

Re-examining the links between policies and fertility

When raising the question of how to increase fertility, policy-makers often assume that there are obstacles that prevent couples from realising their desired number of children. Moreover, it is assumed that if governments can reduce some of these obstacles through specific policies, it would allow more couples to realize their fertility desires, which would therefore result in higher fertility. There are two main elements behind this assumption that need to be considered.

About fertility desires and the fertility gap

First, there is the so-called fertility gap, that is, the difference between individuals' fertility desires and their actual fertility. This gap, it is commonly assumed, represents the window of opportunity for policies and is usually estimated by comparing the individuals' ideal family size and their actual fertility. Figure 16.1 shows the average personal ideal number of children, as captured in the 2006 Eurobarometer Survey, and the actual fertility rate for that year. The difference between these two indicators for the countries represented here is 0.85 children on average. It is larger in countries such as Cyprus, Greece and Ireland (exceeding 1 child), and smaller in countries such as Austria (with less than 0.5 children).

Numerous commentators have used this gap as evidence for the possible impact of policies (European Commission 2005). This gap is however likely overestimated for numerous reasons. First of all, although the survey asks respondents about their own personal ideal number of children,[6] we know that there is a strong social desirability element involved. In other words, people know what is generally considered acceptable in their society and may therefore indicate what they perceive as being the ideal number of children as opposed to what they really think themselves. An indication that this may be the case is the fact that a very small percentage of people usually respond that zero or one child is ideal. Instead, the majority of people answer that having two children is the ideal. Across the 25 countries that participated in

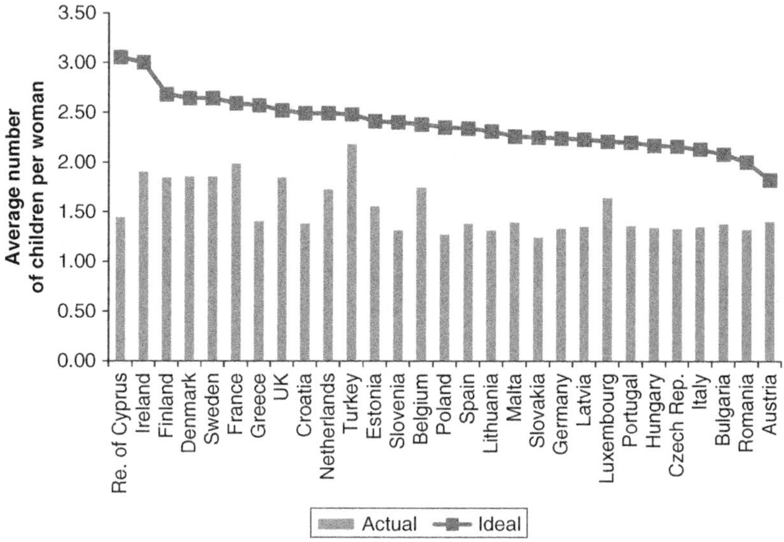

Figure 16.1 Ideal and actual fertility (2006)
Sources: Data on ideal family size come from the 2006 Eurobarometer survey (see Testa 2006, table 4). Data on actual fertility come from the 2008 European Demographic Data Sheet.

the 2006 Eurobarometer Survey, only 1 per cent responded that zero was the ideal and 6 per cent responded that one child was ideal. In contrast 53 per cent responded that two was ideal, and 23 per cent responded that three children was ideal.[7] We obviously do not know the extent to which this social desirability causes a bias in the data. What we however do know from a small experiment carried out in the Netherlands is that respondents are split when confronted with the hypothetical situation of not being able to have their stated ideal number of children. In the experiment, respondents had to choose between having one more child or one fewer child than their ideal number. Among respondents who said that having two children was ideal, 46 per cent said that they would opt for one child if they could not have two, and 54 per cent said that would opt for having three (Hin et al. 2011). The reasons to opt for one child or for three children when confronted to this hypothetical situation were not asked in the survey. But one may interpret these results by saying that the respondents initially stated the fertility ideal that corresponded to what they perceived as socially desirable, while the follow-up question instead tapped more closely into their own preference. Unfortunately, this type of follow-up question is not part of standard fertility questionnaires, thus forcing analysts to rely on the standard question on fertility ideals.

Second, we also know that people's fertility desires and intentions are not stable over time. In fact they are highly volatile in that they change as people mature and face various new circumstances. For example, an analysis based on longitudinal data in West Germany revealed that around half of the respondents modified their total desired fertility over a six-year period (Heiland et al. 2008). Furthermore, evidence from the Netherlands suggests that the majority of people adjust their fertility intentions downwards as they age (Liefbroer 2009). What this means is that the estimation of the fertility gap based on the comparison of fertility ideal and actual fertility, as measured at one point in time, may also be very unstable.

Third, one of the additional reasons why people have less children than they desire may also be because of disagreement between spouses (Thomson 1997). In almost all countries, men's ideal number of children is lower than that of women. In some countries, such as Poland and Portugal, the difference is negligible, but in others, such as Finland, the Netherlands and Sweden, it is larger, reaching around 0.25 children (data from the 2006 Eurobarometer survey not shown here). And while it is difficult to predict how couples resolve such differences regarding fertility desires, studies suggest that the resolution of the disagreement depends on various factors including the level of gender equity in the household and in the society in general (Rosina and Testa 2009).

Finally, what we should also remember is that the data on actual fertility that were used in the previous graph are period fertility rates which are highly sensitive to changes in the timing of birth. If data that correct for changes in the timing of births had instead been used (the so-called tempo-adjusted fertility rate), the gap would have decreased from 0.85 children per woman to 0.62.[8]

Although various obstacles may indeed force some people to have fewer children than they would like, what should be kept in mind is that the fertility gap is probably smaller than what is usually estimated from survey data, and therefore the window of opportunity of governments is also likely to be much smaller.

About the obstacles to fertility

The second assumption made by policy-makers is that there are obstacles that prevent people from fulfilling their fertility desires, namely obstacles of a financial nature and obstacles related to the combination

Table 16.1 Reasons for not wanting a(nother) child, age 20–40 (% identifying these reasons as very important)[a,b]

	Future	Cost of children	Standard of living	Work-family balance	Lifestyle	Leisure
Belgium-Flanders	18	11	n/a	20	12	n/a
Czech Republic	27	12	4	7	4	2
Germany-East	33	25	18	11	12	7
Germany-West	19	14	17	10	13	9
Estonia	33	37	6	15	n/a	3
Cyprus	44	17	8	11	6	5
Lithuania	41	15	7	3	2	1
Hungary	39	22	15	7	3	3
The Netherlands	10	7	10	1	6	3
Austria	25	22	29	19	18	15
Poland	41	23	11	4	5	2
Romania	34	29	13	13	7	4
Slovenia	13	9	7	8	4	3
Finland	7	5	5	2	4	2
Average	27.4	17.7	11.5	9.4	7.4	4.5

n/a: not available.
[a]The exact wording of the items was as follows: (1) Future: 'I am too concerned about the future of my children'; (2) Cost of children: 'A(nother) child would cost too much'; (3) Standard of living: 'I want to maintain my present standard of living'; (4) Work-family balance: 'My job and professional activities would not allow it'; (5) Lifestyle: 'I would not be able to enjoy life as I have so far'; and (6) Leisure: 'I would have to give up leisure time interest'.
[b]Items related to health and partner's situation have been omitted.
Source: Fokkema and Esveldt (2006, table 3.3).

of work and family. It is however worth examining the extent to which people themselves identify such reasons as being obstacles to fertility. The data here come from the 'Population Policy Acceptance Study', which were collected in selected countries in the period 2000–03. Results appear in Table 16.1. Respondents aged 20–40 were asked to identify the reason for not wanting a(another) child.[9]

Very interestingly, the top reason in all countries is not the one related to the work-family combination nor about the cost of children but instead the reason related to the future of children, namely 'I am too concerned about the future of my children'. Across all countries surveyed, more than a quarter of respondents identified this reason as very important. This compares with 18 per cent for the reason related to the cost of children, and 9 per cent for the reason related to work-family combination. Obviously, the reason related to the future of children was phrased very broadly in the survey, and we do not know exactly what participants had in mind when they selected this answer. But it seems to suggest that although helping families financially and helping them combine work and family responsibilities may be welcomed societal goals, there are other reasons why fertility may be lower than people say they desire and reasons why policies appear to have only a small impact on fertility.

Re-examining the nature of family policies

Other possible reasons why policies appear to have only a small impact on fertility may be related to the nature of policies themselves. In particular, and as discussed below, cash transfers are relatively small in most countries, the leave entitlement and related benefits cover only a fraction of the opportunity cost for women, and the cost of childcare continues to be very high for most parents.

Cash support for families with children

In most countries, cash support for families is provided in the form of direct cash transfers (such as child or family allowances) and indirect transfers (such as tax relief). These transfers are universal in some countries and means-tested in others and are usually paid until the child reaches 16 or 18 years old (or until an older age in some countries). The other form of cash support that is provided in some countries is the so-called baby bonus or baby grant which is a lump sum amount paid at the birth of a child. Together these various forms of cash transfers represent an amount that varies widely across countries but that also varies according to the number and age of children, the family's income and the type of family. Figure 16.2 captures the situation for one type of family, namely a married couple with average earnings.[10] The index compares the net income (after taxes and transfers) of one such family with two children aged four and six years with that of an equivalent childless couple. A value of '1' for this index would indicate that the two families have an identical net income and thus that no cash transfer or tax relief was provided for the family with two children. In contrast, a value above '1' indicates the presence of governmental support. Across all 34 countries represented in Figure 16.2, the average value of the index is 1.065, which means that the combined cash transfers and tax relief for children increases the net income of the family with children by 6.5 per cent. In absolute terms, the combination of cash transfers and tax relief averages around US $3000 for two children per year (data not shown

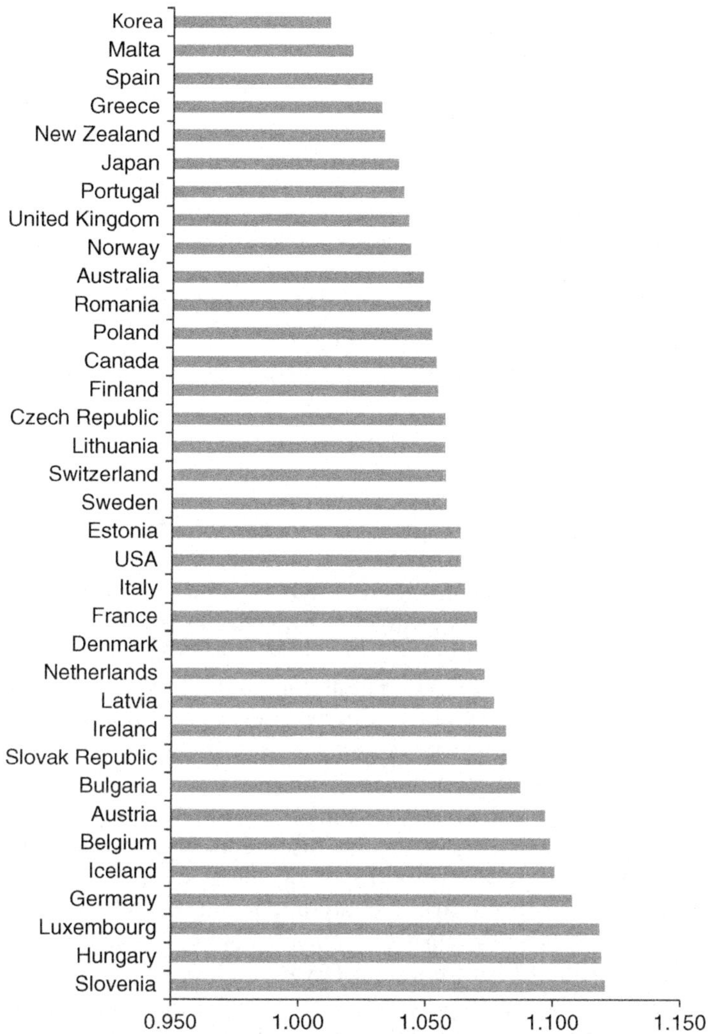

Figure 16.2 Index of disposable income (2009)
Source: Computed by the author using the OECD online cash-benefit calculator.

here). Thus, while not negligible, this amount is very small compared to the actual cost of children.

A similar comment can be made regarding the provision of birth grants (or baby-bonus) hailed by some governments as a good instrument to encourage young adults to have more children. Generous bonuses are currently found in Russia (see Chapter 8) and Australia. In Australia there is payment of A$5294 (in 2010) at the birth of a child.[11] And while this amount would be welcomed by any parent, one could doubt its ability to convince individuals to have an additional child. Yet, the literature generally concludes to a positive effect of such a birth grant on fertility (Drago et al. 2009; Lain et al. 2009; Sinclair et al. 2010). Analyses of the Australian case suggest, however, also the presence of a timing effect, as parents appear to have strategically timed their childbirth in order to take advantage of the policy when it was first introduced (Gans and Leigh 2009). Other studies furthermore point to the symbolic nature of the benefit, which may have contributed to make parents feel more supported (Lee 2011).

Maternity and parental leave

In addition to cash benefits, nearly all countries nowadays also provide parents with maternity and parental leave schemes. In the case of maternity leave, this is not a new development since such schemes were mostly introduced in the early twentieth century (see Gauthier 1996). The introduction of parental leave schemes is however a much more recent development and dates mainly from the 1990s. In recent years, some countries have furthermore introduced specific paternity leaves either as an independent scheme or as part of the parental leave. There are two main elements about these schemes that are important to consider: their duration and the value of their cash benefits. In terms of duration, in most countries, the maternity leave is about 12–16 weeks: the idea being to give time for the child and mother to bond, to recover from childbirth and to provide the mother with an opportunity to breastfeed during the first months of her child's life. In the case of parental leave, the duration is usually much longer and extends until the child's second or third birthday in some countries. Nowadays, these two types of leaves, when combined, have a duration of around 87 weeks (in industrialized countries), so just short of a child's second birthday.

The duration of the leave should however not be examined on its own but in combination with the amount of cash benefits paid during the leave. For the maternity leave, most countries offer a financial compensation of around 80–100 per cent of earnings (although in some countries this is subject to a ceiling). The situation is much more varied regarding parental leave, which varies from unpaid leave to fully compensated leaves.

In Figure 16.3 these two elements, duration and pay, are illustrated. Together, they allow us to distinguish four main clusters of countries

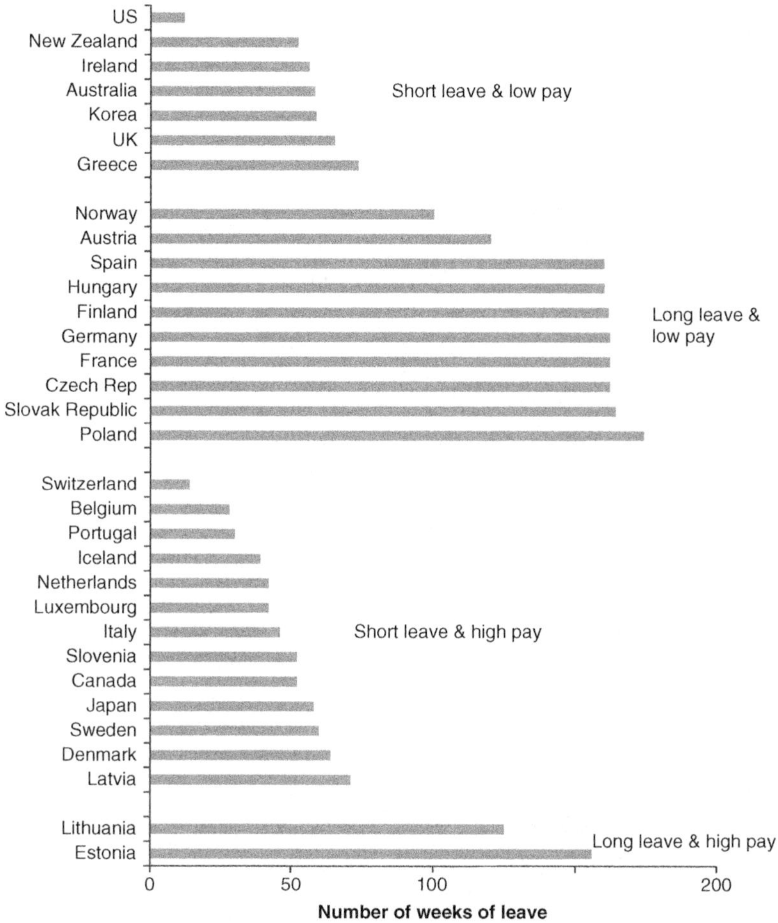

Figure 16.3 Characteristics of parental leave scheme (2007–08)
Source: OECD family policy database. PF2.1: Key characteristics of parental leave systems. Online: http://www.oecd.org/dataoecd/45/26/37864482.pdf

ranging from countries offering leave of short duration with low cash benefits to countries offering leave of long duration accompanied with high cash benefits. From a fertility and financial perspective, it seems that leaves that are not too long and that are well paid offer the best combination in allowing parents to spend time with their young child but also by restricting the so-called opportunity cost of children (i.e. the amount of money foregone while being on leave).

In addition to the duration and pay of maternity and paternity leave, other dimensions of the leaves may also matter. In particular, a few studies have focused on the extent to which the take-up of leave by fathers has an impact on fertility. These studies conclude that fathers' use of parental leave has a positive impact on childbearing at least in Norway and Sweden where the participation of fathers in parental leave has a longer history and is encouraged (Duvander et al. 2010; Lappegard 2010). In most countries, however, although the parental leave may be shared between parents, the take-up by fathers remains quite low (Moss 2010).[12]

As to other dimensions such as the eligibility to maternity and parental leave schemes, their scheduling flexibility, their job protection, their acceptability in the workplace and the right to part-time work, their impact on fertility has not yet been examined systematically in the literature, thus leaving us with a limited understanding of the impact of leave entitlements on fertility.[13]

Childcare provision

In an attempt to help families combine work and family responsibilities, much attention has been given in recent years to the provision of childcare facilities. The nature of such childcare facilities varies largely within and across countries from formal day care centres to family homes, crèches and pre-primary school institutions. As a result, it is relatively difficult to obtain comparable data. Figure 16.4 illustrates the enrolment rates of children under age six in formal care or early education services in various countries.

When it comes to children under the age of three, the enrolment is low in all countries averaging 29 per cent among the countries represented on this chart. In general, the figure tends to be higher in Nordic countries and some other Western European countries (e.g. the Netherlands, Luxembourg, France), while it tends to be very low in Eastern Europe as well as in Austria and Germany. The low level of enrolment of children in formal care in some of these countries is however a reflection of the availability of very long parental leave schemes, which reduce the demand for childcare especially for very young children. For older children, the coverage is much more extensive reaching around 75 per cent for the countries represented in Figure 16.3. Provision for children aged three and above reaches nearly 100 per cent in France, Belgium and Italy but continues to be low in countries such as Greece, Poland and Switzerland.

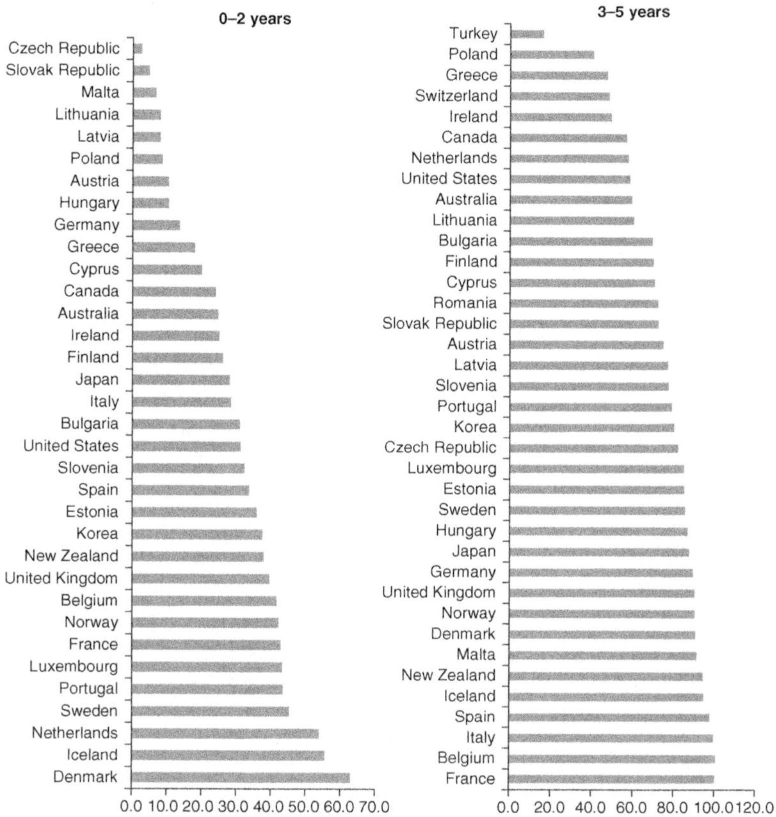

Figure 16.4 Enrolment rates of children under age six in formal care or early childhood education services (in percent)
Source: OECD family policy database. PF3.2: Enrolment in childcare and pre-schools. Online: http://www.oecd.org/dataoecd/46/13/37864698.pdf

In most countries, the provision of childcare has increased rapidly in the past two decades in response to the increased labour force participation of mothers with children. As discussed earlier, the evidence is however quite mixed when it comes to the effect of this type of policies on fertility. Likely, one possible reason for this is that the actual provision of childcare is only one of several elements that matter for parents. Other factors that most likely play a role, and that are usually not considered in studies, include the cost of childcare, its quality, its accessibility, its convenience in terms of opening hours and its rules regarding the admission of siblings.

An heterogeneous impact of policies

A final element to be considered is the possible heterogeneous impact of policies on fertility, in other words, the possibility that the same family policy may have different impacts on different subgroups in a population. There are two such possible sources of heterogeneity. First, numerous studies have shown that women of different parities (i.e. with a different number of children) tend to respond differently to policies. Some studies suggest, for example, that the impact of family policies tends to be largest for women with two or three children as compared to women with no children or only one (Buccuzzo et al. 2008; Gabos et al. 2009). In contrast, other studies conclude that policies have a larger impact on first births (Gauthier and Hatzius 1997). It may well be that the decision to have a first, second or subsequent child is influenced differently by policies, but our knowledge on this type of heterogeneity remains limited.

The second possible source of heterogeneity is the socio-economic status of parents and parents-to-be. Several studies indeed suggest that the effect of policies is largest among less-educated women. This appears, for example, to be the case with the income tax in Spain (Azmat and Gonzales 2010) and the baby bonus in Italy (Buccuzzo et al. 2008). Similarly, the impact of parental and childcare leave schemes appears to be larger on the fertility decision of women with a low level of education and low income (Aassve and Lappegard 2009). This may be explained by the fact that for women with a lower income, the cash benefits cover a relatively higher percentage of the cost of children. Alternatively, it could also be that women with low socio-economic status are more responsive to measures such as the child home care allowance in Norway and the Allocation Parental d'Education in France because of their weaker attachment to the labour market. In contrast, measures that tend to be more beneficial to higher income individuals (such as the tax rebates for children in France) tend to have a larger impact on households with higher incomes (Landais 2003).

Discussion and conclusion

Despite the large interest in academic and governmental circles in the possible impact of policies on fertility, and despite a rapidly growing literature on this topic, our knowledge on this question remains limited. Various factors remain unknown or have not (yet) been properly captured in analyses. First, there is the fact that studies have not been able to convincingly demonstrate whether specific policy measures matter most to families or whether it is instead the whole 'package' of policies that may influence fertility decisions. Although there are good reasons to expect that it is indeed the package of policies that matters most, this is something that we have not so far shown empirically. Second, what we also assume is that what matters is the consistency of policies over time. The assumption here is that parents or parents-to-be need to feel secure in their decision to have a child and need to know that they can rely on governmental support and that this support will not disappear from one day to the other. From this point of view, the lack of consistency in governmental support for families that has been observed in some Eastern and Central European countries in recent years most likely added additional obstacles to fertility (Gauthier 2010).

Third, there is the issue of people's overall confidence in the economy, which may also have an impact on the decision to have a(nother) child, and this overall confidence goes far beyond the possible impact of family policies themselves. Although it may be very important to help families combine work and family responsibilities (which is the objective of many family policies), to start with people need to feel that their job and financial situation are secure. This is perhaps the explanation why worries about the future of children rank so highly among the reasons for not wanting another child as discussed earlier. Fourth, we can expect that what also matters is for policies to be flexible and to accommodate different lifestyles, such as married or cohabiting parents, being in full-time or part-time work, or being a student in higher education. We really do not know much about this, but with the increasing differentiation of the life course, we can expect people to expect policies that can accommodate their specific situation.

Finally, although the empirical evidence suggests that family policies alone are unlikely to have a large direct impact on fertility – at least not without costing a lot of money to governments – it is possible that they may have an indirect impact. Perhaps what policies can do is to act more broadly on the overall context in which young families live, for example, by creating greater happiness with work and with life in general, generating more confidence in the future, and helping create greater gender equality including in paid and unpaid work. Once these conditions are in place, we will perhaps observe a significant effect of policies on fertility. The creation of a more family- or child-friendly environment would however require a concerted action from various ministries within a government and also between the public and private sectors. Basically, what governments need to do is to put in place policies that make prospective parents feel that they are supported in their decision to have a child. Perhaps only then may policies end up having a larger difference on fertility.

Notes

1. Among 49 developed countries surveyed in 2009, 30 stated that they considered their level of fertility as too low, while 19 said it was satisfactory (United Nations 2010).
2. The French *'Code de la famille'* was introduced in 1939. It contains a series of measures to support families and to help boost the fertility rate (Reggiani 1996).
3. For a more detailed review, the reader is referred to Thévenon and Gauthier (2011).
4. However, Lutz and Skirbekk (2005) argue that such a tempo-effect may in the long run also influence the total completed fertility.
5. Numerous studies have also pointed out that long maternity or paternal leaves have a detrimental impact on women's earnings (see, e.g. Gupta et al. 2008).
6. The question asked in the 2006 Eurobarometer survey was: 'And for you personally, what would be the ideal number of children you would like to have or would have liked to have had?'.
7. In addition, 4 per cent responded that four or more children was ideal, and 11 per cent responded that they had no ideal.
8. For the tempo-adjusted fertility rates, I used data from the 2010 European Demographic Data Sheet.
9. Note that this question was only asked to respondents who stated earlier in the survey that they did not intend to have a(nother) child in the future.
10. In this particular case, the main earner is assumed to have an earning equal to 100 per cent of the average wage, while his spouse is assumed to have an earning equal to 67 per cent of the average wage.
11. Using Parity Purchasing Power, this is the equivalent of around US $3500.
12. The take-up rate by fathers appears to be higher when the parental leave scheme includes an individual entitlement element (as opposed to a family entitlement) and when it is relatively well paid (Moss 2010, p. 30).
13. The possibility of taking part-time work appears to have a positive effect on fertility according to D'Addio and D'Ercole (2005).

References

Aassve, A. and Lappegard, T. (2009) Childcare cash benefits and fertility timing in Norway, *European Journal of Population*, 25(1): 413–38.

Azmat, G. and Gonzales, L. (2010) Targeting fertility and female participation through the income tax, *Labour Economics*, 17(3): 487–502.

Blanchet, D. and Ekert-Jaffé, O. (1994) The demographic impact of family benefits: evidence from a micro-model and from macro-data. In J. Ermisch and N. Ogawa (eds) *The Family, the Market and the State in Aging Societies* (Oxford: Clarendon Press), pp. 79–103.

Buccuzzo, G., Caltabiano, M., Dall Zuana, G. and Loghi, M. (2008) The impact of the bonus at birth on reproductive behaviour in a lowest-low fertility contect: Friuli-Venezia Giulia (Italy) from 1989 to 2005, *Vienna Yearbook of Population Research*, 125–48.

Burnett, V. (2007) Low birth rate prompts Spain to approve child bonus, *The New York Times*. Online: http://www.nytimes.com/2007/07/13/world/europe/13iht-spain.4.6652189.html, date accessed 27 April 2011.

Chesnais, J.-C. (1987) Quand un people en devient deux: Une allemagne et l'autre, *Population et Sociétés*, 209, 1–4.

Cowell, A. (1993) Low birth rate is becoming a headache for Italy, *The New York Times*, 28 August 1993.

D'Addio, A. C and D'Ercole, M. M. (2005) Policies, institutions and fertility rates: a panel data analysis for OECD countries, *OECD Economic Studies*, 41: 7–43. Online: http://www.oecd.org/dataoecd/61/44/40505223.pdf, date accessed 13 May 2011.

Drago, R. Sawyer, K., Sheffler, K. Warren, D. and Wooden, M. (2009) Did Australia's baby bonus increase the fertility rate?, *Melbourne Institute Working Paper Series*, no. 1/09 (Melbourne).

Dumont, G.-F. and Descroix, P. (1988) La spécificité du comportement démographique de la France: Mesure de la surfécondité relative de la France par rapport aux autres pays industriels à faible fécondité précoce de 1963 à 1986, *Histoire, Economie et Société*, 7(3): 419–32.

Duvander, A.-Z., Lappegard, T. and Andersson, G. (2010) Family policy and fertility: a comparative study of the impact of fathers' and mothers' use of parental leave and continued childbearing in Norway and Sweden, *Journal of European Social Policy*, 20(1): 45–57.

European Commission (2005) Confronting demographic change: a new solidarity between the generations, *Green Paper COM 2005.94* (Brussels: Communication from the Commission of the European Communities).

Fokkema, T. and Esveldt, I. (2006) Work Package 7: Child-friendly Policies. Report. Online: http://www.bib-demografie.de/cln_090/nn_965290/SharedDocs/Publikationen/EN/Research/DIALOG/ReportsPapers/dialog__ps__no7,templateId= raw,property= publicationFile.pdf/dialog_ps_no7.pdf, date accessed 12 January 2011.

Gabos, A., Gal, R. and Kezdi, G. (2009) Birth order fertility effects of child-related benefits and pensions – a test on Hungarian data, *Population Studies*, 63(3): 215–31.

Gans, J. S. and Leigh, A. (2009) Born on the first of July: an (un)natural experiment in birth timing, *Journal of Public Economics*, 93: 246–64.

Gauthier, A. H. (1996) *The State and the Family* (Oxford: Clarendon Press).

Gauthier, A. H. (2002) Family policies in industrialized countries: is there convergence, *Population*, 57(3): 200.

Gauthier, A. H. (2010) *The Impact of the Economic Crisis on Family Policies in the European Union* (Brussels: European Commission), 18p.

Gauthier, A. and Hatzius, J. (1997) Family benefits and fertility: an econometric analysis, *Population Studies*, 51: 295–306.

Gupta, N. D., Smith, N. and Verner, M. (2008) The impact of Nordic countries' family friendly policies on employment, wages, and children, *Review of Economics of the Household*, 6(1): 65–89.

Hank, K. and Kreyenfeld, M. (2003) A multilevel analysis of child care and women's fertility decisions in Western Germany, *Journal of Marriage and the Family*, 65(3): 584–96.

Heiland, F., Prskawetz, A. and Sanderson, W. C. (2008) Are individuals' desired family sizes stable? Evidence from West German panel data: *European Journal of Population*, 24(2): 129–56.

Hilgeman, C. and Butts, C. (2009) Women's employment and fertility: a welfare regime paradox, *Social Science Research*, 38: 103–17.

Hin, S., Gauthier, A., Goldstein, J. and Buehler, C. (2011) Fertility preferences: what measuring second choices teaches us, *Vienna Yearbook of Population Research*, 135–162.

Kalwij, A. (2010) The impact of family policy expenditure on fertility in Western Europe, *Demography*, 47(2): 503–19.

Lain, S. J., Ford, J. B., Raynes-Greenow, C. H., Hadfield, R. M., Simpson, J. M., Morris, J. M. and Roberts, C. L. (2009) The impact of the baby bonus payment in New South Wales: who is having 'one for the country'?, *The Medical Journal of Australia*, 190(5): 238–41.

Landais, C. (2003) Le quotient familial a-t-il stimulé la natalité francaise, *Economie Publique*, 13: 3–31.

Lappegard, T. (2010) Family policies and fertility in Norway, *European Journal of Population*, 26: 99–116.

Lee, V. (2011) More babies, but was it the bonus? Australia's success in raising its birth rate could offer pointers for Singapore. Online: http://www.todayonline.com/Print/World/EDC110205-0000138/More-babies,-but-was-it-the-bonus, date accessed 13 May 2011.

Liefbroer, A. C. (2009) Changes in family size intentions across young adulthood: a life-course perspective, *European Journal of Population*, 25(4): 363–86.

Lutz, W. and Skirbekk, V. (2005) Policies addressing the tempo effect in low-fertility countries, *Population and Development Review*, 31(4): 699–720.

Moss, P. (ed.) (2010) International Review of Leave Policies and Related Research 2010. Employment Market Analysis and Research Department for Business, Innovation and Skills, United Kingdom.

Reggiani, A. H. (1996) Procreating France: the politics of demography, 1919–45, *French Historical Studies*, 19(3): 725–54.

Rindfuss, R. R., Guilkey, D., Morgan, S. P., Kravdal, O. and Guzzo, K. B. (2007) Child care availability and first-birth timing in Norway, *Demography*, 44(2): 345–72.

Rosina, A. and Testa, M. R. (2009) Couples' first child intentions and disagreement: an analysis of the Italian case, *European Journal of Population*, 25(4): 487.

Sinclair, S., Boymal, J. and de Silva, A. (2010) A re-appraisal of the fertility response to the Australian baby bonus, MPRA paper no. 27580, School of Economics, Finance and Marketing, RMIT University. Online: http://mpra.ub.uni-muenchen.de/27580/, date accessed 13 May 2011.

Testa, M. R. (2006) Childbearing Preferences and Family Issues in Europe. Online: http://ec.europa.eu/public_opinion/archives/ebs/ebs_253_en.pdf, date accessed 12 January 2011.

Thévenon, O. and Gauthier, A. H. (2011) Family policies in developed countries: a 'fertility booster' with side-effects, *Community, Work and Family*, 14(2): 197–216.

Thomson, E. (1997) Couple childbearing desires, intentions and births, *Demography*, 34: 343–54.

United Nations (2010) *World Population Policies 2009*, United Nations Department of Economic and Social Affairs/Population Division, pp. 52.

Zeller, F. (2010) Low birth rates threaten Asia's top economies, *The Jakarta Globe*. Online: http://www.thejakartaglobe.com/business/low-birth-rates-threaten-asias-top-economies/413375, date accessed 26 April 2011.

17
Investing in Early Childhood

Gøsta Esping-Andersen

A major puzzle of our times is the lack of any serious progress in equal opportunities, despite so much effort invested in the pursuit thereof. To fully understand why, we need to identify more precisely the mechanisms at work. What is now well understood is that educational reforms, no matter how progressive and egalitarian in design, are institutionally ill-equipped to break the Gordian Knot of social inheritance. Developmental psychology has shown that the crucial cognitive and behavioural foundations for learning are cemented very early in childhood. What occurs in the *preschool* ages is fundamental for children's ability and motivation to learn when they subsequently embark on formal education. The imprint of social origins is therefore already firmly established before schools play any major role in our lives. The logical conclusion is that we must centre our attention more on what happens within the family than on education policy.

Both cognitive and noncognitive skills are transmitted partially genetically and partially as the result of nurturing – that is, of environmental stimulus (Bjorklund et al. 2005; Bowles et al. 2001). It may be futile to aspire towards an exact differentiation between nature and nurturing effects, but there is little doubt that the impact of the latter is very large. Since cognitive (and noncognitive) abilities influence school success and, subsequently, adults' life chances, the policy challenge is to ensure a strong start for all children. Investing well in our children will yield very large returns both for individuals' life chances and for society at large.

There are two basic 'efficiency' reasons for why we need to ensure minimal inequality of skills and human capital. The first is demographic. Due to prolonged low fertility the coming youth cohorts are, and will continue to be, very small. Over the next decades, the working age population of the EU will shrink by 50 million. These small cohorts must support a large and rapidly growing elderly population. Hence, we need to invest maximally in the productive potential of contemporary youth in order to guarantee a sustainable welfare state over the decades to come.

The second reason has to do with the rapidly rising skill requirements in the knowledge-intensive economies. While everyone agrees that skills are ever more decisive, there is substantial controversy over what types of skills matter most. Formal educational credentials surely remain crucial. We can, as a rule of thumb, pretty much predict that someone with no more than a lower secondary degree will fare very poorly in tomorrow's labour market. In virtually all advanced economies today, early school leavers suffer three times more unemployment than do those with higher degrees, and they are hugely overrepresented among the long-term unemployed. Viewed in life course terms, the low educated are unlikely to accumulate much pension wealth and are, accordingly, at risk of old age poverty.

Any serious consideration of equality and efficiency must realize that children are a positive collective good. It is certainly not easy to arrive at any precise estimate of their social value. Preston's (2004, pp. 263–7) estimate for an average child on a lifetime basis of $100.000 may be indicative of the magnitudes. But the question is whether the high social gains that wonder kids produce are offset by the costs to society of the failures. The Urban Institute in the United States estimates that child poverty creates social costs equivalent to 4 per cent of Gross Domestic Product (GDP) of which 1.3 per cent is attributable to reduced economic output, another 1.3 per cent to crime and 1.2 per cent to health effects.[1] This is in great part caused by the strong link between poverty, school failure and juvenile delinquency.

Rising income inequality influences children's opportunities. At one extreme we see top income households distancing themselves from the middle, in part because of rising returns to skills and, in part, due to concentrations of high-earning dual-career couples at the top. At the bottom of the income pyramid, less-educated couples face strong probabilities of low income and joblessness (Gregg and Wadsworth 2001; Hyslop 2001; Katz and Autor 1999). With the notable exception of France, the Gini coefficient of (market) income inequality has risen throughout the advanced societies, and in some countries such as Germany, Sweden, the United Kingdom and the United States by more than 20 per cent. Perhaps the single most troubling trend lies in the often substantial rise in child poverty. It has doubled in Italy, Germany and the

Netherlands but has remained fairly stable (at about 8 per cent) in France (Esping-Andersen and Myles 2009).

As inequality widens, parents' capacity to invest in their children's fortunes will become more unequal (Solon 1999, pp. 1761–800). This means that social inheritance is reinforced.

Ongoing change in family structure may also contribute to polarization. To begin with, families are more unstable and the share of children growing up in lone mother households is rising. Lone mother families now account for 15–20 per cent of all child families in Northern Europe and the United States. The consequences for children's well-being are decidedly negative in the United States, but the evidence for Europe is more ambiguous. This has undoubtedly something to do with underlying social selection. In the United States (and United Kingdom), lone motherhood and divorce is increasingly concentrated within the lower social strata, while this is less so in most of Europe. There are two main reasons why lone mother families create negative child outcomes. One is that they are at high risk of poverty. In the United States, half of all lone mother families are poor, but as we would expect the risk is lower in Europe: 29 per cent in France, 38 per cent in Germany and a low of 13 per cent in Sweden (Esping-Andersen and Myles 2009). The containment of poverty in Scandinavia is probably less due to generous welfare state support and more to the fact that virtually all lone mothers work. Another reason why children of lone parents fare poorly lies in the potential 'nurturing deficit' due to less parental time dedication. This, of course, is especially likely when lone mothers are employed.

A second trend is the increase in marital selection, particularly with regard to educational homogeny. This is especially pronounced at the top and the bottom of the social ladder so that, at one end, we see a concentration of two parents with strong human capital and, at the other end, a concentration of parents with little education. This should widen inequalities, not only because of the gap in earnings power, but also due to employment patterns.

Marital homogamy is also likely to polarize parental dedication to their children. There is clear evidence that highly educated mothers *and* fathers dedicate much more time to their children, in particular, with regard to what we might call developmental time, that is, active stimulation.

A third demographic challenge comes from large-scale immigration. A curious facet of immigration is that second generation immigrants tend to converge with local populations in terms of demographic behaviour, such as fertility, but not in terms of education and skills.

To illustrate, even in Sweden where the school system is extraordinarily committed to rectify immigrant children's learning disadvantages, the probability of school failure is nevertheless five times higher for immigrants than for natives. A more general illustration comes from the Programme for International Student Assessment (PISA) data which show generally very large gaps in cognitive abilities between native and immigrant youth.

In sum, ongoing societal trends are worrisome and potentially a source of polarization. We know that income inequalities are widening and that child poverty is rising. The gap in parental time investment is, likewise, growing between the high and less educated. Worst of all, there appears to be a strong coincidence between the two, suggesting the possibility of compounding effects.

What can policies do?

How may policy influence positively on children's life chances? In a sense, the question is as old as is our civilization. Plato was seriously worried about the quality of Athenian soldiers and advocated that children of incapable parents should be removed from their family and be raised by the state. The Kibbutz ideology was surely more egalitarian with its stipulation that *all* children should be ensured an identical stimulus and, hence, be raised collectively. Such kinds of measures are clearly excluded from any realistic policy menu in the advanced democratic nations. Parents have children because this is their desire, and our societies are founded on the firm principle that the sanctity of the family is inherently inviolable. How, then, might we design a workable equal opportunities strategy?

Reducing the income effect

The link between low income and children's life chances suggests the relevance of income redistribution. There are both social and individual costs associated with child poverty.

Redistribution can be an effective tool for combating child poverty. Public spending in favour of families is 3–4 per cent of GDP in the Nordic countries and 2.8 per cent in France, compared to 0.4 per cent in the United States and 1.1 per cent in the Netherlands.[2] However, France ends up with a post-transfer child poverty rate around 8 per cent despite dedicating resources of Nordic magnitudes. This is to be expected considering that French poverty before redistributive transfers is about ten percentage points higher.

An income redistribution strategy would seem attractive for a number of reasons. If the objective were to fully eradicate child poverty (defined as less than 50 per cent of equivalent median income), the price tag is actually surprisingly small. For the United States, with record child poverty, I have estimated it to cost only 0.4 per cent of GDP (Esping-Andersen 2002). This happens to be exactly ten times less than the estimated social costs of US child poverty. But such redistribution would have to be repeated year after year and the *net* benefit should be considered against possible second-order effects such as reduced parental labour supply. Also, a targeted transfer approach may fail to command broad citizen support. We should not forget that family transfers are motivated by other concerns, such as collectively recognizing the importance of parenthood. Indeed, the value of parenting in Sweden is equivalent to one-fifth of the GDP (Klevmarken 1998). If children are so beneficial to the economy while most of the costs of children are internalized by the parents, an equity calculus would conclude in favour of universal, non-income graduated, and fairly generous child and family allowances. If those without children are free-riders, they should be made to pay.

Child benefits should therefore not be confused with anti-poverty policies. If our aim is to minimize or, indeed, eradicate child poverty we might introduce some form of a guaranteed minimum to families that supplements standard family benefits. If the cost were, say, 0.4 per cent of GDP we would then need to match this against possible second-order effects. Would parents respond by working less? Would it effectively narrow the school attainment gap of poor kids? As to the latter, there is cause for scepticism since the schooling gap is surely not solely the effect of income but also of unobservable factors, some of which need not be correlated with being poor, and some of which (say, poor health or teenage pregnancy) may provide the explanation of poverty to begin with.

In any case, the burden on income redistribution would be lessened significantly if maternal employment were to increase within low income households. The probability of child poverty drops by a factor of 3 or even 4 when mothers are employed. The effect is potentially strongest in lone parent families. It makes a big difference whether, as in Denmark, the lone mother activity rate is 81 per cent or, as in the United Kingdom, only 35 per cent. Kangas and Ritakallio (1998) provide particularly suggestive evidence in this regard. They simulate what France's poverty rate would be with Scandinavia's transfer system and demographic structure. Considering, as we have seen, that France approximates the Nordic countries in terms of poverty-reduction – but not in terms of post-transfer child poverty – it is not surprising that any serious convergence with Scandinavia's low child poverty would have to come from increments in French mothers' employment rate. But as is well-recognized, maternal employment depends crucially on access to affordable childcare.

Equal opportunities in the learning milieu

We now realize that a truly effective policy needs also to address the family 'culture' effects. But if we exclude any Platonian solution this would, to most, appear as being entirely outside the competence of policy. How, we might ask, can policy induce parents to read with their children or censure television viewing?

One important clue is found in the extensive evaluation research on early childhood intervention that has been conducted in the United States. The main – and very systematic – finding is that high-quality intervention on behalf of at-risk preschool age children has substantial and lasting effects in terms of improved social integration, less delinquency and more schooling (Carneiro and Heckman 2003; Kamerman et al. 2003; Karoly et al. 2005). The Perry preschool programme, which emphasizes early intervention with high quality services targeted to underprivileged children, appears particularly effective in terms of both child outcomes and cost effectiveness. Participation in the ABCedarian programme, widely celebrated for its quality, is associated with a 32 per cent drop in high school dropout risks, and it increases the chance of attending college by a factor of three (Barnett and Belfield 2006). Through age 27, it yields a $5.70 return for every dollar spent – in part due to less criminal behaviour and, in part, due to substantially improved learning abilities among the children (Carneiro and Heckman 2003, p. 165). Early learning begets better learning later on; a poor start translates into persistently inferior learning abilities.

The logic behind this cost-benefit analysis is very compelling, since it incorporates the positive synergy effects (learning begets learning) of early investments into the cost of later ones. The rate of return rises exponentially the child, suggesting that preschool and early-school investments yield disproportionally high net returns. If the standard monetary rate of return to schooling hovers around 10 per cent, we could anticipate returns to preschool investments that are possibly more than twice this magnitude. And if the marginal returns are much greater for those who are most likely to fail in school, then early investments should produce an equal opportunities gain.

Such findings from the United States should not be uncritically generalized to Europe where inequalities in child conditions are less extreme. But the crucial point is that early intervention programmes that include strong behavioural and cognitive stimulus can be effective in equalizing outcomes, especially to the advantage of the most-at-risk. There is accordingly a very strong case to be made in favour of financing early high-quality childcare.

Here again, the experience from the Nordic countries can be of relevance – for good and bad. Denmark and Sweden began in the late 1960s a massive and very rapid expansion of preschool institutions aimed at securing universal access; a goal by and large achieved by the 1980s. The policy was actually not cast in terms of investing in children but rather as an instrument to reconcile motherhood and careers. But in order to cater to the tastes of middle-class families, it ensured that standards were high. For instance, Denmark boasts a ratio of three children per carer for the under- 3 years.

Nordic childcare policy learned many lessons along the way. Until the 1990s, for example, children were not eligible if the mother was on maternity leave or in receipt of unemployment compensation. This had the undesirable consequence that many of those children who might benefit the most were excluded, considering which women are more likely to be unemployed or to have many children. In recent years, policy-makers have tried to make it especially attractive for immigrant and unemployed parents to place their children in public care centres. A second lesson was that parental leaves and childcare needed to be better synchronized. Until the 1990s, the combined maternity-parental leave in Denmark covered little more than six months, which meant that a very large percentage of infants were placed in crèches very early.

For these countries, there are few systematic impact studies of childcare policy. Andersson (1992) shows that, in Sweden, day care has positive consequences for child development, especially in the case of less-privileged families. A more recent comparison between Denmark and the United States shows also that Danish childcare has especially favourable effects for the most at-risk children (Esping-Andersen et al. 2012).

There is also more indirect evidence to suggest that the arrival of universal preschool attendance is associated with a significant equalization of school attainment and, one can argue, also with the quite homogeneous performance on tests of educational outcomes. Using the 2003 PISA data, we can compare the cognitive performance of youth who participated more than one year in preschool education with those who did not participate at all. In Denmark and the United States, participation is associated with a gain of almost 40 points on the literacy test; in most countries, the effect is even larger: a 90-point improvement in Germany and a 60-point gain in the United Kingdom. Additionally, childcare participation diminishes the explanatory importance of socio-economic origins, of parents' 'cultural capital', of being immigrant child, and of having a low-educated mother.

The International Adult Literacy Survey allows us to assess the effects of social origin on the probability of completing upper level secondary education across birth cohorts. I estimated the social origin effect net of children's abilities in order to capture the essence of social inheritance, and controlled for the children's cognitive test scores as well as for sex and immigrant status. The analyses followed three cohorts, the oldest born in the late 1940s and early 1950s; the youngest in the 1970s, and compared social inheritance trends in the three Nordic countries with Germany, the United Kingdom and the United States (Esping-Andersen 2009).

In Germany, the United Kingdom and the United States, there was no decline whatsoever in the impact of origins on educational attainment across the three cohorts – which is to say, over a half century. In the United States, for example, the odds of completing upper secondary education are roughly a tenth of those that come from higher educated parents. In contrast, there was a very significant decline in the association in all three Scandinavian countries. The drop occurs primarily in the youngest cohort, which was the first to enjoy near-universal participation in childcare. To exemplify, in Denmark the probability of attaining higher education was, for the oldest cohort, a fifth as large as for those whose parents had high education. For the youngest Danish cohort, the relative probability has declined to only a half. Or, if we compare across countries, the Danish youth of low-educated fathers now enjoy an almost five times greater chance of finishing upper secondary education as their American or German counterparts.

These results do not, of course, tell us whether equalization was due to childcare, income redistribution or, most likely, a combination of both. But the coincidence of timing is very suggestive. It is evident, especially in Denmark and Sweden, that the big leap in equalization is centred in the youngest cohort. This is, in fact, the first cohort in which the majority of children came to be enrolled in preschool institutions in either country.

High-quality childcare and preschool participation may, accordingly, constitute a truly effective policy in the pursuit of more equal opportunities. Since access to childcare is concomitantly a precondition for maternal employment, which yields positive income effects, the promotion of childcare would appear a perfect win-win policy. We need therefore to examine this nexus in closer detail.

Mothers' employment and child outcomes

The income gain that comes from mothers' employment may be offset by potentially adverse consequences for nurturing their children. We know that motherly employment during the first year can be harmful for child health and cognitive development. Waldfogel et al. (2002) find that such negative effects are especially accentuated within low income families. Thus policy would need to ensure a combination of *paid* maternity and parental leave that approaches the one year duration. In both Denmark and Sweden, leave schemes permit the parents to remain home with the infant over the entire first year with full earnings compensation. The norm in most of the EU is no more than four months.

Very brief leaves can be doubly problematic. They may push mothers back to work very early. To illustrate, 60 per cent of new Dutch mothers return to work within six months of birth (Dutch paid leave is only four months), while virtually all Danish mothers return within 10–14 months (Simonsen 2005). Overly brief leaves may also provoke exit from employment. About one in four of Dutch mothers simply disappear from the labour market, while the Danish per cent is negligible (Gustafsson and Kenjoh 2004).

The cost of providing a one-year leave system is substantial. Using Denmark as a benchmark, it equals 0.6 per cent of GDP. This must be held up against the benefits. According to one study, paid leaves increase female employment rates by 3–4 per cent, and post-leave wages are higher (Ruhm 1998). In part, therefore, the cost of longer leaves is recuperated further on via enhanced career earnings and tax payments. We should also evaluate the cost in terms of the positive child effects of parental presence during infancy.

If we look beyond the first year, the major obstacle to mothers' employment lies in access to childcare. Childcare costs become a *regressive tax* if fees are independent of mothers' (or household) earnings. Tax deductions are commonly used in many nations, but these are unlikely to eliminate the regressive incidence since they are of less relevance for low income families to begin with.

Kindergarten (age 3+) attendance is near universal in many countries and is often defined as integral to the education system and thus free of charge. The key question has to do with children less than three years old. In large parts of Europe, the conventional solution has been familial care – the grandmother. This option is rapidly becoming obsolete because the reservoir of available family carers is in rapid decline. Private childcare markets can thrive, as in the United States, because of high price and quality differentiation. But in most of the EU, the market for quality childcare is very limited due to high costs. The Nordic countries and, to a lesser degree, Belgium and France subsidize childcare for toddlers. But due to design differences, the outcomes vary substantially. For a standard two-earner couple in France, the cost of one child approaches 25 per cent of their earnings, compared to only 10 per cent in Denmark (Immervoll and Barber 2005). This is surely one explanation for why Danish childcare attendance at age one is double the French.

The potential learning impact of early care is also likely to differ. French childcare coverage for the under-three years amounts to approximately 40 per cent. Only half of these children are enrolled in centre-based care, while the other half is placed with individual carers. The Nordic approach (and especially the Danish), in contrast, is premised on high-quality, full-day care with guaranteed access for all children. This requires, unsurprisingly, heavy subsidies: the parental co-payment is only 33 per cent of cost and disappears for lower income parents.

In order to evaluate whether public subsidies for childcare are warranted, we need to examine two distinct cost-benefit logics: how childcare affects female employment and earnings, and how it affects child outcomes. As to the former, we have clear evidence that childcare availability raises maternal employment levels. A Danish study shows that a 100 Euro decrease in childcare costs produces a 0.8 per cent increase in employment (Simonsen 2005). Since childcare allows mothers to return quicker to their jobs, the lifetime income penalty of motherhood is lowered substantially. The lifetime income gains and the associated larger tax payments to the exchequer will, over the years, basically defray the initial public subsidy to childcare.

The cost-benefit calculus in terms of child outcomes may, in one sense, be unnecessary if childcare practically pays its own way due to higher lifetime earnings for women. Any positive learning or behavioural effect that it yields comes, so to speak, gratis. The good news here is that the returns to high-quality early childhood programmes are potentially huge. One US study found that every dollar spent yields a $5.60 return, and more recent estimates suggest a return in excess of $12.00 (Carneiro and Heckman 2003). However, these estimates refer to underprivileged children who we already know will benefit disproportionably.

Targeted or universal measures?

Should we therefore favour a targeted rather than Danish-style universal policy? If our primary aim is to level the playing field, a targeted approach would appear the more cost-effective alternative. The choice for or against targeting depends, first, on the value we place on equity in the broadest sense. Targeting services to the most underprivileged children can, as US experience shows, narrow the performance gap for those at the very bottom. However, unless targeting is very ample it will not necessarily result in overall improvement of life chances. The US Head Start programme reaches only about 7 per cent of three-year-olds and thus falls far short of reaching the entire at-risk population (US child poverty hovers above 20 per cent, and that the share falling below the PISA minimum score is almost as big). The remaining 93 per cent of any child cohort will receive care options that to a large extent mirror parents' purchasing power. The huge unevenness of US early care is well documented (Blau 2001).

More generally, the basic dilemma of targeted policy is how to ensure that it does reach the needy. Here, a comparison of the US approach to Britain's Sure Start is of interest. While the former targets problem families, the latter targets high-risk communities. Neither approach can ensure that need is adequately addressed. Identifying problem families is only easy when their problems are visible; and in the case of Sure Start it is far from certain that all the needy live in high-risk communities. The real obstacle to effective targeting lies in the multiple mechanisms that produce adverse child outcomes. While income poverty is easily identifiable, this is certainly not the case for parental nurturing practices.

Opting in favour of universal coverage has the great advantage of ensuring that all children, irrespective of origin, come to enjoy similar high standards. And if the system helps mix children from different backgrounds, so much the better. US evaluation research shows that disadvantaged children reap very positive effects when mixed with stronger kids (Hanushek et al. 2003). Yet, the obvious shortcoming of an across-the-board universal model of the Nordic variety is that the most underprivileged children might require additional resources and attention. One example of this problem is the lower participation rate of children from immigrant families. Some form of affirmative action, including perhaps special incentives to target groups, may therefore be called for to accompany a universal approach.

Conclusion: helping families to invest in their children

Human capital investments have, over the past half century, been almost exclusively directed at formal education. It is only quite recently that we have come to realize that the foundations of learning – as well as the chief mainsprings of inequalities – lie buried in very early childhood and that schools are generally ill-equipped to remedy a bad start. It is now evident that investments yield the highest returns in the preschool stage and decline exponentially thereafter. The returns are especially high for underprivileged children.

All this suggests that we need to re-evaluate human capital policy. As a starter, educational spending in *all* advanced countries goes in exactly the opposite direction from what the learning-begets-learning perspective prescribes. Per student spending rises monotonically from preschool up to tertiary education. We spend on average twice as much *per student* on tertiary level as on pre-primary education. Moreover, pre-primary spending is, in most countries, concentrated in the ages 3–6. Except for the Nordic countries and, at some distance, Belgium and France, investment in children under three years is truly marginal.

Concerns about equality of opportunities and future productivity coincide in policies that aim to raise the homogeneity of our human capital reservoir. The share of youth that ends up with insufficient skills is very large in many countries, be it in terms of either formal qualifications or cognitive and noncognitive abilities. Here is cause for alarm considering that skill requirements continuously grow.

Departing from the dictum that the key mechanisms lie in very early childhood and are prevalently centred in the family, we need to identify how policy can aid families give their children the best possible chances in life. A core issue lies in the persistence of strong social inheritance. Conventional theory has emphasized monetary effects in general and poverty in particular. This is without any doubt a major contributor to differential school success and, more generally, to unequal life chances. But social scientists as well as policy-makers have paid far less attention to noneconomic factors in the inter-generational transmission of disadvantage. There is a credible case to be made that noneconomic mechanisms may be of equal if not greater importance than income. To a degree, the two coincide: teen-age mothers, immigrants and low-educated parents are also more likely to be income poor. But we are almost certainly tapping two rather distinct dimensions, and this implies that a strategy based narrowly on income redistribution is unlikely to fully succeed.

The evidence suggests, instead, a two-pronged policy that would appear attractive both from the point of view of cost effectiveness and because it can produce a more equal start for all children. In a nutshell, the strategy condenses into an early childhood care policy. The case for income redistribution towards families with children is certainly evident and requires little additional comment save to stress that the burden on redistribution would be eased considerably if mothers were employed. There are multiple reasons why especially less-educated women's activity rates are low and access to affordable childcare is only one. Nevertheless, if accompanied by adequate maternity leave provisions and with a neutral taxation of spousal earnings, such policy should produce a nontrivial employment gain. Any such gain can produce a double advantage because it helps reduce poverty and, if external childcare is of high quality, it may have positive effects on child stimulus. High-quality childcare is also cost efficient in the sense that more female employment together with higher lifetime earnings will enhance the revenue base.

All said, policy that combines paid leave through the child's first year with affordable high-quality external care should yield important dividends in terms of homogenizing children's school preparedness. A major policy dilemma presents itself with regard to design. Since we know that the returns are exceptionally high for less-privileged children a simple cost-benefit calculus would suggest a targeted approach. What, then, would recommend a broad universal model?

In the first place, one should keep in mind the implicitly dual function of childcare: supporting mothers' employment and child socialization. There is also another equity issue at stake. Given the socio-economic importance of parenting, there is a clear case for redistribution in favour of *all* parents alike, rather than redistribution from some parents to others.

This brings us to a second standard argument in favour of universalism, namely that broad citizen support for the policy is considered essential for adequate financing. A third important consideration lies in the high transaction costs and the difficulties of identifying need. Targeting low income families may be fairly simple to administer, but learning deficits are also powerfully related to family 'culture', which is a dimension that is virtually impossible to identify by any public bureaucracy.

At the end of the day, the choice for or against targeting will depend very much on our aspirations regarding skill homogenization. If our aim is limited to 'bringing up the rear', which is how one might describe

US policy in this regard, there is a better case for targeting than if we pursue a more general goal of minimizing, across the board, the impact of inequalities on children's opportunities. The possible shortcoming of a universal approach is that it may not succeed fully in 'bringing up the rear'. Truly disadvantaged children are likely to require an additional effort, and this suggests that universal designs may need to be coupled with some form of interventions.

Notes

1. Testimony by Harry Holzer (Urban Institute) before the US House Committee on Ways and Means, 24 January 2007.
2. Calculated from OECD's SOC-X data.

References

Andersson, B. (1992) 'Effects of day care on cognitive and socio-emotional competence of 13-year old Swedish schoolchildren', *Child Development,* 63: 20–36.

Barnett, W. and Belfield, C. (2006) 'Early childhood development and social mobility', *The Future of Children,* 16: 73–98.

Blau, D. (2001) *The Child Care Problem – An Economic Analysis* (New York: Russell Sage).

Bowles, S., Gintis, H. and Osborne, M. (2001) 'The determinants of earnings: a behavioural approach', *Journal of Economic Literature,* XXXIX: 1137–76.

Bjorklund, A., Jantti, M. and Solon, G. (2005) 'Influences of nature and nurture on earnings variation', in S. Bowles, H. Gintis and M. Osborne (eds) *Unequal Chances* (New York: Russell Sage), pp. 145–64.

Carneiro, P. and Heckman, J. (2003) 'Human capital policy', in J. Heckman and A. Krueger (eds) *Inequality in America* (Cambridge, Mass.: MIT Press), pp. 77–240.

Esping-Andersen, G. (with Gallie, D., Hemerijck, A. and Myles, J.) (2002) *Why We Need a New Welfare State?* (Oxford: Oxford University Press).

Esping-Andersen, G. and Myles, J. (2009) 'The welfare state and redistribution', in W. Salverda, B. Nolan and T. Smeeding (eds) *The Oxford Handbook of Economic Inequality* (Oxford: Oxford University Press), pp. 639–64.

Esping-Andersen, G. (2009) *The Incomplete Revolution* (Cambridge: Polity Press).

Esping-Andersen, G., Garfinkel, I., Jui Han, W., Magnuson, K., Wagner, S. and Waldfogel, J. (2012) 'Child care and school performance in Denmark and the United States', *Children and Youth Services Review,* 34(3): 576–89.

Gregg, P. and Wadsworth, J. (2001) 'Everything you ever wanted to know about worklessness and polarization at the household level but were afraid to ask', *Oxford Bulletin of Economics and Statistics,* 63: 777–806.

Gustafsson, S. and Kenjoh, E. (2004) 'New evidence on work among new mothers', *European Review of Labour and Research,* 10: 34–47.

Hanushek, E. A., Kain, J. F., Markman, J. M. and Rivkin, S. G. (2003). 'Does peer ability affect student achievement?', *Journal of Applied Econometrics*, 18(5): 527–44.

Hyslop, D. (2001) 'Rising U.S. earnings inequality and family labor supply: the covariance structure of intrafamily earnings', *American Economic Review*, 91(4): 755–77.

Immervoll, H. and Barber, D. (2005) 'Can parents afford to work?' OECD-DELSA Working paper, no. 10.

Kamerman, S. B., Neuman, M., Waldfogel, J. and Brooks-Gunn, J. (2003) 'Social policies, family types, and child outcomes in selected OECD countries', Paris, France: OECD, *Working Paper.*

Kangas, O. and Ritakallio, V. (1998) 'Social policy or structure? Income transfers, socioeconomic factors and poverty in the Nordic countries and France', *LIS Working Paper*, 190.

Karoly, L., Kilburn, R. and Cannon, J. (2005) *Early Childhood Interventions: Proven Results, Future Promise* (Santa Monica, CA: RAND Corporation).

Katz, L. and Autor, D. (1999) 'Changes in the wage structure and earnings inequality', in O. Ashenfelter and D. Card (eds) *Handbook of Labor Economics*, Volume 3A (Amsterdam: Elsevier), pp. 1463–555.

Klevmarken, A. (1998) 'Microeconomic analyses of time use data: did we reach the promised land?', unpublished paper, Department of Economics, Uppsala University (May 15).

Preston, S. (2004) 'The value of children', in D. Moynihan, T. Smeeding and L. Rainwater (eds) *The Future of the Family* (New York: Russell Sage), pp. 263–99.

Ruhm, C. (1998) 'The economic consequences of parental leave mandates', *Quarterly Journal of Economics*, 113(1): 285–317.

Simonsen, M. (2005) 'Provision and costs of high quality day care and female employment', unpublished paper, Department of Economics, Aarhus University (April).

Solon, G. (1999) 'Intergenerational mobility in the labor market', in O. Ashenfelter and D. Card (eds) *Handbook of Labor Economics*, Volume 3A (Amsterdam: Elsevier Science), pp. 1761–800.

Waldfogel, J., Han, W. and Brooks-Gunn, J. (2002) 'The effects of early maternal employment on child cognitive development', *Demography*, 39: 369–92.

18
Making Time for Children

Ann Buchanan and Anna Rotkirch

This final chapter sums up some of the key findings and seeks a possible direction in the fast-changing scenarios. In the first part of the chapter, we summarize conclusions to the questions raised in Chapter 1. In the second part, we look into the crystal ball and suggest possible directions for the future.

The key questions

Is the decline in fertility rates just a blip in the ups and downs of population statistics?

The demographers in Part I appear to agree that low fertility rates are here to stay and that this, in time, will lead to population decline. Although there are variations within, and between, different areas, in most parts of the world, fertility is declining rapidly or has stabilized at quite low levels. In many countries, Total Fertility Rates (TFRs) are below replacement levels of 2.1, and it is expected that developing countries, as economies improve, will follow suit. In theory, a new baby boom is possible and, as will be discussed later, there are still areas of uncertainty. For instance, the recent Census in the United Kingdom, as mentioned in chapter one, noted that the TFR in the UK was the highest since 1972 most probably due to immigration (ONS 2011). Changing fertility rates are only one part of population forecasts. Increasing longevity is the other side. Population predictions are notoriously unreliable, but the current consensus appears to be that total world population will be declining before the end of this century and it may be sooner.

Some areas will be more affected than others. As Gavin Jones notes in Chapter 3, fertility in East Asia is now the lowest in the world, and this appears likely to remain the case for some time. TFRs of around

1.1–1.3, which in international public perception is characteristic of China because of publicity given to the one-child policy, are actually even more characteristic of other East Asian countries than of China. Indeed, Taiwan's fertility (a TFR of 0.895 in 2010) was the lowest ever recorded in a country with a population exceeding 10 million. Despite limited pro-natalist policies in recent years, fertility rates in East Asia remain stubbornly low. In India, the fertility ideals of many groups are similar to that of Western countries. This means that the world's most populous nations will probably also soon reach low fertility levels.

Stuart Basten's research (Chapter 11) highlighting the impact of media places a new light on population predictions. One thing is certain, media influences are likely to grow apace. How will they influence childbearing decisions in the future? It could go either way.

Do we need to worry about population decline? Certainly a world with fewer people may be beneficial for the environment and sustainability. Also several other key indicators suggest that smaller populations may outperform bigger ones, as David Coleman and Robert Rowthorn argue. The darker side of a declining workforce supporting a growing aged population and shrinking of economies is more tentative. The pace of decline matters. A given reduction in population will have different implications depending on whether it occurs gradually through the course of centuries or is compressed into a few decades. The conclusion, however, appears to be that the speed of population reduction of the working age population and the speed of change in the dependency ratio is likely to be fast.

Why are women having fewer children?

The main reasons for declining fertility give further support to the argument that current trends are unlikely to change. Not only are women globally having fewer children, but a growing number of women in European countries, as John Haskey notes in Chapter 4, are remaining childless. In East Asia, after divorce, fewer women are remarrying, indicating a growing acceptance of, and perhaps preference for, singlehood.

Whether and when adults have children as discussed in Part II of this book, is shaped by a range of other factors: health and income, economic uncertainty, availability of contraception, use of contraception, political climate, fashions in family size, to name a few. For Mumsnetters who gave their views in Chapter 6, the reasons for having fewer children can be summed by the five C's. *Contraception* is available to them. As a result, they have more *Choice* on how to lead their lives. With increasing education, this has opened up the possibility of rewarding *Careers*. These mothers have had children but the barriers to having more are the comparative *Cost* of providing for children and the availability and expense of paying for *Childcare*.

As we saw in Chapter 1, availability of contraception is now expanding to high fertility regions such as Africa. Girls' education across the globe, although still limited in some developing areas, is opening out previously unimagined opportunities for women with strong economic incentives to enter paid work. In Russia, as we saw in Chapter 8, there had been a particularly dramatic decline in fertility partly due to the economic crisis with women delaying childbearing hoping conditions would improve. Before the fall of the Soviet Union, Russia's TFR was around 1.8. By 1990 it was below 1.2. The improving economic situation and national policies have brought about a marginal increase. In 2011, the TFR was estimated at 1.42 born per woman (CIA 2012) and was partly due to the recuperation effect since women who delayed childbirth in the last decades were now becoming mothers (CIA 2012).

In South Africa (Chapter 10), we still do not really know what impact HIV is having on fertility. Quite apart from the children not born as a result of parents' early death and children themselves not surviving because of HIV, there is now substantial economic growth in many areas of Africa. Gross Domestic Productivity (GDP) rose by 4.9 per cent a year from 2000 through 2008, more than twice its pace in the 1980s and 1990s. From Ghana in the west to Mozambique in the south, Africa's economies were consistently growing faster than those of almost any other region of the world (*McKinsey Quarterly* 2010). Although there are gross disparities between different sectors of society, increasing health, prosperity and opportunity is likely to impact on women's choice in much the same way as in the developed world.

Two of the chapters in Part II, however, illustrate the dilemmas and uncertainties in predicting childbearing decisions. Large numbers of women, as Barber and her colleagues showed, still have unplanned births despite the availability of contraception. Recent figures from the United States show:

> The typical American woman, who wants two children, spends about five years pregnant, postpartum or trying to become pregnant, and three decades – more than three-quarters of her reproductive life – trying to avoid pregnancy. About half of all pregnancies in the United States each year – more than three million – are unintended. By age

> 45, more than half of all American women will have experienced an unintended pregnancy, and three in 10 will have had an abortion.
>
> (The Guttmacher Institute 2012, p. 1)

Jennifer Barber and colleagues in Chapter 7 illustrate that there are many and various reasons for women maintaining they do not want children, yet not using contraceptives. Given this ambiguity, it is hard to predict whether the number of unplanned births will increase or fall. Rising levels of education, however, will probably increase efficacy in contraceptive use.

Stuart Basten's chapter (Chapter 11) highlights another dimension. He demonstrates that media has been influential in changing attitudes to family size in South America. In the developed world he gives examples of how the elite and celebrities can influence families via television documentaries, Internet and the Internet chat vehicles. How will media influences develop in the future? In countries such as India, media is still crucial for spreading propaganda on the value of small families. In parts of the Western world, however, it is becoming fashionable for wealthy families to have three or more children. Some celebrities such as Angelina Jolie and Brad Pitt have huge families, maybe strengthening this trend. Given growing access to the Internet, one can only surmise that these influences will increase.

What is the impact of lower fertility rates?

Possible economic impact

Bob Rowthorn, an economist, in Chapter 5 outlined some of the possible economic consequences of a world in which there are fewer workers. He suggests that population growth increases total GDP as long as additional workers can be employed. However, a declining population may imply slower output growth unless there are increases in productivity. While a growing population provides a growing market for goods and services, a shrinking population may mean a mismatch between production and consumption. Thus, in theory, a larger population can permit economies of scale and division of labour, thereby improving productivity. Technology is likely to reduce the number of labour-intensive industries. With a smaller population, it also may not be economic to produce manufactured products with high development costs.

In low fertility countries, 'replacement migration' is seen as the solution to future labour shortages (United Nations 2000). Replacement migration refers to the international migration that a country would need to prevent population decline and population ageing resulting from low fertility and mortality rates. The argument is that, as populations decline, shortages in the workforce are inevitable in the absence of replacement migration. In the short term, as we have experienced in the developed world, replacement migration fills an important role – in the United Kingdom, for example, the National Health Service (NHS) is heavily dependent on foreign professionals. However, over the next half century, when economies in poorer areas develop, and economic conditions improve in the home country, as has been seen with the Polish migrants, the economic attractions of migration will become less of a draw (Pollard et al. 2008). And if the whole world has low fertility, replacement migration will just shuffle the problem around – that is, it will improve the situation in the receiving country while aggravating it in the sender country. Countries, such as the United Kingdom and the United States of America ,who attract large numbers of skilled migrants, will in the future be relatively advantaged as they may be better able to maintain their workforce and economic output.

The impact on children

For most children, having no or just a few siblings brings lower mortality in childhood, better health, more education and eventually greater economic prosperity (e.g. UNDP 2010) as discussed in Chapter 12. From a psychological research perspective, lone children appear to thrive (see Falbo and Polit 1986). Individual children generally do not turn out to be the 'little emperors' that many feared. Across the life course, the situation may be less positive. Coping with the huge expectations from parents as well as the heavy burden of caring for elderly family members and the lack of support from siblings may place unsustainable pressures on the working generation.

But equally concerning is the gap that is growing between the relatively privileged, upwardly mobile young person receiving huge economic and emotional investments from his parents, and the large numbers of children living in deprivation and poverty, many who may still be part of large families. Many of these children are in the developed world. For both humanitarian and economic reasons, we need to reduce this gap. In future every child will be economically needed, and societies need to find ways to maximize the potential of each and every one of them.

Can policy initiatives support parental decisions?

For many years, the hope of those concerned about fertility decline has been that more family friendly policies may make a difference.

Anne Gauthier (Chapter 16), however, reviewed the empirical evidence regarding the effects of policies on fertility. The overall conclusion of her review is that, while policies appear to have a positive impact on fertility, the magnitude of this impact is not very large. Moreover, the effect of policies is often on the timing of births rather than on the total number of births. She notes, for example, Blanchet and Ekert-Jaffé (1994), using data from 11 European countries for the period 1970–83, estimated that family benefits similar to those provided in France resulted in a higher fertility level of about 0.2–0.3 children per woman. Gauthier and Hatzius (1997) using similar methodology and more countries estimated that a 25 per cent increase in cash benefits would result in an increase in fertility of 0.07 children per woman. Gauthier adds that studies disagree whether generous maternity and paternity leaves have a positive or negative effect. Similarly, when it comes to the provision of childcare, the evidence is also mixed. It is certainly true, as Jones notes in his chapter on the low fertility rates in East Asia (Chapter 3) that simple monetary incentives are not enough. If anything, long-term, comprehensive family friendly policies supporting both women's position in the labour market and work-family balances appear to promote fertility. This appears to happen by enabling parents to have third and fourth children.

The evidence, however, is clearer when it comes to migration. Economic migrants are usually young and many arrive in the host country before forming their families.

In 2008, 24 per cent of all live births occurring within England and Wales occurred to foreign-born mothers, which is the highest ever proportion since recording of the mother's country of birth began in 1969, and compares to 14 per cent of live births ten years previously in 1998 (Tromans et al. 2009). The fertility of the foreign-born population, as we have seen in the 2011 UK Census, is higher than that of the UK-born population, meaning that their increasing share of childbearing will drive increases in UK fertility levels. Indeed, as already noted, the recent rises seen in UK fertility levels are most probably accounted for by foreign-born fertility as well as some UK born mothers delaying childbirth. In Finland, however, migrants coming from areas with already low fertility such as Estonia and Russia marginally increase their fertility rate to that of the local area. All over, most children of migrants appear to adjust quickly to the general childbearing patterns of the country. Thus this effect soon levels out if no new migrants arrive – or the sender countries already have low fertility themselves.

Possible directions for the future

With a smaller population children, will become more valuable?

The central finding from this book, is that, with a declining population, in both the developed and developing world, *all* children will become more valuable, both the privileged few and those who to date have experienced harder times. Quite apart from their relationships with their parents, nation states will need to maximize the potential of the next generation. In a world where the potential workforce is declining, this will be an even greater imperative.

Gøsta Esping-Andersen in Chapter 17 makes a strong case that we need to invest more in the early years of our existing children, particularly children living in poverty. These are the children at the worse end of the spectrum. He evidenced the research that has been important in fostering better early years care and demonstrates that the investment in excluded children has an important economic return.

The distinguished economist, James Heckman (Heckman et al. 2007) showed the possible economic returns from investment in early years education for poorer children. Heckman's work, noted by Esping Andersen, argues that the rate of return from investing in the early years is greater than investing at any other time of a child's life.

Recent research on the brain has added fuel to this debate. Ever since Bowlby (1969), we have been well trained on the importance of emotional 'attachment' and how a baby bonds with his or her primary caregiver in the early months. Research showed us that children who were more or less attached in the early years had very different patterns in later life including their own childbearing and parenting styles (Ainsworth et al. 1978). But it was not until the last two decades that we have had the ability to look inside the living child's brain. Work by Rutter (1998) on the children rescued from the Romanian orphanages opened our eyes. Rutter showed that those children removed to loving adoptive parents before they were six months did just fine, but those who had languished in the orphanages for more than 18 months had ongoing cognitive and other difficulties, despite receiving at a later stage, loving and nurturing adoptive parents.

An even more dramatic finding was that summarized in the paper by Perry (2002).

> Abuse studies from the author's laboratory ... point to the need for children to have both stable emotional attachments with, and touch from, primary adult caregivers and spontaneous interactions with

> peers. If these connections are lacking, brain development both of caring behaviour and cognitive capactities is damaged in a lasting fashion.
>
> (Perry 2002, paper abstract)

A key mechanism is that essential neural systems do not develop without the necessary experiences. The brain is incomplete at birth and is most sensitive to experiences in infancy and childhood. The child's inherited potential is designed to work in a certain kind of environment. The brain has sensitive periods and although this may be marginally different for each child, the most sensitive period is around birth and during the first three years.

> The implications of this are profound. In the development of socio-emotional functioning, early life nurturing appears to be critical. If this is absent for the first three years of life and then a child is adopted and begins to receive attention, love and nurturing, the positive experiences may not be sufficient to overcome the lack of development/damage to the brain.
>
> (Perry 2002, p. 87)

Of course child well-being matters throughout childhood. Perry's stress of the importance of spontaneous peer interaction should also ring some warning bells in societies where the stress to perform and competition levels among children are so high that children sometimes have literally no free time for playing, at least not after starting school.

While, investment in the early years may be a priority, a relatively neglected group of young people are adolescents. UNICEF (2011) has recently made adolescents the target for their endeavours. The argument is although most resources should be devoted to children and young people in the first decade of their life, when they are most vulnerable to disease and death, lasting change in the lives of children and young people can only be achieved by complementing investment in the first decade of life with greater attention and resources applied to the second (UNICEF 2011). The report concludes:

> The accumulated evidence demonstrates that investing in adolescents' second decade is our best hope of breaking the intergenerational cycle of poverty and inequity and of laying the foundation for a more peaceful, tolerant and equitable world.
>
> (UNICEF 2011, p. 2)

The economic recession has been particularly hard on young people on the cusp of entering a working life. In England and Wales, at the end of 2010, 141,800 (7.3 per cent) 16- to 18-year-olds were Not in Education or Employment or Training (NEET). Rates vary considerably with age – 2.3 per cent of 16-year-olds, 6.8 per cent of 17-year-olds and 12.4 per cent of 18-year-olds. Research shows that being out of work, training or employment at this age has a long-term impact on later working patterns. By 42, those who have been frequently unemployed as teenagers are likely to earn up to 15 per cent less than their peers (Department for Education 2012). Particularly vulnerable are those with few or no qualifications and those with a health problem, disability or low aspirations. In England and Wales, special initiatives are being developed to try to get these vulnerable young people into work, but this is likely to be difficult with the ongoing economic recession. The riots in the United Kingdom in 2011 add a special urgency to this agenda. In addition, the sex abuse scandals surrounding the late Jimmy Savile and others, largely impacting teenage girls, have also fuelled the debate that we need to do more to protect our vulnerable adolescents.

The youth unemployment problem is not confined to the United Kingdom. Youth unemployment in the EU rose to 22.4 per cent, or 5.507 million, in January 2012 up from 22.2 per cent, or 5.495 million in December 2011. Across Europe, at 49.9 per cent, Spain has the highest youth unemployment in the EU with Greece not far behind at 48.1 per cent (Eurostat 2012). These high rates of youth unemployment will do little to foster the future skills and work habits necessary for a coming world where workers will be at a premium. In addition, economic uncertainty and the lack of employment security make young people postpone or forego family formation. The current economic recession is already having a negative impact on US and EU fertility. Thus, we have come the full circle: with economic uncertainty, youth fare worse and fertility rates continue their downward trend.

More women will be needed to fill the gaps in a declining workforce

Lee Kuan Yew famously lamented that educating women and giving them opportunities in the labour force had affected their traditional role as mothers.

> It is too late for us to reverse our policies. ... Our women will not stand for it. And anyway, they have already become too important a factor in the economy.
>
> (Lee 2006, p. 115)

In 2006, the *Economist* published an interesting article: 'A guide to womenomics: The future of the world economy lies increasingly in female hands' (Economist 2006a). Their point was that working women were playing an increasing role in the growth of national economies. They noted, for example, that in the emerging East Asian economies, for every 100 men in the labour force there were now 83 women, which was higher than in many OECD countries. They concluded that the increase in female employment had been responsible for much global growth in recent decades. In a further article (Economist 2006b) they added:

> Governments, too, should embrace the potential of women. Women complain (rightly) of centuries of exploitation. Yet, to an economist, women are not exploited enough: they are the world's most under-utilised resource; getting more of them into work is part of the solution to many economic woes, including shrinking populations and poverty.
>
> (Economist 2006b)

Since policy-makers would like women to both work and have children, we witness a certain tension. OECD (2003) has, for instance, criticized the long parental leaves of Scandinavian countries as bad for women's labour market participation. Yet research shows that once a certain amount of maternal or paternal leave becomes the standard, neither parental careers nor economic productivity suffers. In Finland and Sweden, practically all parents take at least one year off for parental leaves per child, and these countries rank relatively high in global productivity (OECD 2012).

If more women enter and remain in the workforce, societies will need to do more to help them balance their work and family

Gauthier in Chapter 16 outlined some of the family friendly policy instruments available to women in Europe. Although work-life 'balance' is an EU policy priority, across Europe there are considerable variations in the nature and extent of supports that national governments have offered to dual-earner families. Overall, the Nordic welfare states offer the highest levels of support. Other countries, such as France, have historically offered extensive childcare supports to working mothers, although their parental leaves are relatively short (Compton and Lyonette 2006).

Compton and Lyonette (2006) found evidence of a 'societal effect' in the cases of Finland and Norway. There were significantly lower levels of work-life conflict reported in these countries even after a range of factors had been controlled for. Surprisingly, childcare in France did not appear to have had a similar impact. The authors surmised that this finding may have been related to the more traditional division of labour in France, notably the low participation of men in domestic chores and child care, which is associated with higher levels of stress.

In the United States a growing number of firms have become aware that the inability of employees to balance work and life responsibilities has a negative impact: higher rates of absenteeism and turnover, reduced productivity, decreased job satisfaction, lower levels of organizational commitment and loyalty and rising healthcare costs (Hobson et al. 2011). They report that an increasing number of progressive firms in the United States have recognized the critical significance of designing corporate policies and programmes to assist employees to achieve a better relationship between their major life and family responsibilities. Among the programmes offered are onsite or subsidized childcare and elder care, flexible work hours, job sharing, easy access to Employee Assistance Programs (EAPs) and supervisory training on the importance of work-life balance.

Hobson et al. (2011) note that there is now considerable evidence that such family friendly initiatives can lead to significant improvements in economic benefits for companies, for example, in recruiting; lower levels of absenteeism and voluntary turnover; increased productivity; organizational commitment and loyalty; job satisfaction; as well as lower stress levels; and health care costs.

In Chapter 14, in the developing world, we noted that siblings often took responsibility for caring for younger brothers and sisters, while their parents worked. For both humanitarian and economic reasons, policies will need to ensure that older siblings, themselves future workers, do not miss out on their education. As Gauthier has shown in Chapter 16, there are a range of maternity protections, leaves and other benefits in Europe, which are valued by parents. The developing world will need to consider how it can develop similar policies to support women and fathers when working. Parents all over the world need reliable and affordable quality preschool and after-school childcare. This care will need to take into account that many parents will be working throughout the children's school holidays.

Family planning clinics will need to include fertility advice or assistance

Looking to a future of declining population, societies may have to take more responsibilities in helping women who want to become mothers to overcome infertility. As Rotkirch pointed out in Chapter 15 the concept of family planning needs to be broadened. Sexual education and health services need to take into account the need for both contraceptive and 'pro-ceptive' advice – when is a suitable time to have a possible child.

In the United Kingdom, one in six UK families is facing infertility problems. Knowledge about when to seek help for difficulties in achieving pregnancies has grown during recent decades as infertility problems have become more widely discussed. Treatment methods and options have also improved so that an increasing proportion of clients end up having the child they wished for. Depending on the country, fertility treatments or surrogate pregnancies are also an alternative way to parenthood for single mothers or homosexual couples. However, the impact of artificially assisted reproduction on fertility rates is limited to a few percentages. Additionally in the United Kingdom over 28,000 women are still failing In-Vitro Fertilization (IVF) every year. Adoption is then one alternative, but the availability of babies is rapidly diminishing. Again, the impact of lower fertility rates and growing wealth in developing countries means that there will be fewer babies who need to find a home from a Western country. There is a very real need for potential prospective parents to become knowledgeable about adoption options. There is growing global awareness of the possible risks of international adoption, although most research does suggest 'adoption works' if the new placement is stable (Rushton and Minnis 1997).

Quite apart from meeting the needs of infertile parents, adoption of children who have been neglected and/or abused is a much better option for promoting their future well-being, than even in advanced welfare countries, spending many years in state care.

Looking into the crystal ball, the importance of assisted reproduction will probably grow, while that of international adoption will diminish. However, facilitating further adoption, where children can no longer safely live with their parents, may be better not only for the adopters and children involved but also society.

Parents will also need time to care for their parents, and family policies will need to facilitate the care of the elderly

We read above how subsidized elder care was highlighted by Hobson et al. (2011) as an important company initiative. Shea (2003) in the United States quotes Timmermann, a gerontologist who tracked the demographic trends of an ageing society as well as employers' responses to their workers' growing elder care responsibilities:

> Child care used to be the topic of discussion at parties .... Now it's aging parents.
>
> (Shea 2003, p. 1)

Shea (2003) points out that as employees' elder care obligations increase, so there will be a cost to employers in lost productivity, absenteeism, workday interruptions, as well as turnover when employees leave the workforce because they feel overwhelmed by their elder care responsibilities.

For example, as Gavin Jones, noted in Chapter 3, in Singapore the percentage of elderly people is expected to treble in the 25 years after 2010. In addition, there is another potential time bomb related to the dependency ratio. The ratio of elderly population who suffer from senile dementia to nonworking women at various ages, for example, is projected to rise substantially over the coming two decades in Japan (Ogawa 2003). The problem of caring for future numbers of elderly who are cognitively impaired will challenge families, carers and societies globally. Parents' employment will be important in raising the income to pay for care for the elderly, both through taxes and through personal budgets. As noted earlier it may be that it is also in the interests of businesses too to share the responsibilities. The growing number of elderly and the 'demographic deficit' highlighted by Harper in Chapter 13 will place extra burdens on the 'sandwich generation' trying to meet the needs of family members both younger and older. Policy initiatives will require more flexibility for workers involved in elder care. But also policy initiatives need to consider how they can facilitate elders to stay healthy and active while at the same time saving for realistic pensions for themselves.

Finally we need to think about the psychological well-being of our future children

In a fast changing world, children and young people will need to be resilient to the many changes that will happen during their lives. They will need to be psychologically strong. There are important links between maternal mental health and that of children (e.g. Burke 2003). If we want our children to be resilient to the pressures of a changing world, to have the steady state and self esteem to cope, we also need to think about the well-being of parents, especially mothers. Mumsnet mothers talked about the stresses of parenthood and the guilt-ridden trip of balancing work and family life. We also need to think how we can better promote the well-being of children (remembering, especially, those children who have not prospered and those who have been intensely pressurized), and do what we can, not only as parents, but also as representatives of societies, to make time for them. In speaking to the Strategy Department of the UK Cabinet, on 'Preparing Children for the 21st Century' the first editor noted that if there was one gift she could give to twenty-first century children, it would be psychological well-being (Buchanan 2009). Modern science has shown that there is much we can do to ensure that our children are not only healthier and better educated to thrive in an increasingly complex world, but they are also more resilient. This, along with the other areas highlighted before in this chapter, must be a future direction.

References

Ainsworth, M. D. S., Blehar, M. C., Waters, E. and Wall, S. (1978) *Patterns of Attachment: A Psychological Study of the Strange Situation* (Hillsdale, NJ: Erlbaum).

Blanchet, D. and Ekert-Jaffé, O. (1994) The demographic impact of family benefits: evidence from a micro-model and from macro-data. In J. Ermisch and N. Ogawa (eds) *The Family, the Market and the State in Aging Societies* (Oxford: Clarendon Press), pp. 79–103.

Bowlby, J. (1969) *Attachment and Loss* (New York: Basic Books).

Buchanan, A. (2009) *Preparing Children for the 21st Century,* Talk to the Strategy Unit of the Cabinet Office. http://webarchive.nationalarchives.gov.uk, office Strategy Unit Seminar, date accessed 25 March 2012.

Burke, L. (2003) The impact of maternal depression on familial relationships, *International Review of Psychiatry*, 15(3): 243–55.

Central Intelligence Agency (2012) The World Factbook, https://www.cia.gov/library/publications/the-world-factbook/fields/2127.html, date accessed 20 March 2012.

Compton, R. and Lyonette, C. (2006) Work-Life 'Balance' in Europe, *Acta Sociologica*, 49(4): 379–93.

Department for Education (2012) 16- to 18-year-olds not in education, employment or training (NEET), http://www.education.gov.uk/a0064101/16-to-18-year-olds-not-in-education-employment-or-training-neet, date accessed 25 March 2012.

Economist (2006a). A guide to womenomics: the future of the world economy lies increasingly in female hands, *The Economist,* http://www.economist.com/node/6802551, date accessed 25 March 2012.

Economist (2006b) The importance of sex. Forget China, India and the internet: economic growth is driven by women, *The Economist,* http://www.economist.com/node/6800723, date accessed 25 March 2012.

Eurostat (2012) News release euroindicators March 12, http://europa.eu/rapid/pressReleasesAction.do?reference= STAT/12/31&format= HTML&aged= 0&language= EN&guiLanguage= en, date accessed 25 March 2010.

Falbo, T. and Polit, D. (1986) Quantitative review of the only child literature: Research evidence and theory development, *Psychological Bulletin,* 100: 176–89.

Gauthier, A. and Hatzius, J. (1997) Family benefits and fertility: an econometric analysis, *Population Studies,* 51: 295–306.

The Guttmacher Institute (2012) *Facts on Publicly Funded Contraceptive Services in the United States,* http://www.guttmacher.org/pubs/fb_contraceptive_serv.html, date accessed 20 March 2012.

Heckman, J., Schultz, H. and Masterov. D. (2007) The productivity argument for investing in young children, *Applied Economic Perspectives and Policy,* 29(3): 446–93, doi: 10.1111/j.1467-9353.2007.00359.

Hobson, C. J., Delunas, L. and Kesic, D. (2011) Compelling evidence of the need for corporate work/life balance initiatives: results from a national survey of stressful life-events, *Journal of Employment Counseling,* 38(1): 38–44.

Lee, Y.-J. (2006) Risk factors in the rapidly rising incidence of divorce in Korea, *Asian Population Studies,* 2(2): 113–32.

McKinsey Quarterly (2010) What's driving Africa's growth? http://www.mckinseyquarterly.com/Whats_driving_Africas_growth_2601, date accessed 20 March 2012.

OECD (2003) Labour force participation of women: empirical evidence on the role of policy and other determinants in OECD countries, OECD Economic Studies, No. 37, http://www.oecd.org/dataoecd/12/39/34562935.pdf, date accessed 25 March 2012.

OECD (2012) Stats extract. Gross domestic product: GDP, volume – annual growth rates in percentage, http://stats.oecd.org/index.aspx?queryid= 26646, date accessed 25 March 2010.

Ogawa, N. (2003) Japan's changing fertility mechanisms and its policy responses, *Journal of Population Research,* 20(1): 89–106.

Office for National Statistics (2011) Frequently asked questions: births & fertility, www.ons.gov.uk/ons/rel/vsob1/ ... of ... /**2010**/faq-births-and-fertility.pdf accessed November 4, 2012

Perry, B. D. (2002) Childhood experience and the expression of genetic potential: what childhood neglect tells us about nature and nurture, *Brain and Mind,* 3: 79–100.

Pollard, N. Latorre, M. and Sriskandarajah, D. (2008) *Floodgates or Turnstiles? Post-EU Enlargement Migration Flows Top and from the UK,* Institute of Public Policy Research, http://www.wsmp.org.uk/documents/wsmp/Migration%20(general)

%20research%20and%20reports/IPPR%20Floodgates%20or%20Turns, date accessed 20 March 2012.

Rushton, A. and Minnis, H. (1997) Trans-racial family placements, *Journal of Child Psychology and Psychiatry*, 38: 157–9.

Rutter, M. (1998) Developmental catch-up, and deficit, following adoption after severe global early privation, *Journal of Child Psychology and Psychiatry*, 39(4): 465–76.

Shea, T. F. (2003) Help with elder care: elder care benefits range from basic to comprehensive as employers help employees cope with this growing need – compensation & benefits agenda, *HR Magazine*, September, http://www.shrm.org/Publications/hrmagazine/EditorialContent/Pages/0903shea.aspx, date accessed 25 March 2012.

Tromans, N., Natamba, E. and Jefferies, J. (2009) Have women born outside the UK driven the rise in UK births since 2001?, *Population Trends*, 136: 28–42.

UNICEF (2011) *Adolescence: An Age of Opportunity*, UNICEF, http://www.unicef.org/publications/files/SOWC_2011_Main_Report_EN_02242011.pdf, date accessed 25 March 2012.

United National Development Programme (2010) *UNDP Report 2010*, http://hdr.undp.org/en/reports/global/hdr2010/chapters/en/, date accessed 25 March 2012.

United Nations (2000) The population division of the Department of Economic and Social Affairs (DESA), *Replacement Migration: Is it a Solution to Declining and Ageing Populations?* http://www.un.org/esa/population/publications/ReplMigED/migration.htm, date accessed 25 March 2012.

Index

Printed in Dunstable, United Kingdom

67512602R00198